D1346818

Handbook of Drug Administration via Enteral Feeding Tubes

DRUG INFORMATION
CENTRE
GLASGOW ROYAL
INFIRMARY

Handbook of Drug Administration via Enteral Feeding Tubes

Rebecca White
BSc (Hons) MSc MRPharmS
Lead Pharmacist; Nutrition and Surgery,
Oxford Radcliffe Hospitals NHS Trust, Oxford, UK

Vicky Bradnam
BPharm (Hons) ClinDip MBA$_{Open}$ MRPharmS
Chief Pharmacist, Bromley Hospitals NHS Trust, Kent, UK

On behalf of the British Pharmaceutical Nutrition Group

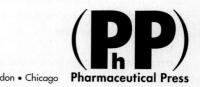

London • Chicago **Pharmaceutical Press**

Published by the Pharmaceutical Press
An imprint of RPS Publishing

1 Lambeth High Street, London SE1 7JN, UK
100 South Atkinson Road, Suite 200, Grayslake, IL 60030-7820, USA

© Rebecca White and Vicky Bradnam 2007

(**P**h**P**) is a trade mark of RPS Publishing

RPS Publishing is the publishing organisation of the
Royal Pharmaceutical Society of Great Britain

First published 2007

Typeset by MCS Publishing Services Ltd, Salisbury, Wiltshire
Printed in Great Britain by Cambridge University Press, Cambridge

ISBN-10 0 85369 648 9
ISBN-13 978 0 85369 648 3

A catalogue record for this book is available from the British Library

Contents

Foreword

The need for this text has been highlighted within the British Pharmaceutical Nutrition Group (BPNG) and the British Association of Parenteral and Enteral Nutrition (BAPEN) by healthcare professionals who are challenged on a daily basis by complex patients whose need for medicines does not fit neatly into the categories used by the pharmaceutical industry as part of their process for licensing medicines. To provide the right level of care for these patients, professionals have to make complex and rational decisions concerning medication, which may mean stepping outside the product licence for the medication needed. As healthcare progresses and becomes more technical, such dilemmas become more commonplace. We hope this book will assist healthcare professionals who have an input into either the patients' medicines or their enteral nutrition to understand the necessary decision process they must enter into and how best to optimise their patient care, thereby ensuring the desired outcomes to meet the patients' medical and personal needs.

The data in the individual drug monographs is based on available evidence supplied by the drug companies, to whom we are very grateful for their support, and also on research undertaken by pharmacists.

The production of this text has raised many questions concerning the data available relating to this method of medication administration; the BPNG will continue to support research in this growing area of practice.

Thanks are due to all the healthcare professionals who have given their time and expertise to ensure the practical applicability of this book. Thanks must also go to Rebecca White who has led tirelessly on this project and undertaken much of the research to produce this comprehensive guide to drugs and enteral feeding tubes.

Vicky Bradnam
Chief Pharmacist
Bromley Hospitals NHS Trust

Preface

The initiative to prepare these guidelines was taken by the British Pharmaceutical Nutrition Group (BPNG) with the support of the British Association of Enteral and Parenteral Nutrition (BAPEN).

This book reflects current practice and the information available at the time of going to press. Although the authors have made every effort to ensure that the information contained in this reference is correct, no responsibility can be accepted for any errors.

It is important to note that owing to the method of administration concerned, most of the recommendations and suggestions in this reference fall outside of the terms of the product licence for the drugs concerned. It must be borne in mind that any prescriber and practitioner administering a drug outside of the terms of its product licence accepts liability for any adverse effects experienced by the patient.

Readers outside the United Kingdom are reminded to take into account local and national differences in clinical practice, legal requirements, and possible formulation differences.

All enquiries should be addressed to:

Rebecca White
British Pharmaceutical Nutrition Group
PO Box 5784
Derby
DE22 32H
UK

About the authors

The British Pharmaceutical Nutrition Group, founded in 1988, is an organisation with a professional interest in nutrition support. The members of this group are pharmacists, technicians and scientists from the health service, academia and industry.

The aims of the group are to promote the role of pharmaceutical expertise and experience in the area of clinical nutrition and to ensure the safe and effective preparation and administration of parenteral nutrition through effective education and research initiatives, and to encourage debate into pharmaceutical aspects of nutritional support.

Rebecca White studied at Aston University, Birmingham, and qualified as a pharmacist in 1994. Experience in aseptic services, intensive care and nutrition support was gained through working at Central Middlesex Hospital, Charing Cross Hospital and UCLH over a period of 10 years in London. During this time Rebecca also completed an MSc, with the School of Pharmacy in London, evaluating opinions, knowledge and protocols relating to drug administration via enteral feeding tubes. Rebecca has been on the executive committee of the BPNG since 1997, currently as Chairman. In 2003 Rebecca chaired the BAPEN multidisciplinary group that produced guidance on the safe administration of medication via enteral feeding tubes.

In 2004 Rebecca qualified with the first wave of pharmacist supplementary prescribers and currently prescribes as part of the nutrition team.

Rebecca is currently Lead Pharmacist for Surgery and Nutrition at the John Radcliffe Hospital in Oxford. She has recently been part of the NPSA group on wrong route errors.

Apart from drug nutrient interactions, her other professional interests include parenteral nutrition and pharmaceutical aspects of surgical and gastroenterological care. She is also enjoys car maintenance, DIY, classical music and a good murder-mystery.

Vicky Bradnam studied at The School of Pharmacy, University of London and qualified as a pharmacist in 1985. Experienced in all aspects of a pharmacy service and specialised in paediatrics in 1990, worked as a lead clinical pharmacist in paediatrics, with an interest in paediatric nutrition, from 1990 to 2000, and has continued to practice clinically in paediatrics despite moving into departmental management. Currently Vicky is the Chief Pharmacist for Bromley Hospitals NHS Trust. She holds a Certificate and Diploma in Clinical Pharmacy, an MBA and PRICE2 foundation level qualifications. Over the 20 years working as a hospital pharmacist Vicky has worked in both large teaching hospitals and DGHs. She has been involved in management, professional development and leadership, lecturing, service planning, budgetary management and clinical practice. Through her specialisation as a paediatric pharmacist, she has an interest in unlicensed drug administration and the importance of standardising practice for the safety and benefit of the patients. Vicky has been an active member of the BPNG and chaired the group between 2002 and 2004, for her services to the group she was awarded life membership in 2006.

Contributors

Authors

Rebecca White BSc MSc MRPharmS, Lead Pharmacist; Nutrition & Surgery, Oxford Radcliffe Hospitals NHS Trust, Oxford, UK

Lynne Colagiovanni RGN, Clinical Nurse Specialist, University Hospitals Birmingham NHS Trust, Birmingham, UK

Kate Pickering RGN DipN BA, Nutrition Nurse Specialist, Leicester General Hospital, University Hospitals of Leicester, Leicester, UK

Dr David Wright, Senior Lecturer in Pharmacy Practice, School of Pharmacy, University of East Anglia, Norwich, UK

Members of the original BAPEN Working Party

Chair: Rebecca White, Oxford Radcliffe Hospitals NHS Trust
Lynne Colagiovanni, University Hospitals Birmingham
Geoffrey Simmonett, PINTT Representative
Fiona Thompson, Glasgow Royal Infirmary
Kate Pickering, Leicester General Infirmary
Katie Nicholls, Princess Alexandra Hospital
Julian Thorne, Torbay Hospital
Julia Horwood, North Thames Medicines Information

Thanks to staff at the pharmacy departments of University College London Hospitals and the John Radcliffe Hospital, Oxford.

Reviewers

Vicky Bradnam BPharm(Hons) ClinDip MBA$_{Open}$ MRPharmS, Chief Pharmacist, Bromley Hospitals NHS Trust, Kent, UK

Lucy Thompson MRPharmS, Principal Pharmacist, Kings Hospital, London, UK

Jackie Eastwood MRPharmS, Pharmacist, St Marks Hospital, London, UK

Ruth Newton MRPharmS, Principal Pharmacist, City Hospital, Stoke-on-Trent, UK
Antonella Tonna MRPharmS, Surgical Emergency Unit Pharmacist, Oxford Radcliffe
Hospitals NHS Trust, Oxford, UK
Mel Snelling MRPharmS, Lead Pharmacist, Infectious Diseases, Oxford Radcliffe
Hospitals NHS Trust, Oxford, UK
Yogini Jani ClinDip, MRPharmS, Medicines Error Pharmacist, University College
London Hospitals NHS Foundation Trust, London, UK
Diane Evans MRPharmS, Lead Pharmacist, Medicine, Oxford Radcliffe Hospitals NHS
Trust, Oxford, UK
Venetia Horn MRPharmS, Specialist Pharmacist – Clinical Nutrition, Great Ormond
Street NHS Trust, London, UK
Scott Harrison MRPharmS, Lead Pharmacist, Neurosurgery, Oxford Radcliffe
Hospitals NHS Trust, Oxford, UK
Mark Borthwick MRPharmS, Lead Pharmacist, Intensive Care, Oxford Radcliffe
Hospitals NHS Trust, Oxford, UK
Dr Allan Cosslett PhD MRPharmS, Lecturer, School of Pharmacy, Cardiff, UK

Contributors from the pharmaceutical industry

The companies listed below have provided information included in the drug
monographs in this handbook. *The information was supplied on the understanding that
these manufacturers do not advocate off-license use of their products.*

Drug information

Alliance Pharmaceuticals Ltd
Alpharma Ltd
AstraZeneca UK Ltd
Aventis Pharma Ltd
Bayer plc
Boehringer Ingelheim Ltd
Bristol-Myers Squibb Pharmaceuticals Ltd
Celltech Pharmaceuticals Ltd
Cephalon UK Ltd
CP Pharmaceuticals Ltd
Eisai Ltd
Elan Pharma Ltd
Ferring Pharmaceuticals (UK)
GlaxoSmithKline
Hawgreen Ltd
Janssen-Cilag Ltd
Leo Pharma
Merck Pharmaceuticals
Napp Pharmaceuticals Ltd
Norgine Ltd
Novartis Pharmaceuticals UK Ltd

Paynes & Byrne Ltd
Pfizer Ltd
Pharmacia Ltd
Procter & Gamble UK
Provalis Healthcare Ltd
Roche Products Ltd
Rosemont Pharmaceuticals Ltd
Sanofi-Synthelabo
Schwartz Pharma Ltd
Servier Laboratories Ltd
Shire Pharmaceuticals Ltd
Solvay Healthcare Ltd
Special Products Limited
UCB Pharma Ltd

Enteral feeding tube information

Baxa Ltd
Fresenius Kabi Ltd
Merck Gastroenterology
Novartis Consumer Health
Tyco Healthcare
Vygon (UK) Ltd

Abbreviations

5-ASA	5-aminosalicylic acid
ACE	angiotensin-converting enzyme
AUC	area under the concentration–time curve
b.d.	twice daily
BAPEN	British Association of Parenteral and Enteral Nutrition
BNF	British National Formulary
BPNG	British Pharmaceutical Nutrition Group
C_{max}	maximum plasma concentration
CSM	Committee on Safety of Medicines (UK)
E/C	enteric coated
EFT	enteral feeding tube
f/c	film-coated
Fr	French gauge (diameter of feeding tube; 1 Fr ~0.33 mm)
GI	gastrointestinal
GP	general practitioner
GTN	glyceryl trinitrate
HETF	home enteral tube feeding
HRT	hormone replacement therapy
i.m.	intramuscular
i.v.	intravenous
ICU	intensive care unit
INR	international normalised ratio
IU	international unit
LDL	low-density lipoprotein
M/R	modified-release
MAOI	monoamine oxidase inhibitor
MIC	minimum inhibitory concentration
NBM	nil by mouth
NCSC	National Care Standards Commission

ND	nasoduodenal
NDT	nasoduodenal tube
NG	nasogastric
NGT	nasogastric tube
NJ	nasojejenal
NJT	nasojejenal tube
NMC	National Midwifery Council
NPSA	National Patient Safety Agency
NSAID	nonsteroidal anti-inflammatory drug
OTC	over the counter
PEG	percutaneous endoscopic gastrostomy
PEGJ	percutaneous endoscopic gastrojejenostomy
PEJ	percutaneous endoscopic jejenostomy
PIL	product information leaflet
PUR	polyurethane
PVC	polyvinylchloride
q.d.s	four times daily
RPSGB	Royal Pharmaceutical Society of Great Britain
s.c.	subcutaneous
s/c	sugar-coated
SPC	Summary of Product Characteristics
SSRI	selective serotonin receptor inhibitor
t.d.s.	three times daily
t_{max}	time to reach maximum plasma concentration
w/w	weight for weight

Notes on the use of this book

The information provided in this resource is intended to support healthcare professionals in the safe and effective prescribing and administration of drugs via enteral feeding tubes. It is a comprehensive guide covering the legal, practical and technical aspects that healthcare professionals should consider before attempting to prescribe or administer drugs via an enteral feeding tube.

The following chapters are intended to provide background knowledge to inform clinical decisions and we recommend that readers familiarise themselves with the contents of these chapters before using the information contained within the monographs.

The individual monographs contain guidance on the safe administration of specific drugs and formulations. Wherever possible, a licensed formulation/route should always be used, and the monographs point the reader to alternatives for consideration. Where alternative routes/formulations are not available, the monographs make recommendations for safe administration via the enteral feeding tube. Any decisions on appropriate drug therapy must be made with the complete clinical condition and wishes of the individual patient in mind. Thought should be given to the care setting the patient is in presently, the future need for administration of medicines via an enteral feeding tube, and the patient's/carer's ability to undertake such administration should care be continued at home.

1

Introduction

Rebecca White

Key Points

- Use of enteral feeding tubes for drug administration is increasing.

- Sizes of feeding tubes are decreasing.

- The range of healthcare professionals involved in drug administration via enteral feeding tubes is increasing.

- Collation of all available information is necessary.

The use of enteral feeding tubes for short- and long-term feeding has increased in both primary and secondary care as a result of a heightened awareness of the importance of adequate nutritional intake. An enteral feeding tube (EFT) provides a means of maintaining nutritional intake when oral intake is inadequate or when there is restricted access to the gastrointestinal (GI) tract, e.g. owing to obstruction. ETFs are now commonly used for a wide range of clinical conditions and across a wide age range of people.

The British Artificial Nutrition Survey[1] published data indicating that the 20% year-on-year growth of the home enteral tube feeding (HETF) market has recently shown definite signs of slowing down. The age distribution of adult patients on HETF, skewed to the older age range with a peak in the 70–80-year age group, has shifted even further towards the older age range, to include patients who are generally more disabled. Now 75% of adult patients on HETF require either some or total support with their HETF. Cerebrovascular accident remains the commonest diagnosis in adults on HETF, but in the last 5 years more cancer patients have been receiving HETF. During 2005 at least 28 095 patients in the UK received HETF.

It can be difficult to find a suitable drug formulation for administration to a patient with limited GI access or with dysphagia. Although parenteral administration can be used and often guarantees 100% absorption, repeated intravenous, subcutaneous or intramuscular injections are associated with complications and are not suitable for continuous long-term use. There are also other routes that can be considered, such as transdermal, buccal, rectal or topical, but the drugs available in these formulations are limited (see chapter 6 for further information). In these patients the feeding tube is often the only means of enteral access and is increasingly being used as a route for drug administration.

The nursing profession has shown an increasing interest in this route of drug administration. More publications cover a number of issues relating to this method of drug administration, not least the implications of administering a drug via an unlicensed route (see chapter 7 for more information). Before any drug is considered for administration via an enteral feeding tube, the patient should be assessed to see whether they can tolerate and manage oral drug administration of appropriate licensed formulations (see chapter 5 for further information).

Administering a drug via an enteral feeding tube usually falls outside of the terms of the drug's product licence. This has implications for the professionals responsible for prescribing, supplying and administering the drug, as they become liable for any adverse event that the patient may experience. When a drug is administered outside of the terms of its product licence (for example, by crushing tablets before adminis-tration)*, the manufacturer is no longer responsible for any adverse event or treatment failure. For further information on unlicensed use of medicines, see chapter 7.

The administration of drugs via enteral feeding tubes also raises a number of other issues – nursing, pharmaceutical, technical and professional. Examples are drug errors associated with the use of i.v. syringes for enteral drug administration; the obstruction of feeding tubes with inappropriate drug formulations; the risk of cross-contamination from sharing of tablet crushing devices; and the risks of occupational exposure to drug powders through inappropriate handling.

There is also a degree of semantics: if the drug is prescribed via the oral route but intended to be given via the feeding tube, then this is a prescribing error. However, if the drug was intended to be given orally but the nurse administered it via the feeding tube, then this is classed as an administration error.

The pharmacist has several key responsibilities and must have access to all the necessary information relating not only to the drug and formulation but also to the patient's condition, the type of feeding tube, and the enteral feed and regimen being used. Pharmacists must be able to assimilate all this information to be able to recommend a suitable formulation for administration via this route. It is also their responsibility to inform the medical practitioner about the use of an unlicensed route. When changing between formulations, the pharmacist must ensure bioequivalence to avoid treatment failure or toxicity. In primary care, pharmacists will not readily have

---

*Crushing of tablets and opening of capsules are the most common ways in which the product licence is breached; using an injection solution for oral or enteral administration is another example.

access to all this information and will need to further discuss the prescriber's intentions with the prescriber before dispensing the prescription.

The pharmacist must also ensure that nursing staff, patients and carers have enough information to give the drug safely. The provision of information by pharmacists on drug charts, in secondary care and nursing homes, is essential to prevent nursing staff crushing tablets unnecessarily or administering inappropriate dosage forms. In primary care the pharmacist should discuss the intended method of administration with the patient/carer so as to ensure that they understand and are competent to undertake the task. The pharmacist should discuss any identified problems with the prescriber before continuing with dispensing.

Two publications have highlighted a number of these issues.[2, 3] Both of these reviews stressed that the administration of drugs via enteral feeding tubes is an area that has implications for each member of the multidisciplinary team; without a holistic view, issues may be overlooked.

This handbook is written *by* practitioners *for* practitioners. It is designed for all healthcare professionals, to provide all the available information in one resource with practical advice and recommendations for the safe and effective administration of drugs via enteral feeding tubes.

References

1. Jones B [Chairman]. Trends in artificial nutrition support in the UK 2000–2005. A report by the British Artificial Nutrition Survey (BANS) a committee of the British Association for Enteral and Parenteral Nutrition; 2006. Worcester: BAPEN, UK. In press.
2. Smith A. Inside story. *Nurs Times*. 1997; 93(8): 65–69.
3. Thomson FC, Naysmith MR, Lindsay A. Managing drug therapy in patients receiving enteral and parenteral nutrition. *Hospital Pharmacist*. 2000; 7(6): 155–164.

2
Types of enteral feeding tubes
Rebecca White

Key Points

- Ensure that you know the type, size and position of the enteral feeding tube before administration of medication via the tube.

- The exit site of the tube may affect drug pharmacokinetics or side-effect profile.

Types of feeding tubes

Enteral feeding tubes come in many different types, lengths and sizes, and exit in a variety of places in the GI tract.

Enteral feeding tubes can be inserted via a number of routes: via the nasopharynx, for example nasogastric (NG) or nasojejunal (NJ), or via direct access to the GI tract through the skin, for example gastrostomy or jejunostomy tubes. These ostomy tubes can be placed surgically, radiologically or endoscopically.

The type of feeding tube used will vary depending on the intended duration of feeding and the part of the GI tract the feed needs to be delivered to. Nasoenteric tubes are used for short- to medium-term feeding (days to weeks), whereas ostomy tubes are used for long-term feeding (months to years).

The external diameter of the feeding tube is expressed using the French (Fr) unit where each 'French' is equivalent to 0.33 mm. Enteral feeding tubes are composed of polyvinylchloride (PVC), polyurethane (PUR), silicone or latex. Silicone and latex tubes are softer and more flexible than polyurethane tubes and therefore require thicker walls to prevent stretching and collapsing. As a result of the differences in rigidity, a silicone or latex tube of the same French size as a polyurethane tube will have a smaller internal diameter. In recent years there has been a trend towards decreasing the size of feeding tubes used for reasons of patient comfort and acceptability.

The different characteristics of the tubing material can also have implications for drug adsorption onto the material; this has been demonstrated with carbamazepine.[1]

Nasogastric tube (NGT)

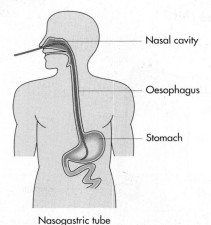

Figure 2.1   Nasogastric tube

This feeding tube is inserted via the nose and exits in the stomach. Tubes used via this route in adults can vary from fine-bore tubes (e.g. 6Fr–12Fr) designed specifically for feeding to the Ryles type tubes, usually 12Fr–16Fr, used for aspiration. In some patients, particularly those in intensive care, a large-bore tube may already be *in situ* when feeding is commenced. In this instance the tube can be used to commence the feed, but should be replaced by a fine-bore tube when tolerance to enteral feeding is established. In adults these tubes are usually 90–100 cm long.

Nasoduodenal tube (NDT)

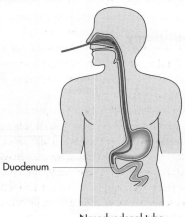

Figure 2.2   Nasoduodenal tube

The nasoduodenal tube feeding tube is inserted in the same manner as the NG tube but is allowed to pass into the duodenum, usually with assistance, either endoscopic or radiological. This is used to overcome the problems associated with gastric stasis. It is also referred to as 'postpyloric'.

Nasojejunal tube (NJT)

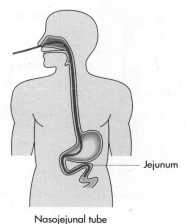

Nasojejunal tube

Figure 2.3 Nasojejunal tube

Nasojejunal tubes are usually inserted endoscopically or radiologically to ensure that they are in the correct position in the jejunum. If being used to minimise pancreatic stimulation, the tube is passed beyond the hepatic flexure (ligament of Trietz).

These tubes are prone to blockage owing to their length, usually more than 150 cm, and should only be used for drug administration in exceptional circumstances because of the lack of evidence relating to drug adsorption from this site.

There are also tubes that have a gastric aspiration port in addition to the jejunal feeding port. This allows for continuous jejunal feeding while the stomach is decompressed.

Percutaneous gastrostomy

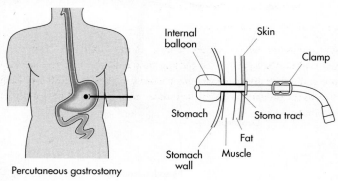

Percutaneous gastrostomy

Figure 2.4 Percutaneous gastrostomy

Percutaneous gastrostomy tubes are inserted into the stomach via the abdominal wall, most commonly endoscopically (percutaneous endoscopic gastrostomy, PEG). A permanent tract (stoma) forms after 3 weeks. The device is held in place with an internal balloon or bumper and an external fixator.

Percutaneous jejunostomy

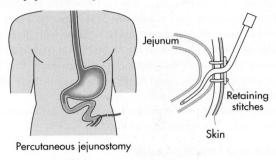

Figure 2.5   Percutaneous jejunostomy

The percutaneous jejunostomy tube is inserted into the jejunum via the abdominal wall, endoscopically (percutaneous endoscopic jejunostomy, PEJ), radiologically or surgically. They are held in place either externally with stitches or internally with a flange or Dacron cuff.

Percutaneous gastrojejunostomy

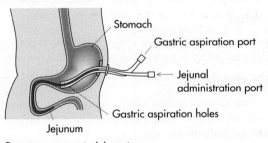

Figure 2.6   Percutaneous gastrojejunostomy

The percutaneous gastrojejunostomy tube is inserted into the stomach via the abdominal wall and the exit of the feeding tube is placed into the jejunum, most commonly endoscopically (percutaneous endoscopic gastrojejunostomy, PEGJ). This can be done as the primary procedure, or a tube can be placed into the jejunum via an existing PEG tube.

Implications of tube type and placement for drug administration

Site of drug delivery

This is of particular concern for feeding tubes exiting in the jejunum. Drug absorption may be reduced owing to effects of pH or delivery beyond the site of drug absorption, as in the case of ketoconazole,[2] or by reduction of the time for which the drug is in contact with the GI tract. Particular care should be taken with drugs with a narrow therapeutic range, although most of these can be effectively monitored through plasma concentrations (e.g. phenytoin or theophylline), or though direct effect (e.g. warfarin). Conversely side-effects can be increased owing to the rapid delivery of drug into the lumen of the small bowel.

Tubes exiting beyond the pylorus usually have different requirements for flushing, e.g. sterile water. Local policy should be consulted.

Size of lumen and length of tube

Narrow tubes and long tubes are more likely to become blocked. Correct choice of formulation and effective flushing are essential to prevent blockage. See chapters 3 and 4 for further information.

Function of enteral tube

Do not administer drugs via tubes that are being used for aspiration or are on free drainage.

Multilumen tubes

Some enteral tubes have two lumens to enable simultaneous gastric aspiration and jejunal feeding. Ensure that the correct lumen is used for drug delivery.

Confirmation of position

Interim advice of the National Patient Safety Agency (NPSA) (February 2005) recommends that all patients being fed using a nasogastric tube should have the position of the tube checked regularly using pH indicator paper.[3]

See chapter 9 for information on syringe size, type and port connection.

References

1. Clark-Shmidt AL, Garnett WR, Lowe DR, Karnes HT. Loss of carbamazepine suspension through nasogastric feeding tubes. *Am J Hosp Pharm.* 1990; 47(9): 2034–2037.
2. Adams D. Administration of drugs through a jejunostomy tube. *Br J Intensive Care.* 1994; 4: 10–17.
3. NPSA (2005) Reducing the harm caused by misplaced nasogastric feeding tubes. Interim advice for healthcare staff – February 2005. NPSA. www.npsa.nhs.uk/advice.

3
Flushing enteral feeding tubes
Kate Pickering

Key Points

- Enteral feeding tubes require regular, effective flushing to prevent tube blockage.

- Tube blockage may occur owing to:
  - Small internal diameter of the tubes
  - Inappropriately prepared medications
  - Poor flushing technique or poor attention to the flushing regimen prescribed
  - Gastric acid, feed and medication interactions
  - Bacterial colonisation within the feeding tube [1]

- Tube flushing is the single most effective action in prolonging the life of any enteral feeding tube.

Syringe size

Small syringes create high intraluminal pressures and may damage the tube. [1, 2] In order to reduce the risk of rupturing the fabric of the enteral feeding tube, the largest functional syringe size should be used; 30–50 mL syringes are recommended. [3] In clinical practice this tends to be a 50 mL syringe. [4]

Documentation

It is essential that flushes are recorded accurately in hospital, on the fluid balance chart, and that in both primary and secondary care the patient's prescribed flush takes account of any renal or cardiac impairment. Assessment to decide upon the necessary flush volume may require a reduction in other fluids to effectively maintain fluid balance. Drug volumes and flushes should always be recorded.

Air flushing

It has been suggested that flushing with air before attempting to obtain gastric aspirate may help to flick the tip of the nasogastric feeding tube into the reservoir of gastric secretion, thereby facilitating gastric aspiration. In pH testing, the tube should be cleared of any substance that will contaminate the sample and affect the pH of the gastric aspirate.[5] Aspirate can then be pH tested according to local policy.

Technique

1. Pre-fill a 50 mL syringe with 30 mL of air.
2. Attach the syringe to the appropriate port of the patient's nasogastric feeding tube.
3. Ensure that any other ports are closed and airtight.
4. Ensure that there is an airtight connection between the syringe and the enteral tube and administer the flush.
5. Listen for any evidence of the air venting into the mouth or upper oesophagus; such venting may suggest misplacement of the tube tip in the upper oesophagus or rupture of the tube.
6. Attempt to aspirate with a 50 mL syringe. This will reduce the likelihood of the inner lumen of the enteral feeding tube collapsing under vacuum.

Frequency

Air flushing should be used for tube placement confirmation each time gastric secretions are required.

It is suggested that tubes are checked for placement at least every 24 hours.[6]

Air flushing on gastric aspiration

Air flushing is not required in patients who are having gastric aspiration to check residual gastric volume. These patients will, however, require the tube to be flushed with water after the residual aspirate is returned, or discarded, to prevent build-up of debris on the internal lumen of the tube that may result in occlusion (blockage of the tube) (see below).

Water flushing

In the USA, carbonated drinks were once heavily favoured as enteral feeding tube flushes,[7] but trials have demonstrated that warm water performs as well as other fluids tested as an enteral feeding tube flush.[8] It should be noted that acidic flushes such as cola can exacerbate tube occlusion by causing feed to coagulate or protein to denaturise.[9]

Water is the most appropriate fluid with which to flush[3, 8] and water is as effective as any flush for reducing the formation of, and for clearing previously established, tube occlusions. A pulsatile flushing action should be used to create turbulence within the inner lumen of the enteral feeding tube, more effectively cleaning the inner walls. Research is limited on the type of water to be used, but it is good practice to use sterile water for patients with tubes beyond the stomach and either tap water or sterile water for gastric tubes, depending on local policy.

Owing to the complexity of the formulations of drugs for enteral administration and the need for accuracy and prompt administration, medication is usually given as a bolus dose preceded and completed with flushing to ensure patency of the enteral feeding tube. This may result in a large gastric residual.

Volume

The volume used should reflect the diameter of the inner lumen of the nasogastric tube. The flush should be adequate to prevent build-up on the inner wall of the tube. A 15–30 mL water flush is recommended,[10, 11] but care should be taken with fluid-restricted patients (see notes below). Water type depends on local policy. Wide-bore enteral tubes may require a higher volume owing to the large diameter of the inner lumen.

Technique

1. Prepare a flush of water (according to local guidelines) in a 50 mL syringe and label if necessary. Place it in a clean tray.
2. Stop or suspend enteral feeding.
3. Ensure that any other ports are closed and airtight.
4. Attach the syringe to a port of the patient's enteral feeding tube. Ensure that there is an airtight connection between the syringe and the enteral tube.
5. Using a pulsatile flushing action, administer the flush.
6. Positioning the patient in a semi-recumbent position can help to prevent regurgitation and possible pulmonary aspiration from gastric flush and/or drug residual.[12]
7. Administer the drug and flush; cap off, or connect further enteral feeding depending on the patient's requirements.

Water flushing and drug administration

Mateo[7] found that although 95% of nurses reported flushing enteral feeding tubes after drug administration, only 47% reported that flushing was undertaken prior to drug administration. Flushing with water helps to prevent interactions between feed and drug in the inner lumen of the tube. It is good practice to flush the tube before and after each drug administered[3, 13] and before recommencing the feed. If the drug is viscous, flushing or dilution with water may be required during administration (see individual monographs for recommendations).

Water flushing and enteral/oral feeding

Whether the enteral feeding tube is to be used for continuous enteral feeding or for supplementary feeding, regular flushing is essential to prolong the life of the tube. Any tube that is not appropriately flushed will have a higher likelihood of occlusion.

Frequency

Flushing should occur before and after each intermittent feed, every 4–6 hours during continuous feeding,[3, 6] and before and after each drug administration. This will help to prevent interactions between the feed and the drugs being administered.

Water flushing after checking residual gastric volume

Gastric aspiration and return of stomach contents via the nasogastric tube in critical care units can increase tube occlusion and bacterial contamination.[14]

Frequency

Feeding tubes should be flushed immediately after gastric aspiration and after the return of the measured gastric contents, in accordance with local policy.

Water flushing after gastric aspiration for pH checking

Air flushing should be used to clear the tube initially each time it is required to obtain gastric secretions. Air flushing removes any liquid from the tube, allowing fresh gastric secretions to be aspirated. This aspirate can then be pH tested according to local policy.[9] Water flushing should be administered promptly after the gastric aspiration and pH testing is complete.

Frequency

It is recommended to check nasogastric feeding tube placement at least once every 24 hours as tubes may be dislodged after vomiting or coughing.[7]

Risks of water flushing and drug administration via enteral feeding tubes

Oesophageal reflux of medication solutions and flushes can occur in any patient. Especially susceptible are those patients with impaired swallowing, heartburn, gastric reflux and oesophagitis. Any patients who have tubes that travel through the cardiac sphincter of the stomach are at risk of oesophageal and pulmonary reflux.

Fluid-restricted patients

In some cases, for example in children or patients with renal or cardiac disease, the flush volumes recommended above will need to be revised to meet the patient's prescribed fluid restriction. Failure to do this could create an overall positive fluid balance and worsen the patient's disease state. Air flushes may be used to replace water flushes[14] in these circumstances.

General recommendations

- The enteral feeding should be stopped and the tube flushed before a drug is administered.
- In the event that the enteral feeding tube tip is placed within the small bowel, reduced flush volumes will be required to prevent distension and possible retrograde fluid flow resulting in an increased risk of regurgitation and possible pulmonary aspiration. Patients who have undergone full gastrectomy are particularly at risk.
- The patient should be nursed semi-recumbent (sitting up) at an angle of 30 degrees or greater to reduce reflux of the medication and flushes. This promotes gravity-assisted progression of the fluid. [12, 15, 16, 17]
- High-osmolality medication boluses administered into the stomach can delay gastric emptying and lead to a higher gastric residual volume and a greater risk of reflux. [18] The patient may therefore need to remain at 30 degrees for some time to facilitate gastric emptying.

References

1. Lord L. Restoring and maintaining patency of enteral feeding tubes. *Nutr Clin Pract.* 2003; 18(5): 422–426.
2. Rollins H. A nose for trouble. *Nurs Times.* 1997; 93(49): 66–67.
3. McAtear CA. *Current Perspectives on Enteral Nutrition in Adults.* Maidenhead, Berks: British Association for Parenteral and Enteral Nutrition; 1999.
4. Cannaby AM. Nursing care of patients with nasogastric feeding tubes. *Br J Nurs.* 2002; 11(6): 366–372.
5. Metheny N, *et al.* Effectiveness of pH measurements in predicting feeding tube placement. *Nurs Res.* 1989; 38(5): 280–285.
6. Colagiovanni L. Taking the tube. *Nurs Times.* 1999; 95(21): 63–67.
7. Mateo M. Nursing management of enteral tube feedings. *Heart Lung.* 1996; 25(4): 318–323.
8. Metheny N, Eisenberg P, McSweeney M. Effectiveness of feeding tube properties and three irrigants on clogging rates. *Nurs Res.* 1988; 37(3): 165–169.
9. Frankle EH *et al.* Methods of restoring patency to occluded feeding tubes. *Nutr Clin Pract.* 1998; 13: 129–131.
10. Bourgault AM, Heyland DK, Drover JW, Keefe L, Newman P, Day AG. Prophylactic pancreatic enzymes to reduce feeding tube occlusions. *Nutr Clin Prac.* 2003; 18(5): 398–401.
11. Keithley JK, Swanson B. Enteral nutrition: an update on practice recommendations. *Medsurg Nurs.* 2004; 13(2): 131–134.
12. Metheny NA, Dahms TE, Stewart BJ, *et al.* Efficacy of dye-stained enteral formula in detecting pulmonary aspiration. *Chest.* 2002; 122(1): 276–281.
13. Scanlan M, Frisch S. Nasoduodenal feeding tubes: prevention of occlusion. *J Neurosci Nurs.* 1992; 24(5): 256–259.
14. Powell KS, Marcuard SP, Farrior ES, Gallagher ML. Aspirating gastric residuals causes occlusion of small-bore feeding tubes. *JPEN J Parenter Enteral Nutr.* 1993; 17(3): 243–246.
15. Drakulovic MB, Torres A, Bauer TT, Nicolas JM, Nogue S, Ferrer M. Supine body position as a risk factor for nosocomial pneumonia in mechanically ventilated patients: A randomized trial. *Lancet.* 1999; 354(9193): 1851–1858.
16. Nagler R, Spiro SM. Persistent gastro-oesophageal reflux induced during prolonged gastric intubation. *N Engl J Med.* 1963; 269: 495–500. JN 480.
17. Metheny NA. Risk factors for aspiration. *JPEN J Parenter Enteral Nutr.* 2002; 26(6 Suppl): S26–S33.
18. Bury KD, Jambunathan G. Effects of elemental diets on gastric emptying and gastric secretion in man. *Am J Surg.* 1974; 127: 59–66. JN 482.

4
Restoring and maintaining patency of enteral feeding tubes
Lynne Colagiovanni

Key Points

- Effective flushing reduces incidence of tube occlusion.

- Feed is the most common cause of tube occlusion.

- Use of inappropriate drug formulations increases the risk of tube occlusion.

Most patients with a functioning gastrointestinal tract can be tube fed if they are unable to take sufficient nutrition orally. The development of soft, flexible fine-bore tubes that are easy to place has increased the popularity of this method of feeding, but tube occlusion, reported to be as high as 23–35%[1,2] is a significant problem.

Many different methods have been tried both to prevent and to clear tube occlusion, but few of these have a strong evidence base. Tubes that cannot be unblocked will need to be replaced, which is distressing for the patient, can increase morbidity, results in lost feeding time and has financial implications.

Aetiology of tube occlusion

Tube occlusions can be classified as either internal lumen obstruction or mechanical failure/problem with the tube. Tubes may become kinked or knotted while *in situ*, but internal lumen obstruction is the most common reason for tube occlusion.

Feeding tubes become occluded for a variety of reasons, which include:

- Feed precipitate from contact with an acidic fluid
- Stagnant feed in the tube
- Contaminated feed

- Cyclical feeding
- Incorrect drug administration
- Feeding tube properties

Consideration of each of these potential causes can help in reducing the incidence of tube occlusion.

Feed precipitate caused by contact with acidic fluid

Precipitation of the feed is responsible for tube occlusion in up to 80% of cases.[3] Occlusions are likely if gastric juices, which have an acidic pH, come into contact with feed solutions. Powell[3] found that tubes that had been aspirated four-hourly to check gastric residual volume had significantly more occlusions than those in the control group that had not been aspirated; however, this study was limited by small numbers and there was failure to record any drug administration via the tube. Occlusion occurred even though the tubes had been flushed with 10 mL water before and after each aspiration. In a study by Hofstetter and Allen,[4] precipitation occurred when intact protein feeds were acidified to less than pH 4.5. Interestingly, the same was not found when elemental or semi-elemental feeds were used. The authors conclude that it is the presence of casein in the whole-protein feeds (which is absent from elemental and semi-elemental feeds) that causes the problem.

Tubes with tips in the jejunum occluded far less frequently in both the Hofstetter and Allen study[4] and that of Marcuard and Stegall,[5] and this was assumed to be due to the higher pH of jejunal secretions.

Stagnant feed in the tube

A feed can easily form a clog in a tube if flushes are not given promptly when the feeding is completed or interrupted. Most enteral feeds are suspensions and, when the feed rate is extremely slow or is stopped, the larger particles (calcium caseinate and soy protein) settle in the horizontal portion of the tube.[6] More viscous feeds and those containing fibre are also more likely to cause occlusion.[7]

Contaminated feed

If there is significant bacterial contamination of the feed (bacterial counts ≥10 cfu/mL) this can cause the feed to precipitate, leading to tube occlusion.[8]

Cyclical feeding

The increased use of cyclical rather than continuous feeding may also be a contributory factor to feeding tube occlusion in the acute care setting. Based on work by Jacobs et al.,[9] many centres choose to give patients an enteral feeding break of 4–6 hours rather than feeding continuously over 24 hours, supposedly to reduce the risk of aspiration pneumonia. Enteral feeds cause a rise in gastric pH, allowing proliferation of Gram-negative bacteria, which may lead to pneumonia if aspirated. The break is thought to allow gastric pH to decrease, thus reducing this risk. Given that many patients now receive proton pump inhibitors, which also cause an increase in gastric pH, it may be time to review the theoretical need for enteral feeding breaks.

Feeding tube properties

Within adult practice 'fine-bore' tubes are now used for nasogastric feeding. Fine-bore is generally taken to mean 6Fr–12Fr. Gastrostomy and jejunostomy tubes vary in size depending on the device used and the preference of the healthcare professional inserting them, and can range from 9Fr to 20Fr.

Tube material may be a factor in the rate of occlusion, with polyurethane being shown to be less prone to occlusion than silicone.[10, 11] This may be because polyurethane tubes have a larger internal diameter than silicone for the same external size.

Wide-bore tubes may be expected to become occluded less frequently than fine-bore tubes, but Metheny et al.[10] found no difference in occlusion rates between polyurethane tubes of three different sizes. This supports the view that material may be more important than diameter.

Silicone has been reported to support the growth of yeasts within the tube, leading to occlusion.[12]

The number of exit holes at the distal tip of the tube may also be important. Tubes with one exit hole have been shown to become occluded less frequently than those with more. This is possibly due to the greater contact between feed and gastric acid.[4]

Incorrect drug administration

The use of enteral feeding tubes to administer drug therapy has increased considerably in recent years and may be a significant factor in tube occlusion. Occlusions can be caused by:

- Particle obstruction from inadequately crushed tablets
- Precipitate formation from interaction between feed and drug formulation
- Precipitate formation from interaction between drugs

Solutions for feeding tube flushes

Maintaining patency of the tube is to a large extent dependent on regular flushing. Various solutions have been used for flushing feeding tubes, including cranberry juice, cola, carbonated water, meat tenderiser, and pineapple juice.[6, 10, 13] However, no solution has been shown to be superior to water in preventing occlusion. Both cranberry juice and cola have a low pH, making precipitation with feed more likely, increasing rather than decreasing the risk of tube occlusion.[8]

Two studies have looked at the use of pancreatic enzymes to reduce feeding tube occlusions.[1, 14] Both of these studies have limitations, which means that although both show a trend towards less occlusions in the study group, it is difficult to recommend the routine use of pancreatic enzymes on the basis of the data presented. More work on the use of pancreatic enzymes in preventing tube occlusion is needed.

There are also practical problems that may limit their use; these are discussed later in this chapter.

Volume of water to be used when flushing

There are no studies looking specifically at what volume is effective in preventing tube occlusion. From the information available,[14, 15] a 15–30 mL flush is recommended, although this may need to be modified in patients with fluid restriction.

Recommendations for preventing feeding tube occlusions

- Use a polyurethane tube.
- Use size 8Fr–12Fr nasogastric tube (adults) and 10Fr or above for gastrostomy/ jejunostomy tubes.
- Follow national and local guidelines for preparation and administration of enteral feeds to minimise bacterial contamination.
- Attend to all pump alarms promptly and flush tubes with water whenever feed is stopped or interrupted.
- If it is safe to do so, keep gastric residual volume checking to a minimum.
- Use 15–30 mL water to flush the tube before and after each feeding episode, and before and after drug administration.
- If giving more than one drug, give each separately and flush with 10 mL water between each one. (Caution is needed in patients with fluid restriction.) See monographs section for specific drug recommendations.

Unblocking occluded tubes

Attempts to clear an occluded tube are more likely to be successful if the process begins as soon as possible after the occlusion occurs. It is therefore important that pump alarms are attended to promptly.[8]

Three main methods can be used in attempting to clear an occlusion:

- Liquid irrigants
- Pancreatic enzymes
- Mechanical devices

Liquid irrigants

Many liquids have been used in attempts to clear occluded feeding tubes. These include water (cold or warm), sodium bicarbonate, cola, other carbonated drinks, and meat tenderiser (which contains the proteolytic enzyme papain). There is little evidence to support the use of many of these. Cola has a pH of 2.5 and is likely to make the situation worse rather than better as it coagulates the protein in a feed. There is no evidence that warm water is any more successful than cold, or that sodium bicarbonate is effective, but as both are harmless and unlikely to make the situation worse, they can be used if individual centres feel they are helpful.

In an attempt to assess the effectiveness of varying irrigants on feed clogs, Marcuard *et al.*[16] tested the following: water, Sprite, Coca Cola, Mountain Dew, Pepsi, papain, and activated Viokase (pancreatic enzymes). Parts one and two of this study were done *in vitro*, so clogs were worked on promptly. Activated Viokase was found to be the most successful and papain the least. In the third, *in vivo*, part of the study, Viokase was compared with water for its ability to unblock the tubes. Water was unsuccessful in all cases, whereas Viokase dissolved the clog in 7 of the 10 tubes studied. This particular study would suggest that pancreatic enzymes may be useful in unblocking tubes. This is discussed further below.

Pancreatic enzymes

The use of pancreatic enzymes to dissolve feed clogs has been studied with differing results. The authors of the above paper went on to study a further 32 patients with a total of 60 tube occlusions over a period of 6 months.[5] In 44 of these occlusions, attempts were made to unblock the tubes. Water was successful in clearing only 12, while activated pancreatic enzymes cleared a further 23. Of the remaining seven, six occlusions were found not to be due to feed. The authors attribute the success of the pancreatic enzymes to the presence of chymotrypsin, a proteolytic agent known to cleave peptide bonds.

Two other studies looked at the use of pancreatic enzymes. Nicholson[17] had little success in freeing the clogs, while the study by Bommarito *et al.*[18] is difficult to evaluate as it contains little information on effectiveness. The differences in the results may be due to the differences in methodology. The type of enzymes used, dilutional volumes, dwell times and method of delivery varied between studies, and these may well be significant factors in success or failure.

Crucial to the success of the pancreatic enzymes is that they are 'activated' by being brought to the correct pH. In the Marcuard studies, sodium bicarbonate was added to achieve a solution with pH 7.9. This study also delivered the activated solution close to the site of the clog by administration via a fine-bore tube passed inside the nasogastric tube to the level of the clog.

Although the above was fairly easy to achieve within the research setting, the practicalities of implementing it in the clinical situation either in acute care or, more problematically, in the community, make its application limited. It is unlikely that pancreatic enzymes would be readily available in a timely manner to unblock an enteral feeding tube on a hospital ward, in a nursing home or within a patient's home, or that staff would know how much sodium bicarbonate to add in what volume. Finding a very fine-bore tube to pass inside a nasogastric tube would also be extremely difficult.

Thus, although pancreatic enzymes do seem to be effective in clearing feed tube occlusions, much work would need to be done in devising protocols/procedures and ensuring supply of relevant solutions and equipment at local level before they could be successfully used in routine practice.

CorPack Medsystems produce a declogging system, Clog Zapper. This is a patented enzyme powder (not pancreatic) within a syringe that is reconstituted with water and administered through a fine-bore tube supplied with the kit and is left to dwell for 30–60 minutes. The powder includes papain, ascorbic acid, maltodextrin and cellulase. Company studies state that Clog Zapper was successful in clearing all tubes on either the first or second attempt in a sample of 17 occluded tubes.[19] The high cost of this product is probably the reason for its low usage, although this should be balanced against the cost of replacing a tube, lost feeding time and the distress that tube replacement causes the patient. Independent studies on the use of this product would be useful.

It should be remembered that pancreatic enzymes, and probably also Clog Zapper, will only be useful if the clog is caused by feed. Clogs due to drug therapy are unlikely to be cleared in this way.

Mechanical devices

Generally it is thought inadvisable to reinsert guidewires or other devices into feeding tubes in an attempt to clear blockages. However, if pre-measured so as not to exceed the length of the tube, and if used with care by an experienced practitioner, they can be helpful. The Enteral Feeding Tube Declogger (Distinctive Medical Products, Cheshire, UK) is a flexible plastic device with a screw thread that is inserted into gastrostomy tubes and rotated to 'bore through' a clog. It is available in a range of French sizes and lengths, and suitable for use with most gastrostomy/jejunostomy tubes. Currently the sizes available make it unsuitable for use with nasogastric tubes. Cost may also be a prohibitive factor in its use.

General recommendations

Many tubes can be unblocked with the use of a 50 mL syringe, water and patience! A withdraw/flush method is the most effective. It can take 30 minutes or more to unblock a tube using this method. The use of small syringes is usually contraindicated as this may result in tube rupture. Should this happen in the oesophagus and go undetected, the consequences could be serious if feeding was recommenced. The risks of tube rupture should be considered against the possible difficulties of repassing the tube when determining the size of syringe used.

Unblocking nasogastric feeding tubes
- Use 15–30 mL water (warm or cold), in a 50 mL syringe, and a pull/push action.
- Do not use cola or other solutions with an acidic pH.
- Use a smaller syringe (5 mL) with caution if the above fails and seek specialist advice.
- Use a mechanical declogging device of the correct size with gastrostomy/jejunostomy tubes (if available).
- Only use pancreatic enzymes if they are activated to the correct pH and you are able to deliver close to the occlusion.

Prevention is nearly always better than cure. Using the correct tube and caring for it properly with prompt attention to pump alarms and protocols for flushing and drug administration should help to reduce the incidence of tube occlusion. If an occlusion is discovered, it should be dealt with as quickly as possible using techniques supported by the available evidence. If this advice is heeded, the amount of feeding time lost and distress caused to patients from occluded feeding tubes can be reduced.

References

1. Sriram K, Jayanthi V, Lakshmi RG, *et al.* Prophylactic locking of enteral feeding tubes with pancreatic enzymes. *JPEN J Parenter Enteral Nutr.* 1997; 21: 353–356.
2. Marcuard SP, Perkins AM. Clogging of feeding tubes. *JPEN J Parenter Enteral Nutr.* 1988; 12: 403–405.
3. Powell KS, Marcuard SP, Farrior ES, *et al.* Aspirating gastric residuals causes occlusion of small bore feeding tubes. *JPEN J Parenter Enteral Nutr.* 1993: 17: 243–246.
4. Hofstetter J. Allen LV. Causes of non medication induced nasogastric tube occlusion. *Am J Health Syst Pharm.* 1992; 49: 603–607.
5. Marcuard SP, Stegall KL. Unclogging feeding tubes with pancreatic enzymes. *JPEN J Parenter Enteral Nutr.* 1990; 14: 198–200.
6. Nicholau DP, Davis SK. Carbonated beverages as irrigants for feeding tubes. *Ann Pharmacother.* 1990; 24: 840.
7. Lord L. Restoring and maintaining patency of enteral feeding tubes. *Nutr Clin Pract.* 2003; 18(5): 422–426.
8. Kohn CL. The relationship between enteral formula contamination and length of enteral delivery set usage. *JPEN J Parenter Enteral Nutr.* 1991; 15: 567–571.
9. Jacobs S. *et al.* Continuous enteral feeding: a major cause of pneumonia among ventilated intensive care unit patients. *JPEN J Parenter Enteral Nutr.* 1990; 14(4): 353–356.
10. Metheny N, Eisenberg P, McSweeney M. Effect of feeding tube properties and three irrigants on clogging rates. *Nurs Res.* 1988; 37: 165–169.
11. Hearne BE *et al.* In vitro flow rates of enteral solutions through nasoenteric tubes. *JPEN J Parenter Enteral Nutr.* 1984; 8(4): 456–459.
12. Marcuard SP, Finley JL, McDonald KG. Large bore feeding tube occlusion by yeast colonies. *JPEN J Parenter Enteral Nutr.* 1993; 17: 187–193.
13. Wilson MF, Haynes-Johnson V. Cranberry juice or water? A comparison of feeding tube irrigants. *Nutritional Support Services.* 1987; 7(7): 23–24.
14. Bourgault AM, Heyland DK, Drover JW, Keefe L, Newman P, Day AG. Prophylactic pancreatic enzymes to reduce feeding tube occlusions. *Nutr Clin Pract.* 2003; 18(5): 398–401.
15. Keithley JK, Swanson B. Enteral nutrition: an update on practice recommendations. *Medsurg Nurs.* 2004; 13(2): 131–134.
16. Marcuard SP, Stegall KL, Trogdon S. Clearing of obstructed feeding tubes. *JPEN J Parenter Enteral Nutr.* 1989; 13: 81–83.
17. Nicholson LJ. Declogging small bore feeding tubes. *JPEN J Parenter Enteral Nutr.* 1987; 11(6): 594–597.
18. Bommarito AA, Heinzelmann MJ, Boysen DA. A new approach to the management of obstructed enteral feeding tubes. *Nutr Clin Pract.* 1989; 4(3): 111–114.
19. Corpak Medsystems. *Clog Zapper.* Clinical Results; 1997.

5
Drug therapy review
Rebecca White

Key Points

- Reduce drug therapy to the minimum necessary.

- Transfer the patient onto once-daily formulations with a long half-life where possible (*not* modified-/slow-release formulations).

- Determine alternative formulations and routes available where possible.

- Make any therapy changes in an environment in which the patient can be effectively monitored.

Regular drug therapy review and rationalisation is an essential part of effective medical treatment. The first step should be to determine the therapeutic rationale for the prescription and to discontinue any therapy for which this cannot be identified, or where there is inappropriate therapeutic duplication.

Drugs can be prescribed unnecessarily, especially within secondary care when many are prescribed 'just in case'. Administering this array of medicines via a feeding tube can often present a daunting challenge to an experienced nurse. The practical and logistical issues become magnified when this dosing regimen is transferred into a home care setting.

The first step should be to determine which of the drugs need to be administered via the feeding tube or whether the patient can still take them orally. The use of alternative routes of administration should be fully explored, but the practical considerations should be borne in mind at all times and offset against using a drug outside the terms of its product licence. Alternative routes such as injections and suppositories are useful for short-term management but are rarely practical in chronic disease management.

Transdermal therapy, sublingual administration and depot injections are useful alternatives for drugs such as GTN, HRT and analgesia. (For further information see chapter 6.)

Where possible, therapy should be changed to drugs with a prolonged therapeutic effect (not modified-/slow-release formulations) to reduce the need for multiple tube manipulations. The choice of drug should be considered in conjunction with local formulary recommendations.

Any changes to therapy should be made in an environment in which the therapeutic response to the change can be monitored. This is particularly important when the therapy will be continued in a different care environment, either by patients themselves or by a carer. As in all aspects of care, discharge planning should start as early as possible, especially if a nonmedical carer is required to administer the medication. A process that is straightforward to the ward nurse can seem an impossible task to a patient or carer. Where possible, document all instructions and ensure that other appropriate healthcare professionals are sent a copy: e.g. district nurses and GPs.

Communication with the wider healthcare team is necessary to ensure continuity of therapy. This is particularly important if the formulation of a drug is prepared extemporaneously or is provided as a manufactured 'special', since inadequate communication may delay supply of medication in the community. It is important to communicate to the prescriber the formulations needed for administration via an enteral feeding tube and that this is an unlicensed use of the medication, thereby providing the prescriber with the full information necessary for them to consider their responsibilities should an adverse event occur. (See chapter 8 for further information.)

6

Choice of medication formulation

Rebecca White

Key Points

- Solutions or soluble tablets are the formulations of choice.

- Do not assume that liquid formulation will be suitable.

- Do not crush tablets or open capsules unless an alternative formulation or drug is unavailable.

When deciding which medication formulation is appropriate for administration via an enteral feeding tube, many factors need to be taken into consideration. It is not necessarily correct to assume that a liquid is preferable to a tablet; unwanted side-effects of the excipients of a liquid formulation must be borne in mind. The needs of the patient or carers must also be considered; it may not be practical for the patient to carry several bottles of liquid medication with them on a daily basis.

In this chapter each of the formulations available will be reviewed. Guidance on how to administer the formulation will be given and advantages and disadvantages listed.

See chapter 9 for further information on appropriate choice of syringe.

Liquid formulations

Solutions

A solution is a homogenous one-phase system consisting of two or more components. The solute is dispersed in the solvent. The solvent is usually present in the greater amount. Syrup is a notable exception with 66.7% w/w sucrose as the solute in 33.3% w/w of water as the solvent.

Because a solution is a homogenous system, the drug will be distributed evenly throughout the system. This is in contrast to a suspension, where inadequate mixing or settling may lead to variable dosing.

Water is the most widely used solvent for pharmaceutical products. Some other solvents can be used in combination with water to act as co-solvents and thereby increase the solubility of the drug in the formulation. Examples of excipients used in solutions are ethanol, sorbitol, glycerol and propylene glycol. Inclusion of these excipients can determine the suitability of a solution for administration via an enteral feeding tube; for example, sorbitol can cause diarrhoea (see disadvantages below).

Administration of solutions

1. Stop the enteral feed.
2. Flush the enteral feeding tube with the recommended volume of water (see p. 11).
3. Check the relevant monograph – can the drug be administered with feed, or should a specific time interval be allowed before administering the drug?
4. Draw the drug solution into an appropriate size and type of syringe.
5. Flush the drug dose down the enteral feeding tube.
6. Finally, flush the enteral feeding tube with the recommended volume of water (see p. 11).
7. Re-start the feed, unless a specific time interval is needed following the administration of the drug.

Alternatively, at step (4) measure the drug solution in a suitable container and then draw into an appropriate size and type of syringe. Avoid syringes that are compatible with parenteral devices. Ensure that the measure is rinsed and that this rinsing water is administered via the enteral feeding tube to ensure the total dose is given. *Do not* measure liquid medicines using a catheter-tipped syringe, as this results in excessive dosing owing to the volume of the tip.

Advantages

- Even drug distribution in the formulation allows accurate dosing.
- Ready to use.
- Easily measured.
- Suitable for administration via an enteral feeding tube without further manipulation.

Disadvantages

- Co-solvents may be present in sufficient quantities to have a pharmacological effect, especially if present in all drug formulations being used; for example, sorbitol ($\geq$15 g/day) will have a laxative effect.
- May not be considered practical for carrying around.
- Cost.
- Stability and a short shelf-life may be impractical.

Suspensions

A suspension formulation is usually developed when the drug is insoluble or if, for reasons of palatability, the drug is formulated into coated microgranules.

Nongranular suspensions can be administered via enteral feeding tubes but may require further dilution owing to the viscosity and osmolarity.

For granular suspensions, granule size and the viscosity of the formulation must be taken into account when assessing the suitability of the formulation for administration via an enteral feeding tube. Examples of granular suspensions are ciprofloxacin, clarithromycin and lansoprazole. Some granular suspensions contain enteric coated granules (e.g. Zoton suspension) or modified-release granules (e.g. MST-continus suspension); caution should be exercised with such formulations to avoid changing the absorption characteristics (see individual monographs).

Administration of a suspension (see notes above)

1. Stop the enteral feed.
2. Flush the enteral feeding tube with the recommended volume of water (see p. 11).
3. Check the relevant monograph – can the drug be administered with feed, or should a specific time interval be allowed before administering the drug?
4. Shake the medication bottle thoroughly to ensure adequate mixing.
5. Draw the medication suspension into the appropriate size and type of syringe.
6. Flush the medication dose down the enteral feeding tube.
7. Finally, flush the enteral feeding tube with the recommended volume of water (see p. 11).
8. Re-start the feed, unless a specific time interval is needed following the administration of the drug.

Alternatively, at step (5) measure the drug suspension in a suitable container and then add an equal volume of water and mix thoroughly. Draw this into an appropriate size and type of syringe. Avoid syringes that are compatible with parenteral devices. Ensure that the measure is rinsed and that this rinsing water is administered via the enteral feeding tube to ensure that the total dose is given. *Do not* measure liquid medicines using a catheter tipped syringe as this results in excessive dosing owing to the volume of the tip.

Advantages

- Ready to use (few exceptions)

Disadvantages

- Granules in suspension may be too large or the suspension may be too viscous to pass through the enteral feeding tube.
- Settling or inadequate shaking may affect the accuracy of dosing.
- May not be practical to carry around.
- Cost.
- Stability and shelf-life may be impractical

Solid dosage formulations

Soluble tablets

A soluble tablet dissolves completely when placed in water to give a solution of the drug; this is usually achieved by using an alternative salt form, e.g. prednisolone sodium phosphate.

Administration of soluble tablets

1. Stop the enteral feed.
2. Flush the enteral feeding tube with the recommended volume of water (see p. 11).
3. Check the relevant monograph – can the drug be administered with feed, or should a specific time interval be allowed before administering the drug?
4. Select an appropriate size and type of syringe for administration.
5. Remove the plunger and place the tablet into the barrel of the syringe.
6. Replace the plunger.
7. Draw 10 mL of water into syringe and allow the tablet to dissolve, shaking as necessary.
8. Inspect the solution to ensure that there are no visible particles.
9. Flush the medication dose down the enteral feeding tube.
10. Draw an equal volume of water into the syringe and also flush this via the enteral feeding tube (this will rinse the syringe and ensure that the total dose is administered).
11. Finally, flush with the recommended volume of water (see p. 11).
12. Re-start the feed, unless a specific time interval is needed following the administration of the drug.

Alternatively, at step (4) place the tablet into medicine pot, add 10 mL of water and allow tablet to dissolve. Draw this into an appropriate size and type of syringe. Ensure that the measure is rinsed and that this rinsing water is administered via the enteral feeding tube to ensure that the total dose is given.

Advantages
- Drug is in solution.
- Long expiry date of original packaged drug.
- Usually less expensive than alternative liquid formulation.
- Easy to carry around.

Disadvantages
- One must allow complete dissolution before administration.
- Fine dose adjustment is difficult.

Effervescent tablets

Effervescent tablets are defined as tablets in which more than 75% of the bulk of the tablet is composed of inert agents intended to make the tablet effervesce. These tablets are created by incorporating sodium or potassium carbonates or bicarbonates with tartaric or citric acid; this produces carbon dioxide when placed in water and rapidly breaks the tablets apart. Owing to the nature of the formulation, these preparations tend to have a high sodium content.

These tablets will effervesce and dissolve or disintegrate when placed in water. The volume suggested is usually $\frac{1}{3}$ to $\frac{1}{2}$ a tumblerful of water; however, for the purposes of administering these formulations via an enteral feeding tube it may be possible to dissolve them in a smaller volume.[1] (See individual monographs for details.)

Administration of effervescent tablets

1. Stop the enteral feed.
2. Flush the enteral feeding tube with the recommended volume of water (see p. 11).
3. Check the relevant monograph – can the drug be administered with feed, or should a specific time interval be allowed before administering the drug?
4. Measure a suitable quantity of water into a container of appropriate size to allow effervescence without spillage.
5. Add the effervescent tablet and allow it to disperse.
6. Draw the contents of the measuring pot into an appropriate size and type of syringe.
7. Inspect the syringe contents to ensure that there are no visible particles that might block the tube.
8. Flush the medication dose down the enteral feeding tube.
9. Rinse the measure and administer this water via the enteral feeding tube to ensure that the total dose is given.
10. Finally, flush with the recommended volume of water (see p. 11).
11. Re-start the feed, unless a specific time interval is needed following the administration of the drug.

Advantages

- Low osmolarity – will not cause diarrhoea.
- Long shelf-life of original packaged drug.
- Easy to carry around/convenient.
- Cheaper than liquids.

Disadvantages

- May require a large volume to be fully dispersed.
- Must be fully dispersed before administration to avoid gas production in the enteral feeding tube.
- Sodium content can be high.
- Excipients may not dissolve and may sediment out.
- Cannot be dispersed in syringe owing to the production of gas.

Dispersible tablets

Although designed to be given orally, dispersible tablets disintegrate in water to give particles that may or may not suspend in water.

These tablets will usually disperse when placed in a small amount of water, e.g. 10–15 mL; however not all are suitable for administration via an enteral feeding tube as the resultant particles or granules may be too large for administration via fine-bore tubes, e.g. Pentasa dispersible tablets.

Administration of dispersible tablets

1. Stop the enteral feed.
2. Flush the enteral feeding tube with the recommended volume of water (see p. 11).
3. Check the relevant monograph – can the drug be administered with feed, or should a specific time interval be allowed before administering the drug?
4. Select an appropriate size and type of syringe for administration.
5. Remove the plunger and place the tablet in the barrel of the syringe.
6. Replace the plunger.
7. Draw 10 mL of water into syringe and allow the tablet to disperse, shaking if necessary.
8. Inspect the syringe contents to ensure that there are no large particles that might block the tube.
9. Flush the medication dose down the enteral feeding tube.
10. Draw an equal volume of water into the syringe and flush this via the enteral feeding tube (this will rinse syringe and ensure that the total dose is administered).
11. Finally, flush with the recommended volume of water (see p. 11).
12. Re-start the feed, unless a specific time interval is needed following the administration of the drug.

Alternatively, at step (4) place the tablet into medicine pot, add 10 mL of water and allow the tablet to disperse. Draw this into an appropriate size and type of syringe. Ensure that the measure is rinsed and that this rinsing water administered via the enteral feeding tube to ensure that the total dose is given.

Advantages
- Cost.
- Convenient to carry around.
- Lower electrolyte content than effervescent tablets.

Disadvantages
- Particles/granules of dispersion may be too large for administration via fine-bore tubes.

Orodispersible tablets

Orodispersible tablets are designed to disperse on the tongue. They are not necessarily absorbed sublingually, merely swallowed with the saliva; however, individual monographs should be consulted. They are intended to be taken without water, examples are Feldene Melts or Zoton FasTab.

Administration of orodispersible tablets

The administration of these formulations via enteral feeding tubes varies depending on the medicine concerned. The formulations and dose equivalences vary depending on the intended site of absorption, for example, Zoton FasTabs are enteric coated micro-granules that, although they disintegrate easily in a small amount of water, may block a very fine-bore enteral feeding tubes. Also, the dose may be inappropriate; for example, Zelaper is a lower dose than the equivalent oral product of selegiline. Individual monographs should be consulted. If the formulation is suitable for administration via an enteral feeding tube, the same method as for dispersible tablets can be used; see individual drug monographs for more details.

Advantages
- Convenient to carry around.
- Cost.

Disadvantages
- Unsuitability of some formulations for fine-bore tubes owing to site of absorption or formulation characteristics.

Buccal/sublingual tablets

Medicines formulated into buccal or sublingual tablets are designed to be absorbed through the oral mucosa and therefore bypass the first-pass metabolism effects of the liver. These formulations are a useful alternative for patients who are 'NBM' or are unable to swallow, providing the patient is able to produce normal quantities of saliva (caution is needed in head and neck surgery patients). However, they are not suitable for administration via enteral feeding tubes as significantly reduced drug absorption will occur, owing to first-pass metabolism.

Compressed tablets

Ordinary-release tablets are usually made by one of two methods: either direct com-pression or wet granulation. Compression pressures are usually higher for tablets made directly from drug powder and bulking agent compared to those used in producing tablets formulated from granules. A variation in the excipients used in the tablet formulation will affect the disintegration time of the tablet when it is placed in water. (See individual monographs for information on disintegration times.)

When a tablet formulated by wet granulation is placed in water, it will usually disintegrate to give visible granules before deaggregating to give primary drug particles.

A large proportion of ordinary-release tablets will disperse sufficiently in water to be suitable for administration via an enteral feeding tube, without the need for crushing.

Advantages
- Cheap.
- Easily obtained.
- Most disintegrate easily when placed in water.
- No need to crush, therefore exposure risk is reduced.

Disadvantages
- Not all tablets will disintegrate easily.
- Variability in dispersion characteristics between generic brands of the same drug.

Administration of compressed tablets
There are several methods of administering compressed tablets.

Tablets that disintegrate
1. Stop the enteral feed.
2. Flush the enteral feeding tube with the recommended volume of water (see p. 11).
3. Check the relevant monograph – can the drug be administered with feed, or should a specific time interval be allowed before administering the drug?
4. Select an appropriate size and type of syringe.
5. Remove the plunger and place the tablet into the barrel of the syringe.
6. Draw 10 mL of water into the syringe and allow the tablet to disintegrate, shaking as necessary (larger volumes may be necessary for some bulky tablets; see individual monographs).
7. Inspect the syringe contents to ensure that there are no large visible particles that might block the tube.
8. Flush the medication dose down the enteral feeding tube.
9. Draw an equal volume of water into the syringe and flush this via the enteral feeding tube; this will rinse the syringe and ensure that the total dose is administered.
10. Finally, flush with the recommended volume of water (see p. 11).
11. Re-start the feed, unless a specific time interval is needed following the administration of the drug.

Alternatively, at step (4) place the tablet into a medicine pot and add 10 mL of water (larger volumes may be necessary for some tablets; see individual monographs) and allow the tablet to disintegrate. Draw this into the syringe. Ensure that the measure is rinsed and that this rinsing water is administered via the enteral feeding tube to ensure that the total dose is given.

Both of the above methods have advantages:

- Allowing the tablet to disintegrate in a small container allows the patient/carer to inspect the dispersion and any particles will be visible when drawn into a syringe; however, there is a risk that some of the dose may be left in the container if it is not rinsed adequately.

- Allowing the tablet to disperse directly in the syringe ensures that the whole dose is given, within a closed system. Particles may not be visible owing to the cloudiness of the dispersion, but using a larger volume for dispersal will usually overcome this problem.

Tablets that do not disintegrate

Several devices are available for crushing tablets. Crushing of tablets should always be considered a last resort as the patient/carer is at risk of exposure to drug powder (see chapter 8 on health and safety and clinical risk management), and there are legal considerations that must be considered (see chapter 7 on the unlicensed use of medications).

Using a mortar and pestle

1. Stop the enteral feed.
2. Flush the enteral feeding tube with the recommended volume of water (see p. 11).
3. Check the relevant monograph – can the drug be administered with feed, or should a specific time interval be allowed before administering the drug?
4. Ensure that suitable protective clothing is worn.
5. Place the tablet(s) in the mortar.
6. Crush the tablet(s) to a fine powder, making sure that the powder is contained in the mortar.
7. Add 5 mL of water and crush further to form a paste.
8. Add a further 5–10 mL of water and continue to crush and mix the paste; this should form a fine suspension. Ensure that there are no visible pieces of coating or large tablet particles.
9. Draw this suspension into an appropriate size and type of syringe and administer via the enteral feeding tube.
10. A further 10–20 mL of water should be added to the mortar and stirred with the pestle to ensure that any drug remaining in the mortar or on the pestle is mixed with the water.
11. Draw this water into the syringe and flush it down the enteral feeding tube. This can be repeated to ensure that all the powder is administered.
12. The tube should then be finally flushed with water to ensure that the whole dose is administered (see p. 11).
13. Re-start the feed, unless a specific time interval is needed following the administration of the drug.

N.b. Care should be taken when using this method in fluid-restricted patients.

The pestle and mortar should be thoroughly cleaned with hot soapy water after each use to avoid cross-contamination.

Using a crushing syringe

1. Stop the enteral feed.
2. Flush the enteral feeding tube with the recommended volume of water (see p. 11).

3. Check the relevant monograph – can the drug be administered with feed, or should a specific time interval be allowed before administering the drug?
4. Place the tablet in the barrel of the crushing syringe and push the plunger down.
5. Put the cap on the crushing syringe and rotate the barrel of the syringe to crush the tablet.
6. Remove the cap and draw 10–15 mL of water into the crushing syringe.
7. Replace the cap and shake the syringe to ensure that the powder is mixed well.
8. Inspect the syringe contents to ensure that there are no large particles that might block the tube.
9. Flush this suspension down the enteral feeding tube.
10. Draw a further 10–30 mL of water into the crushing syringe and shake before flushing down the enteral feeding tube; this will ensure that the whole dose is given.
11. Finally, flush with the recommended volume of water (see p. 11).
12. Re-start the feed, unless a specific time interval is needed following the administration of the drug.

This closed system is preferred for cytotoxics or hormones for which no liquid formulation is available, so as to avoid environmental contamination and exposure of a carer to the medicine.

Modified-release tablets

Modified-release tablets are formulated to release the drug slowly over time. As a rule these are not suitable for administration via enteral feeding tubes because altering the dosage form, for example by crushing, will affect the pharmacokinetic profile of the drug and may result in excessive peak plasma concentrations and side-effects.

Hard gelatin capsules

Some hard gelatin capsules can be opened and the powder mixed with water. There are a number of considerations, including the risk of inhaling powder.

Most capsules are too small to be manipulated and opened, and this should be taken into consideration with elderly or arthritic patients. Some capsules contain granules rather than powder.

Administration of hard gelatin capsules

1. Stop the enteral feed.
2. Flush the enteral feeding tube with the recommended volume of water (see p. 11).
3. Check the relevant monograph – can the drug be administered with feed, or should a specific time interval be allowed before administering the drug?
4. Open the capsule and pour the contents into a medicine pot.
5. Add 15 mL of water.
6. Stir to disperse the powder.
7. Draw into an appropriate size and type of syringe and administer via the enteral feeding tube.

8. Add a further 15 mL of water to the medicine pot; stir to ensure that any powder remaining in the pot is mixed with water.
9. Draw up this dispersion and flush it down the tube. This will ensure that the whole dose is given.
10. Flush the enteral feeding tube with the recommended volume of water (see p. 11).
11. Re-start the feed, unless a specific time interval is needed following the administration of the drug.

Advantages
- Cheap.
- Convenient.

Disadvantages
- Occupational exposure risk.
- Small capsules may be difficult to open.
- Not all capsules are suitable; the contents may not disperse in water owing to the hygrophobic or hydrostatic nature of the powder.

Soft gelatin capsules

Drugs that are presented in soft gelatin capsules are usually poorly soluble in water and are therefore contained in an oily solution within the capsule; an example is ciclosporin in Neoral. Therefore, it is unlikely that these will be suitable for administration via an enteral feeding tube.

In certain circumstances it may be possible to pierce the capsule shell using a pin and squeeze out the contents (for example the contents of a nifedipine capsule for sublingual use); however, accurate dosing cannot be guaranteed. The volume contained in the capsule can vary depending on the brand of capsule used, and the volume expelled will vary depending on the skill of the person expelling the contents; for these reasons this method is unreliable and is not recommended.

Enteric coated tablets

Tablets are given an enteric coating to protect the drug from degradation by the acidic conditions of the stomach or to reduce the incidence of gastric side-effects.

Crushing enteric coated tablets and administering them via feeding tubes is highly likely to cause tube blockage.

Administering enteric coated tablets via an enteral feeding tube with the tip placed in the stomach would necessitate crushing or removing the enteric coat prior to administration; therefore, the drug is likely to be degraded in the stomach. The extent of drug degradation is unpredictable and the practitioner should explore alternative therapies or routes before deciding to administer enteric coated tables via an enteral feeding tube placed in the stomach. If it is decided to administer the drug by this method, the above techniques are applicable but will result in decreased amounts of drug available for absorption and the patient's response to therapy should be monitored carefully. If the patient has a feeding tube with the end in the small intestine (duodenum or jejunum), then crushing or removing the enteric coat prior to administration down the enteral feeding tube is not an issue.

Injectable formulations

Injections vary widely in their suitability for administration via enteral feeding tubes. The injectable formulation may be a different salt form from the oral formulation and therefore the oral bioavailability may be unknown. The pH of injections can also vary widely, making some unsuitable for enteral administration (see chapter 7). Refer to the individual monographs for information about the appropriateness of different injections for use via an enteral feeding tube.

Advantages
- The drug is in a soluble form.

Disadvantages
- Variable salts.
- Cost.

References

1. BPNG Data on file, 2004.

Suggested further reading

Aulton ME, ed. *Pharmaceutics: The Science of Dosage Form Design.* Edinburgh: Churchill Livingstone; 1988.
Protocol produced by Dr David Wright, Senior Lecturer in Pharmacy Practice, University of East Anglia, Norwich; *Swallowing Difficulties Protocol: Achieving Best Practice in Medication Administration-* (March 2005) distributed by Rosemont Pharmaceuticals.

7

The legal and professional consequences of administering drugs via enteral feed tubes

David Wright

Key Points

- Understand the legal implications of manipulating a drug formulation prior to administration.

- Be aware of relevant national guidelines.

- Be aware of relevant local protocols.

When considering the practical and clinical issues associated with the administration of drugs via enteral feeding tubes, the healthcare professional should be aware of legal and professional consequences of altering a drug's formulation prior to administration and the administration of drugs via an unlicensed route. The aim of this chapter is to consider the legal and professional frameworks that govern the practice of healthcare professionals and to relate these specifically to the administration of drugs via enteral feeding tubes. It is appropriate at this point to state that providing the healthcare professional is acting in the patient's best interest, following locally agreed protocols and effecting evidence based practice, it is unlikely that any legal or ethical frameworks will be infringed.

The law and ethics that govern the activities of a healthcare professional are provided in Table 7.1. An activity that transgresses one aspect in Table 7.1 will frequently transgress others and may result in more than one action being taken against the professional. If a pharmacist's action results in serious patient harm or death, then they could find themselves in a court of law to answer a criminal charge, in front of the Royal Pharmaceutical Society of Great Britain's (RPSGB) disciplinary committee, and appropriately sanctioned by their employer. Furthermore, the patient or a relative could take out a civil case in order to obtain compensation for the damage or harm caused.

Table 7.1 Different types of law and ethics that govern healthcare professionals

Type	Description	Relevant standards
Criminal law	Legislation that is used by the state to enforce behaviour; i.e. it is legislation that if contravened generally results in the state becoming the prosecutor and a defendant, if found guilty receiving either imprisonment, community penalty or a fine.	Medicines Act 1968 Misuse of Drugs Act 1972 Data Protection Act 1984
Civil law	Legislation that is used to dispute settlements; i.e. it is used to claim for damages. The claimant is the person or body who has been 'harmed' and the defendant is the person or body who has to prove that they were not liable for the harm caused. The outcome of a successful civil case may be payment of damages by the defendant or an injunction against them.	Applicable to all instances that involve patient care. If you are an employer you may also be liable for any harm that may come to your staff while they are in your employment.
Administrative law	This applies where legislation is devolved from parliament to public bodies to allow them to regulate certain activities. Unlike criminal and civil law, contravention of administrative law will not generally result in a court hearing. It will be dealt with using appropriate mechanisms by the public body and may result in a penalty being imposed, e.g. removal of a care home licence.	The National Care Standards Commission
Ethics	The principles that are accepted in any profession as the basis for proper behaviour. Transgression of the 'ethics' of the profession may ultimately result in the removal of the individual's right to practice.	Nursing and Midwifery Council Code of Professional Conduct, 1 June 2002 RPSGB Code of Ethics

To place the legal and professional issues surrounding administration of drugs via enteral feed tubes in context, a fictitious scenario is provided in Case Study 7.1 and this will be referred to throughout the chapter.

Case Study 7.1

Mr. J.M., 78 years old, has returned to a nursing home from hospital with a PEG tube.

The discharge note states that the medication is as follows:

- Digoxin 62.5 microgram in the morning
- Zopicone 7.5 mg at night
- Warfarin 5 mg in the morning
- Felodipine 5 mg in the morning

There was no guidance provided in the discharge letter as to how to administer these medicines via the PEG tube. The general practitioner prescribes all of the medicines as tablets or capsules and the nurse therefore has to crush or open them all and mix with water before placing them into the tube.

Criminal law

The Medicines Act 1968 governs the supply and administration of all drugs in the UK. The vast majority of drugs prescribed in the UK are 'authorised for marketing' (licensed), under the Medicines Act.[1] A pharmaceutical manufacturer can market the drug solely for the indication for which it has been tested. To remain within the Marketing Authorisation, the drug must be given to the patient in the authorised form, within the authorised dose range and not to a patient with a condition for which the drug has not been tested for safety by the manufacturer. Frequently drugs are not authorised for use in pregnant women or children, not because they are necessarily unsafe but because the manufacturer chooses not to test the drug in these populations.

Administration of drugs via enteral feeding tubes will generally be outside of the marketing authorisation as manufacturers do not tend to test or license drugs to be administered via this route. It could be argued that by circumventing the oral mucosa, the oesophagus in the case of PEGs and additionally the stomach in the case of PEJs, the bioavailability of the drug may be significantly altered. Furthermore, there is limited evidence demonstrating that drug is lost on the tube itself and this again will affect the effectiveness of the therapy.[2]

The crushing of tablets and opening of capsules prior to administration (which in some circumstances is the only option available for administration via this route) will, in the majority of cases, also place the administration outside of the drug's marketing authorisation. This action will alter the release profile of the drug (to a greater or lesser extent depending on the original formulation) and it is this that is perhaps more likely to cause harm to the patient if not fully considered before being undertaken.

The Medicines Act states that without an appropriate marketing authorisation it is unlawful for any person to sell or supply a medicine in the UK. Doctors, dentists and veterinarians, however, are exempted by the Act from this requirement and can request that unauthorised medicines be administered to their patients.[1] If this were not the case, it would be impossible for standard treatments to be tested or used in unusual situations or for pre-marketing authorisation clinical trials to take place.

In the case study provided, in prescribing drugs for administration via a PEG tube the doctor is within the law by authorising an unlicensed use of a medication. It is important to note, however, that if the nurse had chosen to crush the tablets without the doctor's prior consent, i.e. if the doctor was unaware of the newly sited PEG tube and prescribed solid dose formulations inadvertently, then the nurse's actions would have been unlawful as nurses are presently not allowed to authorise the use of drugs outside of their marketing authority. Although it is common for nurses to seek advice from other healthcare professionals before undertaking this action, and such actions are completely appropriate, it must also be recognised that healthcare professionals other than doctors or dentists, e.g. pharmacists, cannot authorise such actions under the Medicines Act 1968.

If the nurse's actions were unlawful, in practice it is unlikely that this would be identified or acted upon unless the patient is actually harmed. In such instances, although the transgression of the Medicines Act would be helpful in demonstrating that the person's actions fell below that of a competent professional in a civil case and could be used by the professional body in deciding on its punishment (both discussed later), in itself it would probably be deemed a lesser offence.

Perhaps the greatest concern for any healthcare professional is the likelihood of their actions causing harm and ultimately resulting in a criminal record. For criminal law cases to be successful, the prosecutor would need to prove 'beyond reasonable doubt' that any harm seen was due to the healthcare professional's actions, i.e. in this case drug being crushed prior to administration or drug being inappropriately administered via an enteral feeding tube.

It might be difficult for a prosecutor to argue that a side-effect was a direct result of crushing when the side-effect is an expected occurrence in a percentage of patients receiving the drug in its licensed state. Similarly, it would be difficult for a prosecutor to prove 'beyond reasonable doubt' that the drug had been ineffective owing to the administration via the enteral feeding tube or to crushing, as it is a normal expectation that drugs are ineffective in a proportion of all patients.

Civil law

Providing the healthcare professional uses the drug exactly as the marketing authorisation states, the liability in any civil case will usually lie with the manufacturer. If a drug is tampered with prior to administration in a way that is not outlined in the marketing authorisation or is administered by an untested route, the administering person will be giving an 'unauthorised drug'. Liability would lie with the doctor, with the pharmacist if they are aware of the method of administration when supplying, and with the nurse or carer administering the drug. If the doctor and administrator had received advice from a third party on the unlicensed administration, then the third party, such as a medicines information unit, would also be partially liable.

In the case scenario provided, there are many reasons for questioning the appropriateness of administration of drugs via this route and whether crushing of drugs is the most appropriate action. Administration of warfarin with enteral feeds can result in a significant reduction in the amount of drug absorbed and hence a reduced clinical effect.[3] Some zopiclone formulations form a gelatinous mass when mixed with water and may block the enteral feeding tube. Crushing of felodipine, which is a slow-release formulation, may result in J.M. receiving a larger than expected dose initially and subsequently a period of time with no drug in the body. Digoxin has a small therapeutic window and therefore adsorption onto the PEG tube may also alter its clinical effectiveness.

In order for a civil case to be successful, the defendant must be proven to have been negligent. This would require the claimant/plaintiff proving that the defendant had a duty of care to them; that duty of care would need to have been breached; and they would have to provide evidence that they had been damaged as a result of the negligent action. Although all three criteria must be met for a civil case to be successful, unlike in criminal law where a case must be proven 'beyond reasonable doubt', within civil law the case would need to be proven only on the 'balance of probabilities'.

The doctor, the pharmacist and the carer all have a duty of care to J.M. with regard to his drug regimen and it would be more likely that any harm that ensued could be proven 'on the balance of probabilities'.

In order to prove that the duty of care had been breached, the actions of the defendant would be compared with those of a reasonably competent person undertaking a similar role. Consequently, it is worth considering what a 'competent' healthcare professional might do in this situation.

Owing to the relatively frequent nature of this problem, a nurse or at least his or her employer might also introduce a protocol for all staff to follow, thus standardising the approach and level of care. However, blindly following a protocol does not necessarily protect healthcare professionals from liability[4] and all protocols must be up-to-date and based on expert evidence.[5]

It can probably be assumed that a 'competent' nurse would first check with a suitable information source as to the best approach for administering drugs via this route and it would be appropriate for the nurse to clarify either with the hospital ward or the hospital pharmacy department from which J.M. was discharged how these medicines were being administered on the ward. If they were unsure about the appropriateness of the described actions or were unable to obtain the information from the hospital in time, then telephoning a medicines information department would be a suitable alternative.

The nurse's actions and the information received from the reference source(s) used would be documented in the patient's care plan. If the advice had been against crushing tablets and the general practitioner had asked for this action to take place, then a competent nurse would provide this information to the prescriber.

The issue whether patient consent had been obtained prior to the administration of the unlicensed medication might also be taken into account when considering the appropriateness of the nurses' actions. In order to minimise liability it is believed to be appropriate when administering unlicensed medicines also to 'tell the person (*patient*) about the risks involved and obtain their consent'.[5]

In summary, therefore, a competent nurse administering drugs to a patient via an enteral feeding tube would be working to an up-to-date protocol, would obtain appropriate guidance, would record their actions and the guidance received, would discuss this with the prescriber, would obtain patient consent, and would then undertake the administration.

If, following the above procedure, J.M. was subsequently harmed by his medication, it might be reasonable to assume that the liability would lie solely with the person authorising the drug administration, i.e. the doctor. There are, however, judgements, that show that this may not be the case.

In Gold v. Essex County Council (1942)[6] the judge stated that 'if a doctor ordered an obviously incorrect and dangerous dosage of a drug a nurse who administered it without obtaining confirmation from a doctor or higher authority might well be found to be negligent'. Furthermore, if the nurse, after confirmation with a higher authority, is still unhappy he or she should refuse to administer any order that is 'manifestly wrong'.[7]

These judgements clearly demonstrate the need for the administrator not to simply accept directions from a doctor, but to question them if unsure and to obtain independent clarification if they are still not happy with what they are being asked to do.

Similarly, the judgements made with respect to nurses could equally be applied to pharmacists when deciding whether or not to supply medication. If the pharmacist believes that administering the drugs according to the doctor's instructions is inappropriate, then there is an opportunity for them to utilise their professional discretion and refuse the supply. In supplying the medication in full knowledge of its intended use, the pharmacist is perhaps accepting a greater share of the liability than the nurse in administering the drug, as they would be deemed to have greater professional competence in this cognitive domain.

In both instances, if the nurse refuses to administer or the pharmacist refuses to supply, they must remember that they still have a duty of care to the patient and should undertake every action possible to resolve the situation and enable appropriate treatment of the patient. Therefore, it is inappropriate simply to refuse to administer or supply. This action should be reserved as a last resort when the healthcare professional feels on balance of all the available evidence that the drug would cause more harm to the patient if administered via the prescriber's intended route/method than if not given.

Administrative law

The body that has been empowered to regulate care in care homes is the National Care Standards Commission (NCSC) and in 2002 it published its national minimum standards.[8] The standards relevant to this case study would mainly be 9.1 and 9.4.

Standard 9.1 states that

> The registered person ensures that there is a policy and staff adhere to procedures for the receipt, storage, handling, administration and disposal of medicines ...

The design of a protocol for the administration of medicines to patients with swallowing difficulties would demonstrate clear adherence to the NCSC guidelines and, providing J.M.'s carer was seen to follow this, there would be no reason for the NCSC to become involved in any dispute that followed.

If the home did not have a protocol, or there was evidence that any protocol was not adhered to by the carer, then NCSC would start to consider the quality of care provided within the home.

Standard 9.4 states that

> Medicines in the custody of the home are handled according to the requirements of the Medicines Act 1968, guidelines from the Royal Pharmaceutical Society (RPSGB), ... and nursing staff abide by the Nursing and Midwifery Council (NMC) standards for the administration of medicines.

The Medicines Act has already been discussed and the NMC standards will be covered when considering professional standards. With respect to crushing of medicines, the RPSGB 'strongly recommends that advice on the storage and administration of medicines should be sought from a community pharmacist, preferably the pharmacist that supplies the home' and has informed pharmacists that 'if a formulation is tampered with then the product will be unlicensed. Pharmacists must consider and advise on the potential for distortion in the bioavailability profile of the medicine and whether there is a need for reduction or increase in the dose and how or whether this can be quantified'. Furthermore, 'pharmacists must consider whether alternative licensed products are available, such as the same drug with a different formulation or a different drug for the same indication'.[9]

In the scenario provided, it would be difficult for a pharmacist to identify other 'licensed' products. Even if a licensed liquid formulation were available as an alternative to crushing tablets, its administration via a PEG or PEJ tube would usually be unlicensed. With little quantitative evidence available to determine whether the liquid formulation or crushed tablet would be better for the patient via this route, the pharmacist would need to identify which option was believed to demonstrate best professional practice.

It would be reasonable for the nurse in this instance to ring the local medicines information department. Although the supplying pharmacist will be able to identify which medicines have special coatings and what alternative formulations are available, they would be less likely to be able to provide specialised advice on administration of medicines by PEG tubes.

Professional standards

The NMC is the responsible body in the UK for reinforcing the standards that nurses are expected to meet and these are broadly outlined in its 'Code of Professional Conduct' published in April 2002.[10] Statements such as 1.3, 'You are personally accountable for your practice. This means that you are answerable for your actions and omissions, regardless of advice or directions from another professional', and 8.1, 'You must work with other members of the team to promote health care environments which are conducive to safe, therapeutic and ethical practice', are relevant in this situation. However, the standards found within 'Guidance for the administration of medicines' that came into effect on 1 June 2002 are perhaps the most pertinent.[11] These start with the guidance:

> The administration of medicines is an important aspect of the professional practice of persons whose names are on the council's register. It is not solely a mechanistic task to be performed in strict compliance with the written prescription of a medical practitioner. It requires thought and exercise of professional judgement.

It would therefore be unprofessional for J.M.'s nurse to accept any direction from a prescriber to crush medication or place it down a PEG tube without first questioning the appropriateness of both of these actions.

Within the principles for the administration of medicines, a nurse is also required to have 'considered the dosage, method of administration, route and timing of the administration in the context of the condition of the patient and co-existing therapies.

Blind administration of medication via a PEG tube, which may require crushing and mixing with water beforehand, may not only result in a civil case, and close consideration of practices within the home by the NCSC, it may also result in the NMC considering the professionalism of the nurse.

Conclusion

This case study demonstrates the need for a good awareness of both professional and legislative guidance with respect to administration of medicines.

For J.M.'s nurse to act both professionally and competently, he or she would need to do the following:

- Ideally work to a protocol written specifically for the administration of medicines outside of their marketing authorisation.
- Seek advice from a pharmacist (preferably working within a medicines information service) on the alternative options available (liquids, alternative routes) and the clinical consequences of crushing and placing medicines down a PEG tube.
- Obtain consent from the patient.
- Record all actions.

- Obtain authorisation, preferably written, from the prescriber if it is decided to administer a medicine outside of its marketing authorisation.

For the pharmacist to act both professionally and competently, they would need to ensure the following:

- That the advice they provided was based on the most up-to-date evidence.
- That the increased risk of harm that would result from administering medicines outside of their marketing authorisation was minimised and justifiable in terms of the potential clinical benefits.

In an ideal world the nurse would have prepared for the meeting with the prescriber in order to have all of the options and relevant information available for this patient at hand and would have obtained this information from an appropriate pharmacist. If the prescriber insisted that the medicines be crushed prior to administration via the PEG tube, it might well be appropriate in this instance for J.M.'s nurse to refuse such a request as it would not be in the patient's best interests and they would not want to be responsible for any harm that ensued.

If the supplying pharmacist was aware of the proposed method of administration and had any concerns regarding its appropriateness, they should also use their professional discretion to refuse the supply. Furthermore, obtaining written authorisation for such action from the prescriber and blindly following it would not be deemed to be professional and would not reduce the level of responsibility that would be attributed to the pharmacist, nurse or carer in a civil court of law.

References

1. Medicines Act 1968 (SI 1994 No. 3144) (For Human Use) (Marketing Authorisations Etc.) Regulations 19.
2. Clark-Schmidt AL, Garnett WR, Lowe DR, Karnes HT. Loss of carbamazepine suspension though nasogastric feeding tubes. *Am J Hosp Pharm.* 1990; 47, 2034–2037.
3. Thomson FC, Naysmith MR, Lindsay A. Managing drug therapy in patients receiving enteral and parenteral nutrition. *Hospital Pharmacist.* 2000; 7(6): 155–164.
4. *Lucy Reynolds* v. *North Tyneside Health Authority* (2002) Lloyds Rep Med 459.
5. Griffiths R. Tablet crushing and the law. *Pharm J.* 2003; 271, 90–91.
6. *Gold* v. *Essex County Council* [1942] 2 KB 293.
7. *Junor* v. *McNicol* (1959) *The Times* 26 March.
8. National Care Standards Commission. *National Minimum Standards for Care Homes for Older People.* London: HMSO; 2001.
9. The Royal Pharmaceutical Society of Great Britain Professional Standards Directorate. Law and Ethics Bulletin: Covert administration of medicines. *Pharm J.* 2003; 270: 32.
10. Nursing and Midwifery Council. *Code of Professional Conduct.* London: NMC; 2002.
11. Nursing and Midwifery Council. *Guidelines for the Administration of Medicines.* London: NMC; 2002.

8
Health and safety and clinical risk management

Rebecca White

Key Points

- Ensure that organisational medicines policy contains specific information relating to safe administration of liquid medicines and medication administration via feeding tubes. (See www.npsa.gov.uk.)

- Use oral or enteral dispensers when administering medicines intended for the oral route or via an enteral feeding tube.

- Used closed-system crushing syringes for hazardous medicines such as cytotoxic drugs or hormones to protect the healthcare professional or carer from exposure.

- Do not crush modified-release formulations; use alternative formulations of drugs with the same therapeutic effect.

- Identify patients who are having medications administered via the enteral feeding tube that may interact with the enteral feed and design a regimen to limit/eliminate such interactions.

- Do not add drugs to the enteral feed bottle/bag.

Wrong-route errors

There have been numerous case reports in the literature of inadvertent parenteral administration of medication intended to be given orally.[1,2] All of these were direct results of the medication being drawn into a syringe with a connector compatible with i.v. devices. A number of these report serious clinical consequences[3] and even fatalities.[4]

Where possible, medicine pots and medicine spoons should be used to measure liquid medicines for oral administration, and specific oral or enteral syringes or dispensers should be used when the degree of accuracy warrants this. Oral or enteral syringes or dispensers should be used to draw up and administer liquid oral medication doses for administration via an enteral feeding tube. Specifically designed oral and enteral syringes and dispensers are available to enable this to be done safely. Ward sisters should ensure that these devices are available on the ward to facilitate administration. Where practical, pharmacists should ensure that these devices are dispensed with medication intended for administration via an enteral feeding tube.

The recent National Patient Safety Agency (NPSA) guidance (see www.NPSA.nhs.uk) has made specific recommendations concerning the prevention of wrong-route errors with oral and enteral medicines, feeds and flushes. Manufacturers are currently reviewing the compliance of enteral feeding tubes, administration sets and other devices.

Until measures are taken to design route-specific connectors and to standardise tube connectors across manufacturers, healthcare providers should endeavour to make purchasing decisions based on best practice. Steps should be taken to ensure that different devices are used for enteral and parenteral administration and that oral or enteral dispensers or syringes are used to draw up medicines and flushes for oral or enteral administration.

Specific recommendations include the following:

- Only oral, enteral or catheter-tip syringes (that are not compatible with intravenous and other parenteral devices) must be used to administer oral/enteral medicines, feeds and flushes to patients. (See chapter 9.)
- Ports on nasogastric and enteral feeding tubes through which medicines, feeds or flushes are administered, or which may be used for aspiration, must be male Luer, catheter or other nonfemale Luer in design.
- Three-way taps and adaptors that connect with parenteral devices must not be used.
- All healthcare organisations should include procedures for preparation and administration of oral/enteral medicines, feeds and flushes in their organisation's medicines policies, and these should be reflected in the organisation's training programmes and competence assessment.

Occupational exposure

Crushing tablets in open containers such as mortars or medicine pots, or opening capsules to obtain the drug powder contained within, will increase the risks of inhalation by the operator. This could potentially lead to sensitisation, allergies, absorption and possible adverse effects. There is also a danger at ward level of exposure of other staff and patients to drug powder resulting from such manipulations. If these operations must be undertaken they should be performed in a room with a closed door and traffic through the room should be limited during the manipulation. It is essential that benches and equipment are thoroughly cleaned following such manipulations to remove any drug residues and to ensure the safety of others.

Under the Control of Substances Hazardous to Health Regulations (COSHH)[5] every employer must provide employees with information, instruction and training to ensure that the employee knows the risks created by exposure to substances hazardous to health and the precautions that should be taken. Employers should also provide the necessary equipment to protect the employee from exposure due to necessary manipulation.

Medicines such as corticosteroids, hormones, antibiotics, immunosuppressants, cytotoxics and phenothiazines are irritant or very potent and extra precautions should be taken when handing these medicines. Exposure to such substances is highly dangerous; therefore, contact with the skin and inhalation of dust should be avoided[6] and protective equipment/devices should be used, e.g. crushing syringes.

Crushing inappropriate formulations

Crushing tablets in order to administer them via an enteral feeding tube not only increases the incidence of tube occlusion but also increases the risks of adverse effects.

There are many modified-release formulations that are marketed for their once-daily convenience. Crushing these tablets and administering them via enteral feeding tubes can have fatal consequences when the entire daily dose is administered as an immediate-release bolus.[7] Wherever possible, the healthcare professional should consider an alternative formulation of the same drug or a different drug that can be administered via an enteral feeding tube that has the same therapeutic effect.

Minimising interactions

Enteral feeds can have a significant effect on the absorption of medication, particularly if they are administered concurrently via an enteral feeding tube. However, in order for the pharmacist to be in a position to intervene and advise, it must be evident that the medication is being administered via the enteral feeding tube – therefore it must be prescribed correctly.

A number of institutions have developed systems to identify patients receiving their medication via enteral feeding tubes, for example coloured sticker systems to alert nurses to the drugs that have significant interactions with food and enteral feed.[8]

Many members of the healthcare team, especially pharmacists[9] and dietitians,[10] are in a position to raise the awareness of potential drug–nutrient interactions. However, it is equally important to empower the patient and carer, and information is now available to support patients and their GPs.[11]

Under no circumstances should drugs be added to the enteral feed bottle/bag. If the feed were to stop or the full volume were not to be delivered, the patient would not receive the prescribed dose of medication, which could have clinically significant consequences.

References

1. Cousins D, Upton D. Wrong route is used yet again. *Pharm Pract.* 2000; 10(2): 63.
2. Cousins D, Upton D. More wrong route problems. *Pharm Pract.* 1999; 9(1): 18–19.
3. Cousins D, Upton D. Oral paracetamol liquid administered intravenously. *Pharm Pract.* 2001; 11(7): 221.
4. Cousins D, Upton D. Inappropriate syringe use leads to fatalities. *Pharm Pract.* 1998; 8(5): 209–210.
5. Control of Substances Hazardous to Health Regulations (1988) (SI No.1657) Department of Health.
6. *BNF 47*, March 2004.
7. Schier JG, Howland MH, Hoffmann RS, Nelson LS. Fatality from administration of labetalol and crushed extended-release nifedipine. *Ann Pharmacother.* 2003; 37(10): 1420–1423.
8. Gaulthier I, Malone M, Lesar TS, Aronovitch S. Comparisons of programs for preventing drug–nutrient interactions in hospitalised patients. *Am J Health Syst Pharm.* 1997; 54: 405–411.
9. Teresi ME, Morgan DE. Attitudes of healthcare professionals toward patient counselling on drug–nutrient interactions. *Ann Pharmacother.* 1994; 28: 576–580.
10. Jones CM, Reddick JE. Drug–nutrient interaction counselling programs in upper Midwestern hospitals: 1986 survey results. *J Am Diet Assoc.* 1989; 89: 243–245.
11. British Association of Parenteral and Enteral Nutrition. Resources on Drug Administration via Enteral Feeding Tubes; 2003. Available at: www.bapen.org.uk/drugs-enteral.htm.

9
Syringes and ports
Rebecca White

Key Points

- Ensure that drugs are administered using the correct type of syringe.

- Do not use syringes compatible with parenteral devices for the administration of enteral drugs.

- Choose the appropriate size of syringe to accurately measure the drug concerned.

Syringe/dispenser types recommended for enteral drug administration

Oral

- The tip of the syringe is wider than Luer fit to prevent wrong-route errors.
- Dead-space volume of the tip is approximately 0.05 mL.

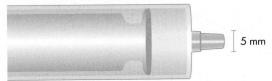

Figure 9.1 Oral syringe

Female Luer/reverse Luer

- The tip of the syringe is designed to connect to a male Luer or male Luer lock ports and devices.
- Dead-space volume of the tip is approximately 0.05–0.15 mL

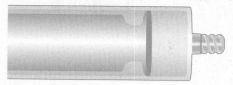

Figure 9.2 Female Luer/reverse Luer syringe

Catheter

- The tip is designed to fit catheters and catheter ports and devices.
- Dead-space volume is approximately 1–1.5 mL.

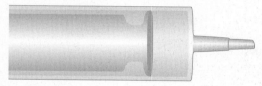

Figure 9.3 Catheter-tipped syringe

Syringe types *not* recommended for medication administration

Male Luer and Luer lock

- The tip is designed to fit female ports and devices (parenteral devices).
- Dead-space volume of the tip is approximately 0.05 mL.

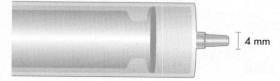

4 mm

Figure 9.4 Male Luer syringe

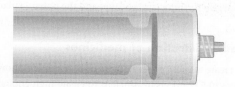

Figure 9.5 Male Luer lock syringe

Ports recommended for enteral devices

Male Luer port

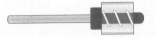

Figure 9.6 Male Luer port

Catheter port

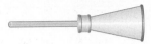

Figure 9.7 Catheter port

Oral port

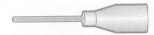

Figure 9.8 Oral port

Ports *not* recommended for enteral devices

Female Luer

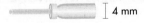

⊺ 4 mm

Figure 9.9 Female Luer

Female locking port

Figure 9.10 Female locking port

Syringe size

The major concerns relating to the size of syringe used are tube fracture and potential damage to local tissues on flushing, and vacuum and the potential damage to tissues on aspiration.

Flushing and administration of medicines

Large syringes will create a lower pressure than smaller syringes; however, the volume in very small syringes (0.5–2 mL) is insufficient to create high enough pressures in the feeding tube because of the internal volume of the tube itself.

Aspiration

Smaller syringes create a lower vacuum pressure than larger syringes; therefore, for aspiration a smaller syringe size is preferable.

Specific manufacturer recommendations

Merck Gastroenterology recommend that care be exercised when using syringes smaller than 50 mL as this can create a pressure greater than the bursting pressure of 80 psi (550 kilopascals). However, they will still permit smaller syringes to be used especially for the administration of small quantities of medicines. This applies to the entire range above. No minimum syringe sizes are set for PEGs or balloon gastrostomies.

Novartis Consumer Health recommend the use of a 20–50 mL syringe for flushing and feed administration. Under no circumstances should syringes less than 5 mL be used for attempting to clear an occluded tube.

Vygon UK do not recommend specific syringe sizes for administration of feeds and medication through enteral feeding tubes; for delivery of medication, select the biggest that can be used while maintaining the accuracy necessary for measurement of the dose. In general, it is suggested that no undue force should be used either to flush or administer any feed, medication or flush. If a tube runs freely it is virtually impossible to deliver sufficient force to cause the tube to burst. If resistance is felt, a gentle push–pull technique should be employed to overcome the blockage. If this is not successful, further clinical advice should be sought. Some drugs are recognised as causing tube blockage, for example granular formulations. If this type of medication is administered through an enteral feeding tube, flushing procedures need to be rigorously enforced and any resistance must result in immediate cessation of the delivery until the blockage can be cleared.

10
Defining interactions
Rebecca White

Key Points

- Drugs can interact with nutritional therapy and nutrients in many ways.

- Steps should be taken to avoid or minimise the effects of significant interactions.

- In the absence of any data, monitor closely for loss of drug effect or increased side-effects.

- The resulting drug and nutrition regimen should be practical and acceptable to the patient/carer.

Introduction

The interrelationship between drugs and nutrients is complex. There are many ways in which drugs and nutrients or nutritional therapy can interact, for example:

- Chemical interaction, binding the drug and reducing its absorption.
- Physical interaction between the drug formulation and the feed formulation, causing a change in the feed consistency and potentially resulting in blockage of the feeding tube.
- Interaction between the drug and a specific nutrient involved in the metabolism of that drug.
- Loss of drug effect due to impaired absorption, increased drug clearance or blocking of pharmacological action.

Effect of drug therapy on nutrient intake

Drug therapy can affect nutrient intake by altering taste, reducing appetite or inducing gastrointestinal (GI) side-effects such as nausea, vomiting, constipation or diarrhoea. These should always be borne in mind when a patient's voluntary nutritional intake changes.[1]

Pharmacokinetic interactions

Interactions between food, feed, nutrients and drugs affect the absorption, distribution, metabolism or elimination of the drug or nutrient.

Factors affecting drug or nutrient absorption

Interactions affecting the absorption of drugs are the most common.

Physiological

The majority of drugs are absorbed via a passive process of diffusion from the gut lumen across the mucosa into the splanchnic circulation. There are a few notable exceptions that utilise existing active transport systems used for nutrients; these include methyldopa and levodopa, whose absorption is decreased by a high-protein diet.[2] The process of passive diffusion is based on contact time and lipophilicity, the latter being influenced by intraluminal pH. Weakly acidic drugs are absorbed from the GI tract at a lower pH because more of the drug is in an unionised form and therefore is more lipophilic; the converse is true for basic drugs.[3] It is unsurprising, therefore, that the absorption of drugs can be increased, decreased or delayed by the physiological affect of food or feed on the GI tract, owing to the ability of food and feeds to alter the pH of the GI tract. Enteral feeds do not have the same effect on gut physiology as food because they are in liquid form and the pH can be very different. Interactions with feed are easier to predict owing to the consistency of the feed compared to a varied diet a patient may eat. Therefore, it cannot be assumed that interactions of this type will be of the same clinical significance for patients on a normal diet or on enteral feeding. Hot food and fatty meals delay gastric emptying to a greater extent than high-protein or carbohydrate meals. This has two principal effects:

- Firstly it increases the time the drug spends in the stomach. The time for disintegration and dissolution of the drug is thereby increased and possibly also the degradation of acid-sensitive drugs
- Secondly it delays the time to peak concentrations for drugs absorbed from the small bowel.

However, the combined effect may be to increase the overall absorption of drugs with saturable uptake mechanisms. This delay and reduction in peak plasma concentrations can be beneficial; for example, taking nifedipine with a meal delays and reduces the peak plasma concentrations and subsequently decreases the flushing reaction.

The presence of food or enteral feed in the small bowel increases splanchnic blood flow and this may enhance drug absorption, and may also increase bioavailability owing to the decreased portal blood flow. This has been purported to be the mechanism by which concentrations of propranolol and metoprolol are higher when it is taken with food compared to dosing in the fasted state.[4] Bile salts released in response to ingestion of fat may promote the absorption of highly lipid-soluble drugs, for example griseofulvin.[5]

Drugs can also affect the absorptive capacity of the GI tract – for example, the diarrhoea caused by colchicine or the effect of metformin on intrinsic factor production, which reduces vitamin B_{12} absorption in 30% of patients – and this side-effects of drugs should always be considered when nutritional intake is being assessed.[6]

Physical interactions

A physical interaction between the drug and a component of the feed or the feed formulation itself may result in a physical change in the consistency of the feed and can result in blockage of enteral feeding tubes or in extreme cases in physical obstruction of the GI tract.

The most commonly reported interaction is that between sucralfate and enteral feed. There is also a potential interaction with the ions in tap water and mineral water (for example, ciprofloxacin can chelate with such ions[7]), but as yet there have been no publications on the significance of these interactions.

Chemical interactions

There are reported interactions between many drugs and individual components of the diet (for example, elements such as calcium and iron) which bind to the drug and change its molecular size or solubility and thereby reduce absorption.

- Tetracyclines readily chelate with divalent and trivalent metal cations such as calcium, magnesium and iron – these are present in higher concentrations in enteral feed and milk-based diets than in a normal diet and therefore the potential for interaction is greater. Tetracycline absorption is decreased by 80% by co-administration with feed, whereas for doxycycline the reaction is not considered clinically important.
- Ciprofloxacin absorption is decreased 50% by enteral feed; the reaction with levofloxacin and ofloxacin is less significant, and food does not have any effect on the absorption of moxifloxacin.
- The interactions reported with phenytoin[8] and warfarin highlight the potential for a drug to bind to protein in the diet, with a reduction in drug absorption. As yet there are no reports comparing the interaction with whole protein as opposed to amino acid-based feeds.
- Pectin and fibre have also been reported to affect drug absorption. Paracetamol absorption is reduced by pectin, which is present in apples and pears, although the significance is unknown. The absorption of digoxin is reduced by the presence of high amounts of fibre in the diet, but the significance of this is negligible for patients

on a normal diet.[9] For drugs such as digoxin with a narrow therapeutic index, close monitoring should be undertaken if major changes in diet occur – for example, a patient being switched from a high-fibre normal diet to a low-fibre enteral feed – as this potential change in the absorption could cause a rise in the therapeutic level.

- Drugs can also affect nutrient absorption. Antacids containing aluminium or magnesium hydroxide bind to dietary phosphate to form insoluble phosphate salts, which cannot be absorbed. Osteomalacia has been reported secondarily to phosphate depletion due to antacid abuse.

Factors affecting drug distribution

Malnutrition affects drug distribution. A severely malnourished individual will have:

- Reduced plasma proteins for drug binding, increasing the free circulating drug concentrations
- An increase in total body water, increasing the volume of distribution of water-soluble drugs
- Decreased fat stores, decreasing the volume of distribution for fat-soluble drugs
- Reduced microsomal enzyme activity and reduced substrates available for metabolism.[10]

All of these factors should be considered for enterally tube-fed patients. As they are already receiving nutritional support, they could be malnourished and have altered drug distribution characteristics. Only normal-release formulations can be given via the enteral feeding tube, resulting in higher peak plasma concentrations than with modified-release formulations. This could be exacerbated by the potential for decreased protein binding and the altered volume of distribution; for example, higher peak concentrations of nifedipine will lead to more flushing reactions.

Factors affecting drug or nutrient metabolism

The hepatic mixed-function oxidase enzyme system is the predominant pathway by which drugs are metabolised. A low-protein diet has been demonstrated to reduce the function of this enzyme system; in contrast, a high-protein/low-carbohydrate diet has been shown to induce this enzyme system and so significantly enhance the clearance of drugs such as theophylline.[11]

It is known that malnutrition per se reduces the ability to effectively metabolise drugs and increases the incidence of adverse effects.[12]

Drugs can affect the storage, utilization and excretion of nutrients in a number of ways. The pharmacological activity of a number of drugs is dependent on interaction with a specific nutrient, for example warfarin with vitamin K or methotrexate with folate; also, a substantial number of nutrients are essential co-factors in drug metabolism.

There are reports of significant interactions between drugs and pyridoxine, folate, vitamin D and many other nutrients;[1] these could be both desirable and undesirable.

Grapefruit juice contains a psoralen that inhibits the cytochrome P450 enzyme subfamily, CYP3A. This effect reduces the metabolism of ciclosporin, simvastatin, terfenadine and calcium-channel blockers (excluding diltiazem and amlodipine), which can cause a clinically significant rise in plasma concentrations.

Changes in the diet can affect gut flora, which in turn can influence the pharmacokinetics of drugs broken down by bacteria in the colon, for example methotrexate.[13] It is predominantly changes in protein source and fibre intake that alter the balance of gut flora.

Monoamine oxidase inhibitors (MAOIs) such as phenezine enhance the cardiovascular effects of phenylethylamines such as tyramine. Diets that are rich in tyramine-containing foods such as mature cheese, broad bean pods, meat or yeast extracts, or fermented soya bean extract cause hypertension, headaches and palpitations, the scale of the reaction being determined by drug dose and tyramine intake. Dietary advice recommending an intake of less than 5 mg of tyramine per day ensures the safe use of these drugs.[14]

Factors affecting drug or nutrient excretion

The most common group of drugs that affect nutrient excretion are the diuretics. However, there are other drugs that cause an increase in electrolyte excretion: for example, the nephrotoxicity of cisplatin leads to increased magnesium and zinc excretion. Amphotericin is also associated with increased electrolyte excretion.[15]

Physical interaction of drug with delivery device

When administering drugs via an enteral feeding tube, there is the potential for an interaction to occur between the drug and the tubing material. It is therefore important for the healthcare professional to know what type of enteral feeding tube a patient has *in situ* before advice is given or decisions are made as to the appropriateness of using the enteral feeding tube for drug administration.

The apparent loss of carbamazepine suspension during administration through polyvinyl nasogastric tubes was studied *in vitro* to determine whether this effect was reproducible. The investigators demonstrated that administration of undiluted suspension via the tube resulted in a loss of drug dose, whereas a 50% diluted suspension resulted in no drug loss.[16]

Summary

This chapter touches on the complex interactions that can occur between drugs and nutritional therapy. Healthcare professionals should consider such possibilities when reviewing both the nutritional and drug therapy. Because the significance of these interactions is not always clear and patient variation can occur, both clinical knowledge of the patient and technical knowledge of the interaction must be used effectively to monitor the patient's pharmaceutical and nutritional progress. The healthcare team must understand potential and actual problems that may diminish the therapeutic success on an individual basis.

References

1. White R, Ashworth A. How drug therapy can affect, threaten and compromise nutritional status. *J Hum Nutr Diet*. 2000; 13: 119–129.
2. Gillespie NG, Cotzias GC, Bell MA, *et al*. Diets affecting treatment of parkinsonism with levodopa. *J Am Diet Assoc*. 1973; 62: 525.
3. Goodman AG, Gilman LS. *The Pharmacological Basis of Therapeutics*, 7th edn. New York: McMillan.
4. Melander A, Danielson K, Scherstein B, Wahlin E. Enhancement of the bioavailability of propranolol and metoprolol by food. *Clin Pharmacol Ther*. 1977; 22: 108.
5. Welling PG. Influence of food and diet on gastrointestinal drug absorption: a review. *J Pharmacokinet Pharm*. 1977; 5: 291–333.
6. Adam JF, Clark JS, Ireland JT, Kesson CM, Watson WS. Malabsorption of vitamin B_{12} and intrinsic factor secretion during biguanide therapy. *Diabetologia*. 1983; 24: 16–18.
7. Dorrian I. Cost-effectiveness – is it always effective? J Antimicrob Chemother. 1997; 39: 286–288.
8. Bauer IA. Interference of oral phenytoin absorption by continuous nasogastric feeding. *Neurology*. 1982; 32: 570–575.
9. Stockley IH. *Stockley's Drug Interactions*, 6th edn. London: Pharmaceutical Press; 2002.
10. Krishnaswamy K. Drug metabolism and pharmacokinetics in malnutrition. *Clin Pharmacokinet*. 1978; 3: 216–240.
11. Kappas A, Anderson KE, Conney AH, Alvares AP. Influence of dietary protein and carbohydrate on antipyrine and theophylline metabolism in man. *Clin Pharmacol Ther*. 1976; 20: 643–653.
12. Campbell TC, Hayes JR. Role of nutrition in the drug metabolism enzyme system. *Pharmacol Rev*. 1974; 26(3): 176.
13. Shen DD, Azarnoff DL. Clinical pharmacokinetics and methotrexate. *Clin Pharmacokinet*. 1978; 3: 1–13.
14. McCabe BJ. Dietary tyramine and other pressor amines in MAOI regimens: a review. *J Am Diet Assoc*. 1986; 86(8): 1059–1064.
15. Boullata JI, Armenti VT, eds. *Handbook of drug-nutrient interactions*. Totowa, NJ: Humana Press; 2004.
16. Clark-Schmidt A, Garnett WR, Lowe DR, Karnes HT. Loss of carbamazepine suspension through nasogastric feeding tubes. *Am J Hosp Pharm*. 1990; 47(9): 2034–2037.

Abacavir

Formulations available

Brand name (Manufacturer)	Formulation and strength	Product information/Administration information
Ziagen (GSK)	Tablet Film-coated 300 mg[1]	Film-coated tablet containing 300 mg abacavir sulfate. Food delays absorption and reduces C_{max} but does not reduce AUC and therefore abacavir can be taken with or without food.[1] However, there is no theoretical reason why crushing the tablets would create stability concerns, as long as administration occurred immediately. Furthermore, the ingredients are uniformly distributed throughout the tablet and have not been formulated in a time-dependent matrix.[4]
Ziagen (GSK)	Oral solution 20 mg/mL[2]	Contains sorbitol 5 g per 15 mL dose.[4] The use of Ziagen oral solution is advised for administration via feeding tubes. Although GSK have no data to support administration via this route, they are aware of anecdotal reports of patients having been successfully treated in this manner.[4]
Trizivir (GSK) Combined with lamivudine and zidovudine	Tablet Film-coated[3] Abacavir: 300 mg Lamivudine: 150 mg Zidovudine: 300 mg	Food decreased the rate of absorption of Trizivir and increased the t_{max} but did not affect AUC, therefore no food restrictions are recommended.[3] GSK have no stability or pharmacokinetic data to support crushing Trizivir tablets. However, there is no theoretical reason why crushing the tablets would create stability concerns, as long as administration occurred immediately. Furthermore, the ingredients are uniformly distributed throughout the tablet and have not been formulated in a time-dependent matrix.[4]

Site of absorption (oral administration)

Specific site of absorption is not documented. Peak plasma concentration occurs 1.5 hours following oral administration for the tablets and 1 hour for the liquid formulation.[1]

Alternative routes available

No alternative route is available for abacavir.

Interactions

The bioavailability of abacavir has been assessed in the fed and fasted state;[5] although peak plasma concentrations were reduced by 35%, there was no significant difference in total bioavailability. The interaction with food is clinically insignificant.[1, 2, 3]

Health and safety

Standard precautions apply.

Suggestions/recommendations

- The liquid formulation is preferable owing to ease of manipulation.
- Monitor total daily intake of sorbitol.
- No break in feeding is necessary as bioavailability is not significantly affected when the drug is given with food.

Intragastric administration

1. Stop the enteral feed.
2. Flush the enteral feeding tube with the recommended volume of water.
3. Draw the medication solution into the appropriate size and type of syringe.
4. Flush the medication dose down the feeding tube.
5. Finally, flush with the recommended volume of water.
6. Re-start the feed, unless a prolonged break is required.

Alternatively, at step (3) measure the medicine in a suitable container and then draw into an appropriate syringe. Ensure that the measure is rinsed and that this rinsing water is administered also to ensure that the total dose is given. **Do not** measure liquid medicines using a catheter-tipped syringe as this results in excessive dosing owing to the volume of the tip.

Intrajejunal administration

There are no specific data relating to the jejunal administration of abacavir. Administer using the above method. Monitor for increased side-effects or loss of efficacy.

References

1. Ziagen 300 mg Tablets, Summary of Product Characteristics; 7 November 2005.
2. Ziagen Oral Solution, Summary of Product Characteristics; 7 November 2005.
3. Trizivir, Summary of Product Characteristics; 5 January 2005.
4. Personal communication, Medical Information Department, GSK; 22 January 2003.
5. Chittick GE, Gillotin C, McDowell JA, et al. Abacavir: absorption, bioavailability, and bioequivalence of three oral formulations, and effect of food. *Pharmacotherapy*. 1999; 19: 932–942.

Acamprosate

Formulations available

Brand name (Manufacturer)	Formulation and strength	Product information/Administration information
Campral EC (Merck)	Tablet Enteric coated 333 mg[1]	Campral tablets are enteric coated and therefore unsuitable for crushing.[2]

Site of absorption (oral administration)

Specific site of absorption is not documented. Oral bioavailability is low with significant interpatient variability. Following oral administration, peak plasma concentration occurs 5.2 hours post dose.[3]

Alternative routes available

No alternative routes are available for acamprosate. Injection is used for clinical studies only, no licensed product.

Interactions

Food reduces bioavailability.[1]

Health and safety

Standard precautions apply.

Suggestions/recommendations

- Acamprosate should only be used under the supervision of a suitably qualified practitioner and supported by counselling. The specialist should be consulted to recommend alternative therapy.
- Disulfiram is unlikely to be suitable owing to the risk of interaction with the small quantities of alcohol present in liquid medicines.[4]

References

1. Campral EC, Summary of Product Characteristics; 14 April 2003.
2. Personal communication, Merck Pharmaceuticals; 23 January 2003.
3. Dollery C. *Therapeutic Drugs*, 2nd edn. London: Churchill Livingstone; 1998.
4. *BNF 50*, September 2005.

Acarbose

Formulations available

Brand name (Manufacturer)	Formulation and strength	Product information/Administration information
Glucobay (Bayer)	Tablet 50 mg, 100 mg	Tablets should be chewed with the first mouthful of food or swallowed whole with a little liquid immediately before food.[1] Tablets do not disperse easily in water but require gentle agitation for approximately 5 minutes. Disperse to give a fine suspension that flushes down an 8Fr NG tube without blockage.[3] Acarbose is insoluble in water.[4] Acarbose in powdered form, obtained by crushing the tablets, and mixed directly with food, has been shown to be more effective than the tablets administered whole.[5, 6]

Site of absorption (oral administration)

Specific site of absorption is not documented. Following oral administration, the first peak plasma concentration occurs after approximately 1 hour, the second peak is a result of breakdown and absorption in the colon and occurs after approximately 20 hours.[2]

Alternative routes available

No alternative routes are available for acarbose. Acarbose does not exhibit a systemic effect; therefore delivery by another route would be ineffective.[4]

Interactions

The mechanism of action is dependent on its interaction with food. Acarbose is a reversible, competitive inhibitor of the alpha-glycoside hydrolases of the small-intestinal brush border.

Health and safety

Standard precautions apply.

Suggestions/recommendations

- Owing to its mechanism of action, acarbose is unlikely to be suitable for diabetic patients on continuous enteral feeding regimens as distribution throughout the meal produces a better response and would not be achievable on a continuous feed. Alternative means of controlling blood sugars should be explored.
- Its use may be suitable for bolus feeding.

Intragastric administration

1. Stop the enteral feed.
2. Flush the enteral feeding tube with the recommended volume of water.
3. Place the tablet in the barrel of an appropriate size and type of syringe.
4. Draw 10 mL of water into the syringe and allow the tablet to disperse, shaking if necessary.
5. Flush the medication dose down the feeding tube.
6. Draw another 10 mL of water into the syringe and also flush this via the feeding tube (this will rinse the syringe and ensure that the total dose is administered).
7. Finally, flush with the recommended volume of water.
8. Re-start the feed immediately.

Alternatively, at step (3) place the tablet into a medicine pot, add 10 mL of water and allow the tablet to disperse. Draw this into an appropriate syringe. Ensure that the measure is rinsed and that this rinsing water is administered also to ensure that the total dose is given.

Intrajejunal administration

As the mode of action is locally within the small bowel, jejunal administration should not affect efficacy of therapy. Administer using the above method.

References

1. *BNF 50*, September 2005.
2. Glucobay 50, Glucobay 100 (Bayer), Summary of Product Characteristics; July 2005.
3. BPNG data on file 18 June 2004.
4. Dollery C. *Therapeutic Drugs*, 2nd edn. London: Churchill Livingstone; 1998.
5. O'Dea K, Turton J. Optimum effectiveness of intestinal alpha-glucosidase inhibitors: Importance of uniform distribution though a meal. *Am J Clin Nutr*. 1985; 41; 511–516.
6. Jenney A, Proietto J, O'Dea K, Nankervis A, Traianedes K, D'Embden H. Low-dose acarbose improves glycaemic control in NIDDM patients without changes in insulin sensitivity. *Diabetes Care*. 1993; 16(2); 499–502.

Acebutolol

Formulations available[1]

Brand name (Manufacturer)	Formulation and strength	Product information/Administration information
Sectral (Akita)	Capsules 100 mg, 200 mg	Acebutolol is very soluble in water.[2] Capsule contents pour easily from opened capsule and disperse readily in water to give almost clear very fine dispersion, flushes via an 8Fr NG tube without blockage.[3] Excipients include starch and lactose.[4]
Sectral (Akita)	Tablets 400 mg	Film-coated tablets. No specific data on enteral tube administration are available for this formulation.
Secadrex (Akita)	Tablets 200 mg/12.5 mg	Film-coated tablets. Acebutolol 200 mg + hydrochlorothiazide 12.5 mg No specific data on enteral tube administration are available for this formulation.

Site of absorption (oral administration)

Specific site of absorption is not documented. Peak plasma concentrations occur 2–3 hours after oral dosing.[2] Acebutolol and its active metabolite undergo biliary excretion with 50% of the dose recovered in the faeces.[4]

Alternative routes available

No alternative routes are available for acebutolol; the parenteral route is available for other beta-blockers.

Interactions

No documented interactions with food.[2]

Health and safety

Standard precautions apply.

Suggestions/recommendations

- Consider changing to an alternative beta-blocker that does not require manipulation to administer.
- If an alternative therapy is not appropriate, open the capsule and disperse the contents in water immediately prior to administration.
- A prolonged break in feeding is not necessary.

Intragastric administration

1. Stop the enteral feed.
2. Flush the enteral feeding tube with the recommended volume of water.
3. Open the capsule and pour the contents into a medicine pot.
4. Add 15 mL of water.
5. Stir to disperse the powder.
6. Draw into an appropriate size and type of syringe and administer via feeding tube.
7. Add a further 15 mL of water to the medicine pot; stir to ensure that any powder remaining in the pot is mixed with water.
8. Draw up this dispersion and flush down the tube. This will ensure that the whole dose is given.
9. Flush the tube with water.
10. Re-start the feed, unless a prolonged break is required.

Intrajejunal administration

There are no specific data relating to the jejunal administration of acebutolol. Administer using the above method and monitor for increased side-effects or loss of efficacy.

References

1. *BNF* 50, September 2005.
2. Dollery C. *Therapeutic Drugs*, 2nd edn. London: Churchill Livingstone; 1998.
3. BPNG data on file 2005.
4. Sectral Capsules (Aventis), Summary of Product Characteristics; January 2005.

Aceclofenac

Formulations available

Brand name (Manufacturer)	Formulation and strength	Product information/Administration information
Preservex (UCB Pharma)	Tablet 100 mg	Film-coated tablet.[1] No specific data on enteral tube administration are available for this formulation.

Site of absorption (oral administration)

Specific site of absorption is not documented. Peak plasma concentrations occur 1.25–3 hours following ingestion.

Alternative routes available

None available for aceclofenac. Diclofenac is an equivalent NSAID available as suppositories or injection.

Interactions

No significant interaction with food has been noted. The rate of absorption was increased in fasted subjects but the AUC was unaffected; it is therefore recommended that aceclofenac be taken after food to reduce GI adverse effects.[1]

Health and safety

Standard precautions apply.

Suggestions/recommendations

- Aceclofenac has a similar action to naproxen and diclofenac.[2]
- Diclofenac is available as dispersible tablets, suppositories and injection and should be considered an appropriate alternative.

References

1. Preservex (UCB Pharma), Summary of Product Characteristics; May 2005.
2. *BNF* 50, September 2005.

Acenocoumarol (Nicoumalone)

Formulations available[1]

Brand name (Manufacturer)	Formulation and strength	Product information/Administration information
Sinthrome (Alliance)	Tablets 1 mg	The manufacturer has no data to support the administration of Sinthrome via enteral feeding tubes. Acenocoumarol is insoluble in water.[2] Tablets disperse in 10 mL of water within 5 minutes to give a very fine white dispersion, which flushes via an 8Fr NG tube without blockage.[3]

Site of absorption (oral administration)

Acenocoumarol is almost completely absorbed from the upper GI tract,[2] although the specific site is not documented. Peak plasma concentrations occur 1–3 hours following oral dosing.[4]

Alternative routes available

None available for acenocoumarol. Heparin can be used as a parenteral alternative.

Interactions

No specific interaction between food and acenocoumarol is documented.[4] However, variable quantities of vitamin K in the diet will have a pharmacological influence on INR.

Health and safety

Standard precautions apply.

Suggestions/recommendations

- Disperse the tablet in water immediately prior to administration.
- A prolonged break in feeding is not required.

Intragastric administration

1. Stop the enteral feed.
2. Flush the enteral feeding tube with the recommended volume of water.
3. Place the tablet in the barrel of an appropriate size and type of syringe.
4. Draw 10 mL of water into the syringe and allow the tablet to disperse, shaking if necessary.
5. Flush the medication dose down the feeding tube.
6. Draw another 10 mL of water into the syringe and also flush this via the feeding tube (this will rinse the syringe and ensure that the total dose is administered).
7. Finally, flush with the recommended volume of water.
8. Re-start the feed, unless a prolonged break is required.

Alternatively, at step (4) place the tablet into a medicine pot, add 10 mL of water and allow the tablet to disperse. Draw this into an appropriate syringe. Ensure that the measure is rinsed and that this rinsing water is administered also to ensure that the total dose is given.

Intrajejunal administration

There are no specific data on jejunal administration of acenocoumarol. Administer as above. Adjust the dose depending on response.

References

1. *BNF* 50, September 2005.
2. Personal communication, Alliance; January 2003.
3. BPNG data on file 2005.
4. Sinthrome (Alliance), Summary of Product Characteristics; July 2005.

Acetazolamide

Formulations available[1]

Brand name (Manufacturer)	Formulation and strength	Product information/Administration information
Diamox (Goldshield)	Tablet 250 mg	Uncoated tablet.[2] Tablets disintegrate very quickly in 10 mL of water to give a coarse dispersion that settles quickly and flushes down an 8Fr NG tube without blockage, but container and syringe must be rinsed thoroughly to ensure that the total dose is given.[6]
Diamox (Goldshield)	Injection 500 mg	For i.v. or i.m. administration. I.m. administration is painful owing to the alkaline pH (9.1) of the injection.[3] The injection contains the active drug (as acetazolamide sodium), sodium hydroxide and hydrochloric acid. The reconstituted injection can be stored in a refrigerator for up to 24 hours.[3] There is no theoretical reason to preclude the use of the injection via a feeding tube. There are anecdotal reports of this practice. Extended stability data for the injectable preparation are available.[5]

Formulations available[1] (continued)

Brand name (Manufacturer)	Formulation and strength	Product information/Administration information
Diamox SR (Goldsheild)	Capsule 250 mg	Capsule contains slow-release pellets ranging from 0.25 mm to 1.68 mm diameter. Unsuitable for tube administration.[4]

Site of absorption (oral administration)

Specific site of absorption is not documented. Peak plasma concentrations occur after 1 hour in fasted patients[4] following administration of the immediate-release product.

Alternative routes available

The parenteral route is available.

Interactions

No recorded evidence of interaction with food.[4]

Health and safety

Standard precautions apply.

Suggestions/recommendations

- Disperse the tablets in water immediately prior to administration.
- Because of cost, only use injection when doses smaller than 250 mg are to be given.
- A prolonged break in feeding is not required.

Intragastric administration

1. Stop the enteral feed.
2. Flush the enteral feeding tube with the recommended volume of water.
3. Place the tablet in the barrel of an appropriate size and type of syringe.
4. Draw 10 mL of water into the syringe and allow the tablet to disperse, shaking if necessary.
5. Flush the medication dose down the feeding tube.
6. Draw another 10 mL of water into the syringe and also flush this via the feeding tube (this will rinse the syringe and ensure that the total dose is administered).
7. Finally, flush with the recommended volume of water.
8. Re-start the feed, unless a prolonged break is required.

Alternatively, at step (3) place the tablet into a medicine pot, add 10 mL of water and allow the tablet to disperse. Draw this into an appropriate syringe. Ensure that the measure is rinsed and that this rinsing water is administered also to ensure that the total dose is given.

Intrajejunal administration

No specific data relate to the jejunal administration of acetazolamide. Administer using the above method. Monitor for increased side-effects or loss of efficacy.

References

1. *BNF 50*, September 2005.
2. Diamox Tablets, Summary of Product Characteristics; 31 July 2002.
3. Diamox Sodium Parenteral, Summary of Product Characteristics; 16 February 2004.
4. Dollery C. *Therapeutic Drugs*, 2nd edn. London: Churchill Livingstone; 1998.
5. Trissel LA, ed. *Stability of Compounded Formulations*, 2nd edn. Washington, DC: American Pharmaceutical Association; 2000.
6. BPNG data on file 2004.

Acetylcysteine

Formulations available

Brand name (Manufacturer)	Formulation and strength	Product information/Administration information
Parvolex (Celltech)	Injection 200 mg/mL [1]	The injection solution can be given orally but is very bitter. [2] The injection solution has a pH of 6–7.5. [4] The injection solution has been administered orally for the prevention of radiocontrast-induced nephropathy. [5]

Other formulations not licensed in the UK are available through IDIS.

Site of absorption (oral administration)

Specific site of absorption is not documented. Extensive absorption occurs, with peak plasma concentration occurring 1 hour after oral ingestion. [3]

Alternative routes available

Injection can be given parenterally; it has also been used as mouthwash, topically and as a bladder washout.

Interactions

No documented interaction with food.

Health and safety

Standard precautions apply.

Suggestions/recommendations

- Use injection orally.
- A prolonged break in feeding is not required.

Intragastric administration

1. Stop the enteral feed.
2. Flush the enteral feeding tube with the recommended volume of water.
3. Draw the injection solution into an appropriate size and type of syringe.
4. Flush the medication dose down the feeding tube.
5. Finally, flush with the recommended volume of water.
6. Re-start the feed, unless a prolonged break is required.

Intrajejunal administration

No specific data. Administer using the above method.

References

1. Parvolex Injection, Summary of Product Characteristics; June 2005.
2. Personal communication, Celltech; 17 February 2006.
3. Dollery C. *Therapeutic Drugs*, 2nd edn. London: Churchill Livingstone; 1998.
4. Trissel LA, ed. *Stability of Compounded Formulations*, 2nd edn. Washington, DC: American Pharmaceutical Association; 2000.
5. Shalansky SJ, Pate GE, Levin A, Webb JG. N-Acetylcysteine for prevention of radiocontrast induced nephrotoxicity: the importance of dose and route of administration. *Heart*. 2005; 91(8): 997–99.

Aciclovir

Formulations available[1]

Brand name (Manufacturer)	Formulation and strength	Product information/Administration information
Zovirax (GSK)	Dispersible film-coated tablets 200 mg, 400 mg, 800 mg	Zovirax tablets may be dispersed in a minimum of 50 mL of water or swallowed whole with a little water.[2] Oral liquid and dispersible tablets have a variable bioavailability.[3]
Zovirax (GSK)	Suspension 200 mg/5 mL, 400 mg/5 mL	Both formulations contain sorbitol.[4]
Zovirax (GSK)	Infusion 250 mg, 500 mg	Not suitable for enteral tube administration.
Aciclovir (Alpharma)	Tablets 200 mg, 400 mg, 800 mg	Disperse in water to administer via feeding tube.[5]
Aciclovir (CP, Opus, Sovereign, Zurich)	Tablets 200 mg, 400 mg, 800 mg	No specific data on enteral tube administration are available for this formulation.

Formulations available[1] (continued)

Brand name (Manufacturer)	Formulation and strength	Product information/Administration information
Aciclovir (Sterwin)	Tablets 200 mg, 400 mg, 800 mg Dispersible tablets 200 mg, 400 mg, 800 mg	No specific data on enteral tube administration are available for this formulation.
Aciclovir (Hillcross, IVAX)	Dispersible tablets 200 mg, 400 mg, 800 mg	No specific data on enteral tube administration are available for this formulation.
Aciclovir (Pharmacia)	Dispersible tablets 200 mg, 400 mg, 800 mg	Tablets should be taken after meals. The tablets may be dissolved in a quarter glass of water.[7] Tablet are dispersible in water.[6]
Aciclovir (Ranbaxy)	Dispersible tablets 200 mg, 400 mg, 800 mg	Tablets disintegrate in less than 1 minute in 10 mL of water. Forms a milky coarse dispersion that flushes easily down an 8Fr tube.[9]
Aciclovir (Sanofi-Synthelabo)	Dispersible tablets 200 mg, 400 mg, 800 mg	Tablets disperse in water.

Site of absorption (oral administration)

Aciclovir is only partly absorbed from the GI tract. A specific site of absorption is not documented. Peak plasma concentration occurs 1–2 hours following oral dosing.[7]

Alternative routes available

The parenteral route is available.

Interactions

No specific interactions with food have been documented.

Health and safety

Standard precautions apply.

Suggestions/recommendations

- In critical situations it is recommended that the injection be used to ensure therapeutic concentrations.[8]
- Use dispersible tablets.
- A prolonged break in feeding is not required.

Intragastric administration

1. Stop the enteral feed.
2. Flush the enteral feeding tube with the recommended volume of water.
3. Place the tablet in the barrel of an appropriate size and type of syringe.
4. Draw 10 mL of water into the syringe and allow the tablet to disperse.
5. Flush the medication dose down the feeding tube.
6. Draw an equal volume of water into the syringe and also flush this via the feeding tube (this will rinse the syringe and ensure that the total dose is administered).
7. Finally, flush with the recommended volume of water.
8. Re-start the feed, unless a prolonged break is required.

Alternatively, at step (3) place the tablet into a medicine pot and add 10 mL of water and allow the tablet to disperse. Draw this solution into the syringe with an appropriate adapter for the tube connector. Ensure that the measure is rinsed and that this rinsing water is administered also to ensure that the total dose is given.

Intrajejunal administration

There are no specific data on the jejunal administration of aciclovir. Administer using the above method.

References

1. *BNF* 50, September 2005.
2. Zovirax 200 mg Tablets, Summary of Product Characteristics; 2 July 2003.
3. Tanna *et al*. Competition studies to elucidate the mechanisms of aciclovir uptake in the small intestine. *J Pharm Pharmacol*. 1992; 449(Suppl); 1047.
4. Zovirax Suspension (GSK), Summary of Product Characteristics; 29 November 2004.
5. Personal communication, Alpharma Ltd; 21 January 2003.
6. Personal communication, Pharmacia Ltd; 11 March 2003.
7. Aciclovir 400 mg tablets, Pharmacia, Summary of Product Characteristics; June 2001.
8. Personal communication, GSK Ltd, 22 January 2003.
9. BPNG data on file 2004.

Acitretin

Formulations available

Brand name (Manufacturer)	Formulation and strength	Product information/Administration information
Neotigason (Roche)	Capsules[1] 10 mg, 25 mg	Retinoids are not water-soluble and are degraded by light, so it is not possible to make an extemporaneous suspension. However, some centres have suggested that patients open the capsules immediately before use and take the contents with food. Neotigason capsules contain a powder formulation. Roche do not know of any technical reasons why this process will alter the bioavailability or efficacy of the drug, but as it is not a published procedure they have no data to support this practice.[2]

Site of absorption (oral administration)

Specific site of absorption is not documented. Time to peak plasma concentration is 1–4 hours following an oral dose.[1]

Alternative routes available

None available for acitretin. Topical therapy is available for milder forms of psoriasis.

Interactions

Food increases the bioavailability of acitretin; there is no information on clinical significance because of the wide interpatient variability in oral absorption.[1] The ingestion of food results in a twofold increase in C_{max} and AUC.[3]

Health and safety

Acitretin is highly teratogenic.[1] Women of childbearing age should not be exposed to the powder if the capsules are opened. Protective clothing should be worn.

Suggestions/recommendations

- As treatment would only be initiated under the supervision of a dermatologist, their opinion should be sought for alternatives. Systemic steroids have been used in severe psoriasis but a rebound flare can occur on discontinuation.[4]
- If continued treatment with acitretin is essential, the capsules should be opened and mixed with water and administered immediately.
- A prolonged break in feeding is not necessary.

Intragastric administration

1. Stop the enteral feed.
2. Flush the enteral feeding tube with the recommended volume of water.
3. Open the capsule and pour the contents into a medicine pot.
4. Add 15 mL of water.
5. Stir to disperse the powder.
6. Draw into an appropriate size and type of syringe and administer via the feeding tube.
7. Add a further 15 mL of water to the medicine pot; stir to ensure that any powder remaining in the pot is mixed with water.
8. Draw up this dispersion into the syringe and flush down the tube. This will ensure that the whole dose is given.
9. Flush the tube with water.
10. Re-start the feed, unless a prolonged break is required.

Intrajejunal administration

No specific data are available relating to the jejunal administration of acitretin. If indicated, administer using the above method. Monitor for signs of toxicity or loss of efficacy.

References

1. Neotigason Capsules, Summary of Product Characteristics; August 2004
2. Personal communication, Roche Products Ltd; 25 March 2003.
3. Dollery C. *Therapeutic Drugs*, 2nd edn. London: Churchill Livingstone; 1998.
4. *BNF 50*, September 2005.

Alendronic acid

Formulations available[1]

Brand name (Manufacturer)	Formulation and strength	Product information/Administration information
Fosamax (MSD)	Tablet 5 mg, 10 mg	Alendronate sodium, 6.53 mg equivalent to 5 mg alendronic acid. Fosamax must be taken at least 30 minutes before the first food, beverage or medication of the day with plain water only. Other beverages (including mineral water), food and some medications are likely to reduce the absorption of Fosamax.[2] Alendronic acid solubility in water is 1 in 25.[6] No specific data on enteral tube administration are available for this formulation.
Fosamax Once Weekly (MSD)	Tablet 70 mg	Licensed for treatment of postmenopausal osteoporosis only.[3] Tablets disperse in 10 mL of water within 2–5 minutes to give very fine particles that disperse easily. The particles settle quite quickly but flush down an 8Fr feeding tube without blockage.[4] In a small retrospective chart review (5 patients), 70 mg alendronate was administered via feeding tubes for an average of 18 months; a reduction in bone turnover markers was noted and there were no reported adverse effects. The authors conclude that alendronate and residronate delivered through feeding tubes in developmentally disabled patients appears to be well tolerated.[5]
Fosavance (MSD)	Tablet[7] 70 mg/70 microgram	Contains alendronate sodium equivalent to 70 mg alendronic acid and 70 micrograms (2800 IU) cholecalciferol (vitamin D_3). There is no specific information available on enteral tube administration of this product.

Site of absorption (oral administration)

The specific site of absorption is not documented; 60–70% of absorption occurs in the first hour. Elevation of gastric pH above 6 is associated with a twofold increase in alendronate absorption.[6]

Alternative routes available

None for alendronic acid. Calcitonin (salmon) nasal spray is licensed for use in postmenopausal osteoporosis (see BNF for details).

Interactions

Absorption of alendronic acid is reduced significantly if food is ingested within 30 minutes of oral dosing. Absorption is negligible if it is taken with or after food.[2]

Health and safety

Standard precautions apply.

Suggestions/recommendations

- Alendronate is contraindicated in patients with oesophageal disease. Owing to the risks of oesophageal damage, alendronate should be used with caution via an enteral feeding tube, especially in patients with delayed gastric emptying at risk of oesophageal reflux and those patients unable to sit or stand upright.
- If alendronate is administered via a feeding tube, the once-weekly formulation should be used. The tablet should be dispersed in water and administered immediately, then flushed with at least 50 mL of water. This should be administered first thing in the morning after rising and the patient should remain sitting upright or standing for 30 minutes after the dose is given, this allows for the longest break without food; if the patients is on an overnight feed it may be appropriate to dose in the evening. Enteral feed should be stopped prior to administration for as long as practicable, and should not be re-started for at least 30 minutes after the dose.

Intragastric administration

1. Stop the enteral feed.
2. Flush the enteral feeding tube with the recommended volume of water.
3. Allow as long a break as is feasibly possible.
4. Place the tablet in the barrel of an appropriate size and type of syringe.
5. Draw 10 mL of water into the syringe and allow the tablet to disperse, shaking if necessary.
6. Flush the medication dose down the feeding tube.
7. Draw another 10 mL of water into the syringe and also flush this via the feeding tube (this will rinse the syringe and ensure that the total dose is administered).
8. Finally, flush with at least 50 mL of water.
9. Ensure that the patient is upright or standing for 30 minutes after the dose.
10. Re-start the feed after the 30 minutes has passed.

Alternatively, at step (4) place the tablet into a medicine pot, add 10 mL of water and allow the tablet to disperse. Draw this solution into an appropriate syringe. Ensure that the measure is rinsed and that this rinsing water is administered also to ensure that the total dose is given.

Intrajejunal administration

There are no data on the jejunal administration of alendronate. If indicated, administer using the above method. Monitor for loss of efficacy or increased side-effects.

References

1. *BNF* 50, September 2005.
2. Fosamax, Summary of Product Characteristics; January 2006.
3. Fosamax Once Weekly, Summary of Product Characteristics; January 2005.
4. BPNG data on file 2004.
5. Tanner S, Taylor HM. Feeding tube administration of bisphosphonates for treating osteoporosis in institutionalised patients with developmental disabilities. *Bone*. 2004; 34(Suppl. 1): S97–98.
6. Dollery C. *Therapeutic Drugs*, 2nd edn. London: Churchill Livingstone; 1998.
7. Fosavance (MSD), Summary of Product Characteristics; August 2005.

Alfacalcidol

Formulations available[1]

Brand name (Manufacturer)	Formulation and strength	Product information/Administration information
One-Alpha (Leo)	Capsules 250 ng, 500 ng, 1 microgram	Soft gelatin capsules. Dose is titrated to biological response.[2] Leo do not recommend opening the capsules owing to the risk of administering an incomplete dose.[3]
One-Alpha (Leo)	Oral drops 2 microgram/mL	1 drop = 100 nanograms.[4]
One-Alpha (Leo)	Injection 2 microgram/mL	One-Alpha injection can be administered orally or via a feeding tube.[3]
Alfacalcidol (APS)	Capsules 250 ng, 500 ng, 1 microgram	No specific data on enteral tube administration are available for this formulation.

Site of absorption (oral administration)

Vitamin D substances are absorbed throughout the GI tract. Absorption is partly dependent on the presence of bile salts.[5]

Alternative routes available

Parenteral formulation.

Interactions

No specific interaction with feed.[6]

Health and safety

Standard precautions apply.

Suggestions/recommendations

- Use oral drops.
- A prolonged break in feeding is not required.

Intragastric administration

1. Stop the enteral feed.
2. Flush the enteral feeding tube with the recommended volume of water.
3. Put the required number of drops into a medicine pot and add a small amount of water (e.g. 10 mL).
4. Draw this into an appropriate size and type of syringe.
5. Flush the medication dose down the feeding tube.
6. Finally, flush with the recommended volume of water.
7. Re-start the feed, unless a prolonged break is required.

Intrajejunal administration

Administer as above.

References

1. *BNF* 50, September 2005.
2. One-Alpha Capsules (Leo), Summary of Product Characteristics; April 2000.
3. Personal communication, Leo Pharmaceuticals; February 2003.
4. One-Alpha drops (Leo), Summary of Product Characteristics; March 2000.
5. Dollery C. *Therapeutic Drugs*, 2nd edn. London: Churchill Livingstone; 1998.
6. Sweetman SC, ed., *Martindale*, 34th edn. London: Pharmaceutical Press; 2005.

Allopurinol

Formulations available

Brand name (Manufacturer)	Formulation and strength	Product information/Administration information
Zyloric (GSK)	Tablet 100 mg, 300 mg	GSK have no information on the administration of Zyloric via PEG or NG tube.[5]
Allopurinol (Alpharma)	Tablet 100 mg, 300 mg	Tablets can be crushed, but drug is very insoluble.[2, 3]
Allopurinol (APS)	Tablet 100 mg, 300 mg	Tablets will disperse if shaken in 10 mL of water for 5 minutes, to form a milky dispersion that flushes via an 8Fr NG tube without blockage.[4]
Allopurinol (Arrow, Generics, Hillcross, IVAX, Sovereign)	Tablet 100 mg, 300 mg	No specific data on enteral tube administration are available for this formulation.
Xanthomax (Ashbourne)	Tablet 100 mg, 300 mg	No specific data on enteral tube administration are available for this formulation.
Caplenal (Berk)	Tablet 100 mg, 300 mg	No specific data on enteral tube administration are available for this formulation.
Allopurinol (CP)	Tablet 100 mg, 300 mg	100 mg tablets do not disperse readily in water but crush easily and form a milky suspension when mixed with water. This suspension flushes down an 8Fr NG tube without blockage.[4]
Cosuric (DDSA)	Tablet 100 mg, 300 mg	No specific data on enteral tube administration are available for this formulation.
Rimapurinol (Ranbaxy)	Tablet 100 mg, 300 mg	Tablets will disperse if shaken in 10 mL of water for 5 minutes; the milky dispersion flushes via an 8Fr NG tube without blockage.[4]

Site of absorption (oral administration)

The specific site of absorption is not documented. Peak plasma concentration occurring $1\frac{1}{2}$ hours post dose.[1]

Alternative routes available

None available for allopurinol. Rasburicase (Fasturtec) injection is licensed for prophylaxis and treatment of acute hyperuricaemia.[3]

Interactions

There are no reports of reduced bioavailability of allopurinol on co-administration with food. The half-life of the active metabolite, oxypurinol, is increased in patients on a low-protein diet and may also be prolonged in malnourished patients. This may increase the risk of toxicity.[6]

Health and safety

Standard precautions apply.

Suggestions/recommendations

- Disperse the tablets in water immediately prior to administration.
- Administer after food.[1]

Intragastric administration

1. Stop the enteral feed.
2. Flush the enteral feeding tube with the recommended volume of water.
3. Place the tablet in the barrel of an appropriate size and type of syringe.
4. Draw 10 mL of water into the syringe and allow the tablet to disperse, shaking if necessary.
5. Flush the medication dose down the feeding tube.
6. Draw another 10 mL of water into the oral syringe and also flush this via the feeding tube (this will rinse the syringe and ensure that the total dose is administered).
7. Finally, flush with the recommended volume of water.
8. Re-start the feed, unless a prolonged break is required.

Alternatively, at step (3) place the tablet into a medicine pot, add 10 mL of water and allow the tablet to disperse. Draw this into an appropriate syringe. Ensure that the measure is rinsed and that this rinsing water is administered also to ensure that the total dose is given.

Intrajejunal administration

No specific data. Administer using the above method. Monitor for increased side-effects or loss of efficacy.

References

1. Zyloric Tablets 100 mg, 300 mg (GSK), Summary of Product Characteristics; 11 August 2004.
2. Personal Communication, Medical Information, Alpharma Limited, 21 January 2003.
3. *BNF 50*, September 2005.
4. BPNG data on file 2004/05.
5. Personal communication, Medical Information, GlaxoSmithKline Ltd; 22 January 2003.
6. Dollery C. *Therapeutic Drugs*, 2nd edn. London: Churchill Livingstone; 1998.

Alverine citrate

Formulations available[3]

Brand name (Manufacturer)	Formulation and strength	Product information/Administration information
Spasmonal (Norgine)	Capsule 60 mg	Norgine have no supporting data for alverine being administered via enteral feeding tubes. Administered directly into the mouth, the active ingredient in Spasmonal capsules may cause numbing of the lips and tongue.[2]
Spasmonal Forte (Norgine)	Capsule 120 mg	No specific data on enteral tube administration are available for this formulation.

Site of absorption (oral administration)

The specific site of absorption is not documented. Peak plasma concentration occurs $1-1\frac{1}{2}$ hours after oral administration.[1]

Alternative routes available

No other routes are available

Interactions

No documented interaction with food

Health and safety

Usual precautions apply.

Suggestions/recommendations

- Owing to lack of data, consider changing to mebeverine liquid (see monograph).

References

1. Spasmonal 60 mg, Summary of Product Characteristics; 6 April 2004.
2. Personal Communication, Medical Information, Norgine Ltd; 24 January 2003.
3. *BNF* 50, September 2005.

Amantadine hydrochloride

Formulations available[1]

Brand name (Manufacturer)	Formulation and strength	Product information/Administration information
Symmetrel (Alliance) Also available as Lysovir	Capsules 100 mg	Once daily dosing.[2] Amantadine is highly soluble in water (1 : 2.5). The capsules may be opened and mixed with water and administered immediately via an enteral feeding tube.[4]
Symmetrel (Alliance)	Syrup 50 mg/5 mL	Contains sorbitol,[3] 4.65 g/5 mL dose.[5] pH range of Symmetrel syrup is 4.8–5.3.[4]

Site of absorption (oral administration)

Specific site of absorption is not documented. Amantadine is absorbed slowly and almost completely following oral administration. Peak plasma concentration occurs 3–4 hours following oral dose.[2]

Alternative routes available

None for amantadine.

Interactions

No documented interaction with food.

Health and safety

Standard precautions apply.

Suggestions/recommendations

- Use liquid formulation. Monitor total daily intake of sorbitol.
- A prolonged break in feeding is not required.

Intragastric administration

1. Stop the enteral feed.
2. Flush the enteral feeding tube with the recommended volume of water.
3. Draw the medication solution into an appropriate size and type of syringe.
4. Flush the medication dose down the feeding tube.
5. Finally, flush with the recommended volume of water.
6. Re-start the feed, unless a prolonged break is required.

Alternatively, at step (3) measure the medicine in a suitable container and then draw into the syringe. Ensure that the measure is rinsed and that this rinsing water is administered also to ensure that the total dose is given. **Do not** measure liquid medicines using a catheter-tipped syringe as this results in excessive dosing owing to the volume of the tip.

Intrajejunal administration

There is no specific information relating to jejunal administration of amantadine. Administer using the above method. Monitor for increased side-effects or loss of efficacy.

References

1. *BNF* 50, September 2005.
2. Symmetrel Capsules, Summary of Product Characteristics; October 2001.
3. Symmetrel Syrup, Summary of Product Characteristics; October 1999.
4. Personal communication, Alliance Pharmaceuticals; January 2003.
5. Personal communication, Alliance Pharmaceuticals; July 2005.

Amiloride hydrochloride

Formulations available[1]

Brand name (Manufacturer)	Formulation and strength	Product information/Administration information
Amiloride (Alpharma)	Tablet 5 mg	Tablets can be crushed, partly insoluble.[2]
Amiloride (APS)	Tablet 5 mg	Tablet disintegrates rapidly when placed in 10 mL of water; the resulting dispersion flushes easily via an 8Fr NG tube without blockage.[3]
Amiloride (CP)	Tablet 5 mg	No specific data on enteral tube administration are available for this formulation.
Amiloride (Hillcross)	Tablet 5 mg	No specific data on enteral tube administration are available for this formulation.
Amiloride (IVAX)	Tablet 5 mg	No specific data on enteral tube administration are available for this formulation.
Amilamont (Rosemont)	Oral solution 5 mg/5 mL	Sugar-free oral solution. Does not contain sorbitol.[4]

Site of absorption (oral administration)

Amiloride is incompletely absorbed from the gastrointestinal tract.[5] Specific site is not documented. Peak plasma concentration occurs 3–4 hours following oral dosing.[5]

Alternative routes available

None available for amiloride.

Interactions

No documented interaction with food.[4, 5]

Health and safety

Standard precautions apply.

Suggestions/recommendations

- Use liquid formulation.
- A prolonged break in feeding is not required.

Intragastric administration

1. Stop the enteral feed.
2. Flush the enteral feeding tube with the recommended volume of water.
3. Draw the medication suspension into an appropriate size and type of syringe.
4. Flush the medication dose down the feeding tube.
5. Finally, flush with the recommended volume of water.
6. Re-start the feed, unless a prolonged break is required.

Alternatively, at step (3) measure the medicine in a suitable container. Draw this into an appropriate syringe. Ensure that the measure is rinsed and that this rinsing water is administered also to ensure that the total dose is given. **Do not** measure liquid medicines using a catheter-tipped syringe as this results in excessive dosing owing to the volume of the tip.

Intrajejunal administration

There are no specific data relating to the jejunal administration of amiloride. Administer using the above method. Monitor for increased side-effects or loss of efficacy.

References

1. *BNF* 50, September 2005.
2. Personal communication, Alpharma Ltd; 21 January 2003.
3. BPNG data on file 2004.
4. Amilamont (Rosemont), Summary of Product Characteristics; 22 December 2000.
5. Dollery C. *Therapeutic Drugs*, 2nd edn. London: Churchill Livingstone; 1998.

Amiodarone hydrochloride

Formulations available[1]

Brand name (Manufacturer)	Formulation and strength	Product information/Administration information
Cordarone X (Sanofi-Synthelabo)	Tablets 100 mg, 200 mg	Tablets can be crushed.[2]
Cordarone X (Sanofi-Synthelabo)	Injection 50 mg/mL	Cannot be administered via a feeding tube.[2] The injection contains Tween 80, which is an irritant.
Amiodarone (Alpharma)	Tablets 100 mg, 200 mg	Tablets can be crushed. Very bitter taste, if taking orally mix with jam.[3]
Amiodarone (APS, Generics, Hillcross, IVAX, Lexon, Sterwin)	Tablets 100 mg, 200 mg	No specific data on enteral tube administration are available for this formulation. See notes below.

Site of absorption (oral administration)

The specific site of absorption is not documented. Peak plasma concentration occurs 3–7 hours following oral dosing.[4]

Alternative routes available

In the acute setting the parenteral route can be used.

Interactions

No specific interaction with food is documented.[4]

Health and safety

Standard precautions apply.

Suggestions/recommendations

- Tablets do not disperse well but can be crushed and mixed with water to form a suspension.[5] An extemporaneous formulation can be made (contact Nova Laboratories for current stability data).
- Owing to the long half-life of amiodarone (in excess of 50 hours), the omission of occasional doses does not significantly influence the therapeutic effect.[6]

Intragastric administration

1. Stop the enteral feed.
2. Flush the enteral feeding tube with the recommended volume of water.
3. Place the tablet in a mortar and crush to a fine powder using the pestle.
4. Add a few millilitres of water and mix to form a paste.
5. Add up to 15 mL of water and mix thoroughly, ensuring that there are no large particles of tablet.
6. Draw this into an appropriate size and type of syringe.
7. Flush the medication dose down the feeding tube.
8. Add another 15 mL of water to the mortar and stir to ensure any remaining drug is rinsed from the container. Draw this water into the syringe and also flush this via the feeding tube (this will rinse the mortar and syringe and ensure that the total dose is administered).
9. Finally, flush the enteral feeding tube with the recommended volume of water.
10. Re-start the feed, unless a prolonged break in feeding is required.

Intrajejunal administration

There are no specific data relating to jejunal administration of amiodarone. Administer as above.

References

1. *BNF* 50, September 2005.
2. Personal communication, Sanofi-Synthelabo; 3 February 2003.
3. Personal communication, Alpharma Ltd; 21 January 2003.
4. Dollery C. *Therapeutic Drugs*, 2nd edn. London: Churchill Livingstone; 1998.
5. BPNG data on file 2005.
6. Cordarone X (Sanofi-Synthelabo), Summary of Product Characteristics; May 2004.

Amitriptyline hydrochloride

Formulations available[1]

Brand name (Manufacturer)	Formulation and strength	Product information/Administration information
Amitriptyline (Alpharma)	Tablets 10 mg, 25 mg, 50 mg	Film-coated Tablets can be crushed. Bitter taste, Film coat may not pulverise.[2] Tablets do not disperse readily in water but can be crushed and dispersed in 10 mL of water prior to administration.[3] Owing to the lack of stability data, this should be done immediately prior to administration.
Amitriptyline (APS)	Tablets 10 mg, 25 mg, 50 mg	Film-coated Tablets do not disperse readily in water but can be crushed and dispersed in 10 mL of water prior to administration.[3] Owing to the lack of stability data, this should be done immediately prior to administration.
Amitriptyline (Rosemont)	Oral solution 25 mg/5 mL, 50 mg/5 mL	Sugar-free liquid.[4] Golden yellow, slightly viscous liquid. Does not contain sorbitol.[4] pH approx. 4.5. Mixes easily with an equal volume of water, flushes down tube with very little resistance.[3]

Site of absorption (oral administration)

The specific site of absorption is not documented. Amitriptyline is absorbed slowly from the GI tract with peak plasma concentration occurring 4–8 hours following oral dosing.[5]

Alternative routes available

None commercially available for amitriptyline. A case report of buccal administration of amitriptyline using crushed tablets demonstrated effective absorption.[6]

Interactions

No documented interaction with food.

Health and safety

Standard precautions apply.

Suggestions/recommendations

- Use the liquid formulation.
- A prolonged break in feeding is not required.

Intragastric administration

1. Stop the enteral feed.
2. Flush the enteral feeding tube with the recommended volume of water.
3. Draw the medication suspension into the appropriate size and type of syringe.
4. Flush the medication dose down the feeding tube.
5. Finally, flush with the recommended volume of water.
6. Re-start the feed.

Alternatively, at step (3) measure the medicine in a suitable container. Draw this into the syringe with an appropriate adapter for the tube connector. Ensure that the measure is rinsed and that this rinsing water is administered also to ensure that the total dose is given. **Do not** measure liquid medicines using a catheter-tipped syringe as this results in excessive dosing owing to the volume of the tip.

Intrajejunal administration

There are no specific data relating to jejunal administration of amitriptyline. Administer using the above method. Monitor for increased side-effects or loss of efficacy.

References

1. *BNF 50*, September 2005.
2. Personal communication, Alpharma Ltd, 21 January 2003.
3. BPNG data on file 2004.
4. Amitriptyline Oral Solution (Rosemont), Summary of Product Characteristics; May 2004.
5. Dollery C. *Therapeutic Drugs*, 2nd edn. London: Churchill Livingstone; 1998.
6. Robbins B, Reiss RA. Amitriptyline absorption in a patient with short bowel syndrome. *Am J Gastroenterol*. 1999; 94(8): 2302–2304.

Amlodipine

Formulations available[1]

Brand name (Manufacturer)	Formulation and strength	Product information/Administration information
Istin (Pfizer)	Tablets 5 mg, 10 mg	Amlodipine besilate. Once-daily dosing in hypertension and angina.[1] Solubility 1 : 500 in water.[2] Crushing Istin tablets does not alter their efficacy or pharmacokinetics. Crushed tablets will form a suspension in about 30 seconds. This can be taken by mouth or administered via a feeding tube and should be washed down with water.[4] Pfizer does not have any stability data on Istin tablets in suspension and therefore recommends the suspension be prepared immediately before use. Tablet disintegrates within 2 minutes when placed in 10 mL of water, to give a very fine dispersion that settles quickly but flushes via an 8Fr NG tube without blockage.[5] *Extemporaneous preparations* *Amlodipine 1 mg/mL suspension (90 days stability):*[6] Amlodipine 5 mg tablets 24 tablets Ora-Sweet/Ora-Plus (equal volumes) to 120 mL *Amlodipine 1 mg/mL suspension* *(56 days stability – RT):*[6] Amlodipine 5 mg tablets 20 tablets 1% methylcellulose in syrup (1 : 1) to 100 mL
Amlodipine (Qualiti)	Tablets 5 mg, 10 mg	Amlodipine maleate. Tablets do not disperse in water, but do crush easily and disperse in water.[5]
Amlodipine (IVAX, Norton)	Tablets 5 mg, 10 mg	Amlodipine maleate. Tablets disperse in 10 mL of water within 2 minutes to give a very fine dispersion that settles quickly; this flushes easily down an 8Fr NG tube without blockage.[5]

Site of absorption (oral administration)

The specific site of absorption is not documented. Peak plasma concentration occurs 6–12 hours post dose.[3]

Alternative routes available

None

Interactions

No significant interactions with food.[4]

Health and safety

Standard precautions apply.

Suggestions/recommendations

- Some brands of amlodipine tablets disperse readily in water (see above) and can be safely administered via a feeding tube; this should be done immediately prior to administration.
- A stable suspension can also be prepared.

Intragastric administration

Either the tablets dispersed in water or the extemporaneous suspension can be used for intragastric administration.

Tablet administration

1. Stop the enteral feed.
2. Flush the enteral feeding tube with the recommended volume of water.
3. Place the tablet in the barrel of an appropriate size and type of syringe.
4. Draw 10 mL of water into the syringe and allow the tablet to disperse, shaking if necessary.
5. Flush the medication dose down the feeding tube.
6. Draw another 10 mL of water into the syringe and also flush this via the feeding tube (this will rinse the syringe and ensure that the total dose is administered).
7. Finally, flush with the recommended volume of water.
8. Re-start the feed, unless a prolonged break is required.

Alternatively, at step (3) Place the tablet into a medicine pot, add 10 mL of water and allow the tablet to disperse. Draw this into an appropriate syringe. Ensure that the measure is rinsed and that this rinsing water is administered also to ensure that the total dose is given.

Intrajejunal administration

The tablet dispersion should be used for intrajejunal administration as this will have a lower osmolarity than the suspension formulation. Follow the guidance above. There are no specific data relating to the administration of amlodipine via the jejunum. Monitor for loss of efficacy or increased side-effects.

References

1. *BNF 50*, September 2005.
2. Dollery C. *Therapeutic Drugs*, 2nd edn. London: Churchill Livingstone; 1998.
3. Istin (Pfizer), Summary of Product Characteristics; October 2005.
4. Personal communication, Pfizer Pharmaceuticals; 23 June 2003.
5. BPNG data on file 2004.
6. Nahata MC, Morosco RS, Hipple TF. Stability of amlodipine besylate in two liquid dosage forms. *J Am Pharm Assoc (Wash)*. 1999; 39(3): 375–377.

Amoxicillin

Formulations available[1]

Brand name (Manufacturer)	Formulation and strength	Product information/Administration information
Amoxil (GSK)	Syrup SF 125 mg/5 mL, 250 mg/5 mL	Contains sorbitol.[2] Quantities unlikely to be clinically important.
Amoxil (GSK)	Paediatric suspension 125 mg/1.25 mL	Sucrose based powder for reconstitution.[3]
Amoxil (GSK)	Sachets SF 3 g/sachet	No specific data on enteral tube administration are available for this formulation.
Amoxicillin (Alpharma, APS, Arrow, Ashbourne, Berk, Bristol, Eastern, Galen, Hillcross, IVAX, Kent, Ranbaxy)	Suspension 125 mg/5 mL, 250 mg/5 mL	When reconstituted forms a viscous liquid. Flushes with some resistance. Mixes easily with an equal volume of water.[4]
Amoxicillin (Hillcross, IVAX, Kent)	Sachets 3 g/sachet	No specific data on enteral tube administration are available for this formulation.

Site of absorption (oral administration)

Amoxicillin is absorbed in the upper intestine, although the specific site is not documented. Peak plasma concentration occurs 1–2 hours after oral dosing.[5]

Alternative routes available

Parenteral route should be used in serious infections.

Interactions

Food has no significant influence on the absorption of amoxicillin.[5]

Health and safety

Standard precautions apply.

Suggestions/recommendations

- Liquid formulations can be administered via feeding tubes. Use the parenteral route for serious infections.
- A prolonged break in feeding is not required.

Intragastric administration

1. Stop the enteral feed.
2. Flush the enteral feeding tube with the recommended volume of water.
3. Draw the medication suspension into the appropriate size and type of syringe.
4. Flush the medication dose down the feeding tube.
5. Draw an equal volume of water into the syringe and also flush this via the feeding tube (this will rinse the syringe and ensure that the total dose is administered).
6. Finally, flush with the recommended volume of water.
7. Re-start the feed, unless a prolonged break is required.

Alternatively, at step (3) measure the medicine in a suitable container and then draw into an appropriate syringe. Ensure that the measure is rinsed and that this rinsing water is administered also to ensure that the total dose is given. **Do not** measure liquid medicines using a catheter-tipped syringe as this results in excessive dosing owing to the volume of the tip.

Intrajejunal administration

Administer using the above method.

References

1. *BNF 50*, September 2005.
2. Amoxil Syrup sugar-free/dye-free (GSK), Summary of Product Characteristics; 5 July 2005.
3. Amoxil Paediatric Suspension (GSK), Summary of Product Characteristics; February 2005.
4. BPNG data on file 2004.
5. Dollery C. *Therapeutic Drugs*, 2nd edn. London: Churchill Livingstone; 1998.

Amphotericin

Formulations available[1]

Brand name (Manufacturer)	Formulation and strength	Product information/Administration information
Fungilin (Squibb)	Tablets 100 mg	Amphotericin is practically insoluble in water.[2] No specific data on enteral tube administration are available for this formulation.
Fungilin (Squibb)	Suspension 100 mg/mL	Fungilin suspension should not be diluted prior to oral use as it is designed to adhere to oral lesions.[3] Fungilin is a viscous suspension, for administration via an enteral feeding tube dilution with water may be necessary.
Fungilin (Squibb)	Lozenge 10 mg	Designed for oral use only. No specific data on enteral tube administration are available for this formulation.

Site of absorption (oral administration)

Little or no absorption occurs through the normal or ulcerated GI tract.[4]

Alternative routes available

Amphotericin is not absorbed via the oral route and therefore the oral route is indicated for topical effect only. Systemic treatment with amphotericin would not be appropriate in these circumstances.

Interactions

As amphotericin is not absorbed when administered orally, there is no documented interaction with food.

Health and safety

Standard precautions apply.

Suggestions/recommendations

- Amphotericin suspension can be used via a feeding tube but will only have a topical effect below the point of delivery.
- Fluconazole could be considered an alternative for oral and intestinal candidosis as it is secreted in sputum.[5]

Intragastric administration

See notes above.

1. Stop the enteral feed.
2. Flush the enteral feeding tube with the recommended volume of water.
3. Draw the medication suspension into the appropriate size and type of syringe.
4. Flush the medication dose down the feeding tube.
5. Finally, flush with the recommended volume of water.
6. Re-start the feed, unless a prolonged break is required.

Alternatively, at step (3) measure the medicine in a suitable container and then draw into an appropriate syringe. Ensure that the measure is rinsed and that this rinsing water is administered also to ensure that the total dose is given. **Do not** measure liquid medicines using a catheter-tipped syringe as this results in excessive dosing owing to the volume of the tip.

Intrajejunal administration

See notes above. Administer using the above method.

References

1. *BNF* 50, September 2005.
2. Personal communication, Bristol-Myers Squibb Pharmaceuticals Ltd; 24 January 2003.
3. Fungilin Oral Suspension, Summary of Product Characteristics; 24 June 2005.
4. Dollery C. *Therapeutic Drugs*, 2nd edn. London: Churchill Livingstone; 1998.
5. Diflucan, Summary of Product Characteristics; July 2000.

Amprenavir

Formulations available[1]

Brand name (Manufacturer)	Formulation and strength	Product information/Administration information
Agenerase (GSK)	Capsules 50 mg, 150 mg	Soft gelatin capsules.[2] Excipients include vitamin E 36 units/50 mg No specific data on enteral tube administration are available for this formulation.
Agenerase (GSK)	Oral solution 15 mg/mL	Excipients include vitamin E 46 units/mL.[1] The oral solution is 14% less bioavailable than the capsules, therefore the dose is 17 mg/kg three times a day (maximum 2.8 g/day).[3] The liquid formulation contains significant quantities of propylene glycol (550 mg/mL).[3]

Site of absorption (oral administration)

Specific site of absorption is not documented. Following oral administration the mean time to reach peak plasma concentration is 1–2 hours for the capsules and $\frac{1}{2}$–1 hour for the oral solution,[2] suggesting absorption high in the intestine. A second peak at 10–12 hours could be the result of delayed absorption or enterohepatic circulation.[2]

Alternative routes available

None available for amprenavir.

Interactions

Administration of amprenavir with food reduces AUC; however, steady-state trough concentrations are unaffected.

Health and safety

Standard precautions apply.

Suggestions/recommendations

- The bioavailability of Agenerase oral solution is lower than that of capsules; the two formulations are not interchangeable on a milligram-for-milligram basis.[1]
- GSK have no information on the administration of Agenerase via enteral feeding tubes.[4]
- If treatment with amprenavir is indicated, use the liquid formulation. A prolonged break in feeding is not required.

Intragastric administration

1. Stop the enteral feed.
2. Flush the enteral feeding tube with the recommended volume of water.
3. Draw medication solution into the appropriate size and type of syringe.
4. Flush the medication dose down the feeding tube.
5. Finally, flush with the recommended volume of water.
6. Re-start the feed, unless a prolonged break is required.

Alternatively, at step (3) measure the medicine in a suitable container and then draw into an appropriate syringe. Ensure that the measure is rinsed and that this rinsing water is administered also to ensure that the total dose is given. **Do not** measure liquid medicines using a catheter-tipped syringe as this results in excessive dosing owing to the volume of the tip.

Intrajejunal administration

There are no specific data relating to the jejunal administration of amprenavir. Where indicated, administer using the above method. Monitor for increased side-effects or loss of efficacy.

References

1. *BNF* 50, September 2005.
2. Agenerase Capsules, Summary of Product Characteristics; 17 November 2005.
3. Agenerase oral solution, Summary of Product Characteristics; 17 November 2005.
4. Personal communication, GlaxoSmithKline Ltd, 22 January 2003.

Anastrazole

Formulations available[1]

Brand name (Manufacturer)	Formulation and strength	Product information/Administration information
Arimidex (AstraZeneca)	Tablets 1 mg	Anastrazole is moderately soluble in water.[3] Anastrazole tablets disperse in 10 mL of water to give an almost clear dispersion that flushes down an 8Fr NG tube without blockage. However, the tablets are slow to disperse and take in excess of 5 minutes.[4]

Site of absorption (oral administration)

Specific site of absorption not documented. Peak plasma concentration occurs within 2 hours of dosing.[2]

Alternative routes available

None for anastrazole.

Interactions

Food slightly decreases the rate but not the extent of absorption.[2] Average time to peak plasma concentrations in fed individuals is 5 hours (range 2–12 hours).[3]

Health and safety

Standard precautions apply. However, owing to the class of drug, crushing is not recommended: a closed system should be used.

Suggestions/recommendations

- Disperse tablet in water, agitating to aid dispersion, and flush via the feeding tube.

Intragastric administration

1. Stop the enteral feed.
2. Flush the enteral feeding tube with the recommended volume of water.
3. Place the tablet in the barrel of an appropriate size and type of syringe.
4. Draw 10 mL of water into the syringe and allow the tablet to disperse, shaking if necessary.
5. Flush the medication dose down the feeding tube.
6. Draw another 10 mL of water into the syringe and also flush this via the feeding tube (this will rinse the syringe and ensure that the total dose is administered).
7. Finally, flush with the recommended volume of water.
8. Re-start the feed, unless a prolonged break is required.

Alternatively, at step (3) place the tablet into a medicine pot, add 10 mL of water and allow the tablet to disperse. Draw this into an appropriate syringe. Ensure that the measure is rinsed and that this rinsing water is administered also to ensure that the total dose is given.

Intrajejunal administration

There are no specific data relating to jejunal administration. Administer using the above method. Monitor for increased side-effects.

References

1. *BNF* 50, September 2005.
2. Arimidex, Summary of Product Characteristics; 10 August 2005.
3. Dollery C. *Therapeutic Drugs*, 2nd edn. London: Churchill Livingstone; 1998.
4. BPNG data on file 2004.

Ascorbic acid

Formulations available[1]

Brand name (Manufacturer)	Formulation and strength	Product information/Administration information
Ascorbic Acid (Alpharma)	Tablets 50 mg, 100 mg, 200 mg, 500 mg	Chewable tablets.[1] No specific data on enteral tube administration are available for this formulation.
Ascorbic Acid (Roche Consumer Health)	Tablets 50 mg, 100 mg, 200 mg, 500 mg	Chewable tablets.[1] No specific data on enteral tube administration are available for this formulation.

Formulations available[1] (continued)

Brand name (Manufacturer)	Formulation and strength	Product information/Administration information
Ascorbic Acid (Various)	Effervescent tablets 1 g	Effervescent tablets are available for general sale, but not prescribable on FP10. This formulation should be suitable for enteral tube administration.

Site of absorption (oral administration)

Ascorbic acid is readily absorbed by active transport from the intestine.[2]

Alternative routes available

The parenteral formulation can be used in acute situations.

Interactions

Ascorbic acid may increase the absorption of iron in iron-deficiency states.[3]

Health and safety

Standard precautions apply.

Suggestions/recommendations

- Use effervescent tablets.
- A prolonged break in feeding is not required.

Intragastric administration

1. Stop the enteral feed.
2. Flush the enteral feeding tube with the recommended volume of water.
3. Measure 20–50 mL of water into a measuring pot.
4. Add the effervescent tablet and allow to dissolve.
5. Draw into an appropriate size and type of syringe.
6. Flush the medication dose down the feeding tube.
7. Rinse the measure and administer this also to ensure that the total dose is given.
8. Finally, flush with the recommended volume of water.
9. Re-start the feed, unless a prolonged break is required.

Intrajejunal administration

Jejunal delivery of ascorbic acid should not affect bioavailability. Administer using the above method.

References

1. *BNF* 50, September 2005.
2. Dollery C. *Therapeutic Drugs*, 2nd edn. London: Churchill Livingstone; 1998.
3. Sweetman SC, ed. *Martindale*, 34th edn. London: Pharmaceutical Press; 2005.

Aspirin

Formulations available[1]

Brand name (Manufacturer)	Formulation and strength	Product information/Administration information
Aspirin (Alpharma)	Dispersible tablets 75 mg, 300 mg	Suitable for use via enteral feeding tube.[2]
Angettes (BMS)	Tablets 75 mg	Very slightly soluble in cold and hot water.[3]
Micropirin (Dexcel)	Dispersible tablets 75 mg	Disperse readily in water.
Aspirin (Aurum)	Suppositories 300 mg, 150 mg	Rectal absorption is less reliable.[5]
Aspav Alpharma	Dispersible tablets Aspirin 500 mg, Papaveretum 7.71 mg	One or two tablets dispersed in water every 4–6 hours. Max: 8 tablets in 24 hours.[4]
Co-codaprin (Alpharma)	Dispersible tablets 400 mg aspirin plus 8 mg codeine	Suitable for use via enteral feeding tube.[2]

Site of absorption (oral administration)

Absorption of nonionised aspirin occurs in the stomach and small intestine.[5]

Alternative routes available

Rectal.

Interactions

No specific interaction is documented.

Health and safety

Standard precautions apply.

Suggestions/recommendations

- Use dispersible tablets. If oral absorption is compromised, consider using suppositories.
- A prolonged break in feeding is not required.

Intragastric administration

1. Stop the enteral feed.
2. Flush the enteral feeding tube with the recommended volume of water.
3. Place the tablet in the barrel of an appropriate size and type of syringe.
4. Draw 10 mL of water into the syringe and allow the tablet to dissolve.
5. Flush the medication dose down the feeding tube.
6. Draw an equal volume of water into the syringe and also flush this via the feeding tube (this will rinse the syringe and ensure that the total dose is administered).
7. Finally, flush with the recommended volume of water.
8. Re-start the feed, unless a prolonged break is required.

Alternatively, at step (3) place the tablet into a medicine pot and add 10 mL of water and allow the tablet to dissolve. Draw this into an appropriate syringe. Ensure that the measure is rinsed and that this rinsing water is administered also to ensure that the total dose is given.

Intrajejunal administration

Administer using the above method.

References

1. *BNF* 50, September 2005.
2. Personal Communication, Alpharma Ltd; 21 January 2003.
3. Personal Communication, Bristol-Myers Squibb; 24 January 2003.
4. Aspav, Summary of Product Characteristics; January 2003.
5. Sweetman SC, ed. *Martindale*, 34th edn. London: Pharmaceutical Press; 2005.

Atenolol

Formulations available[1]

Brand name (Manufacturer)	Formulation and strength	Product information/Administration information
Tenormin '25' (AstraZeneca)	Film-coated tablet 25 mg	No specific data on enteral tube administration are available for this formulation.
Tenormin LS (AstraZeneca)	Film-coated tablet 50 mg	No specific data on enteral tube administration are available for this formulation.
Tenormin (AstraZeneca)	Film-coated Tablet 100 mg	No specific data on enteral tube administration are available for this formulation.
Tenormin (AstraZeneca)	Syrup Sugar-free 25 mg/5 mL	Contains sorbitol. Protect from light.[2] Clear liquid, nonviscous, flushes easily via an 8Fr NG tube without significant resistance. Mixes well with equal volume of water.[5]
Tenormin (AstraZeneca)	Injection 500 μg/mL	No specific data on enteral tube administration are available for this formulation.

Formulations available[1] (continued)

Brand name (Manufacturer)	Formulation and strength	Product information/Administration information
Atenolol (Alpharma)	Film-coated tablets 25 mg, 50 mg, 100 mg	Film coat may clog tube.[3]
Atenolol (Alpharma, APS, Ashbourne, CP, Hillcross, IVAX, Sterwin, Tillomed)	Tablets 25 mg, 50 mg, 100 mg	Most brands are film-coated tablets, which do not disperse readily in water.[5]
Co-tenidone (Alpharma)	Tablets 50/12.5 mg, 100/25 mg	Film-coated tablets. May clog tube.[3]

Site of absorption (oral administration)

Peak plasma concentration occurs 2–4 hours post oral dose.[4] There are data to demonstrate that atenolol is absorbed in the jejunum and ileum, providing similar bioavailability data to oral absorption.[6]

Alternative routes available

The parenteral route is available.

Interactions

No documented interaction with food.[4]

Health and safety

Standard precautions apply

Suggestions/recommendations

- Use liquid formulation for gastric administration; no further dilution is necessary. For administration into the jejunum, dilute the liquid with an equal volume of water prior to administration to reduce osmolarity.
- A prolonged break in feeding is not necessary.

Intragastric administration

1. Stop the enteral feed.
2. Flush the enteral feeding tube with the recommended volume of water.
3. Draw medication solution into the appropriate size and type of syringe.
4. Flush the medication dose down the feeding tube.
5. Finally, flush with the recommended volume of water.
6. Re-start the feed, unless a prolonged break is required.

Alternatively, at step (3) measure the medicine in a suitable container and then draw into an appropriate syringe. Ensure that the measure is rinsed and that this rinsing water is administered also to ensure that the total dose is given. **Do not** measure liquid medicines using a catheter-tipped syringe as this results in excessive dosing owing to the volume of the tip.

Intrajejunal administration

Jejunal administration will not affect the therapeutic effect of atenolol.

1. Stop the enteral feed.
2. Flush the enteral feeding tube with the recommended volume of water.
3. Draw the medication suspension into the appropriate size and type of syringe.
4. Draw an equal volume of water and a little air into the syringe and shake to mix thoroughly.
5. Flush the medication dose down the feeding tube.
6. Finally, flush with the recommended volume of water.
7. Re-start the feed, unless a prolonged break is required.

Alternatively, at step (3) measure the medicine in a suitable container and then add an equal volume of water and mix thoroughly. Draw this into an appropriate syringe. Ensure that the measure is rinsed and that this rinsing water is administered also to ensure that the total dose is given. **Do not** measure liquid medicines using a catheter-tipped syringe as this results in excessive dosing owing to the volume of the tip.

References

1. *BNF* 50, September 2005.
2. Tenormin Syrup, Summary of Product Characteristics; 31 October 2003.
3. Personal Communication, Alpharma Ltd; 21 January 2003.
4. Dollery C. *Therapeutic Drugs*, 2nd edn. London: Churchill Livingstone; 1998.
5. BPNG data on file 2005.
6. Adams D. Administration of drugs through a jejunostomy tube. *Br J Intensive Care*. 1994; 4(1): 10–17.

Atorvastatin

Formulations available[1]

Brand name (Manufacturer)	Formulation and strength	Product information/Administration information
Lipitor (Parke-Davis)	10 mg, 20 mg, 40 mg, 80 mg	Atorvastatin calcium trihydrate. Film-coated tablets. 10 mg, 20 mg and 40 mg tablets disperse within 2–5 minutes when placed in 10 mL of water, to produce a very fine milky, white dispersion that does not settle quickly. This suspension flushes via an 8Fr NG tube without blockage.[2] Atorvastatin is only slightly soluble in water and is light sensitive.[3]

Site of absorption (oral administration)

Exact site of absorption is unknown but likely to be the upper intestine as peak plasma concentration is reached 1–2 hours post dose.[3]

Alternative routes available

No alternative routes for any of the 'statins'.

Interactions

No significant interaction with food. Food reduces the AUC and delays absorption of atorvastatin; however, the clinical effect on LDL cholesterol and total cholesterol is not significantly affected.[4, 5]

Health and safety

Standard precautions apply.

Suggestions/recommendations

- Disperse the tablet in water and immediately administer via feeding tube.
- No break in feeding is necessary.
- Atorvastatin can be given at any time during the day.[6]

Intragastric administration

1. Stop the enteral feed.
2. Flush the enteral feeding tube with the recommended volume of water.
3. Place the tablet in the barrel of an appropriate size and type of syringe.
4. Draw 10 mL of water into the syringe and allow the tablet to disperse, shaking if necessary.
5. Flush the medication dose down the feeding tube.
6. Draw another 10 mL of water into the syringe and also flush this via the feeding tube (this will rinse the syringe and ensure that the total dose is administered).
7. Finally, flush with the recommended volume of water.
8. Re-start the feed, unless a prolonged break is required.

Alternatively, at step (3) place the tablet into a medicine pot, add 10 mL of water and allow the tablet to disperse. Draw this into an appropriate syringe. Ensure that the measure is rinsed and that this rinsing water is administered also to ensure that the total dose is given.

Intrajejunal administration

No specific data relating to jejunal administration of atorvastatin. Administer using the above method. Monitor for increased side-effects or loss of efficacy.

References

1. *BNF 50*, September 2005.
2. BPNG data on file, 2004.
3. Dollery C. *Therapeutic Drugs*, 2nd edn. London: Churchill Livingstone; 1998.
4. Whitfield LR, Stern RH, Sedman AJ, Abel R, Gibson DM. Effect of food on the pharmacodynamics and pharmacokinetics of atorvastatin, an inhibitor of HMG-CoA reductase. *Eur J Drug Metab Pharmacokinet.* 2000; 25(2): 97–101.
5. Radulovic LL, Cilla DD, Posvar EL, Sedman AJ, Whitfield LR. Effect of food on the bioavailability of atorvastatin, an HMG-CoA reductase inhibitor. *J Clin Pharmacol.* 1995; 35(10): 990–994.
6. Lipitor (Parke-Davis), Summary of Product Characteristics; March 2005.

Auranofin

Formulations available[1]

Brand name (Manufacturer)	Formulation and strength	Product information/Administration information
Ridaura (Yamanouchi)	Tablets 3 mg	Film-coated. No specific data on enteral tube administration are available for this formulation.
Myocristin (JHC)	Sodium aurothiomalate Injection 10 mg/0.5 mL, 20 mg/0.5 mL, 50 mg/0.5 mL	Intramuscular (i.m.) administration only. Pharmacokinetics, distribution and metabolism are different from oral gold therapy.[2]

Site of absorption (oral administration)

Specific site is not documented. Peak plasma concentration occurs 1.8 hours after oral dosing.[3]

Alternative routes available

The i.m. route could be used in the short term to maintain therapy. I.m. gold is given weekly, specialist advice should be sought from a rheumatologist before transferring from oral to i.m. gold therapy.

Interactions

No documented interaction with food.

Health and safety

Gold is teratogenic in some animal species. Women of child-bearing age should avoid handling crushed tablets.[2]

Suggestions/recommendations

- Other treatments should be considered. Gold therapy should only be used under specialist advice.
- Diarrhoea is a common side-effect of oral gold therapy and treatment should be discontinued if diarrhoea develops.[2]

References

1. *BNF 50*, September 2005.
2. Ridaura Tiltab Tablets 3 mg (Yamanouchi), Summary of Product Characteristics; 4 November 2005.
3. Dollery C. *Therapeutic Drugs*, 2nd edn. London: Churchill Livingstone; 1998.

Azathioprine

Formulations available[1]

Brand name (Manufacturer)	Formulation and strength	Product information/Administration information
Imuran (GSK)	Tablets 25 mg, 50 mg	Film-coated. Tablets disperse in 10 mL water within 5 minutes, to give a pale yellow milky dispersion that flushes easily via an 8Fr NG tube.[3]
Imuran (GSK)	Injection 50 mg	Azathioprine as sodium salt. Injection pH 10–12, when diluted pH 8.5–9.[5] No specific data on enteral tube administration are available for this formulation.
Azathioprine (Alpharma, Hillcross, IVAX, Kent)	Tablets 25 mg, 50 mg	No specific data on enteral tube administration are available for this formulation.
Immunoprin (Ashbourne)	Tablets 25 mg, 50 mg	No specific data on enteral tube administration are available for this formulation.
Azathioprine (Generics)	Tablets 25 mg, 50 mg	Both 25 mg and 50 mg tablets disintegrate within 3 minutes when agitated in a syringe with 10 mL of water. Gives a pale milky yellow dispersion that flushes easily down an 8Fr NG tube.[3]
Oprisine (Opus)	Tablets 25 mg, 50 mg	No specific data on enteral tube administration are available for this formulation.
Azamune (Penn)	Tablets 25 mg, 50 mg	No specific data on enteral tube administration are available for this formulation.
Azathioprine (Nova labs)	Suspension 2.5–100 mg/5 mL	Manufactured 'special'. One month expiry. Viscosity suitable for administration via feeding tube.[7]
Azathioprine (extemporaneous suspension)	Suspension 50 mg/mL	*Extemporaneous suspension:* Azathioprine 50 mg tablet 100 tablets Cherry syrup to 100 mL Sixty days expiry at room temperature.[6]

Site of absorption (oral administration)

Peak plasma concentration occurs 1–2 hours after oral dosing.[2]

Data available from animal studies indicate that azathioprine is absorbed mainly through the epithelium of the stomach and ileum. Although no data are available in humans, this information suggests that jejunal delivery of the drug should not adversely affect dosing.[4]

Alternative routes available

Intravenous injection is alkaline and very irritant; the parenteral route should be used only if the oral route is not feasible.[1]

Interactions

No documented interaction with food has been noted. However, administration after food reduces side-effects of nausea.[2]

Health and safety

Azathioprine is a cytotoxic. The tablets should not be crushed owing to the risk of inhaling the powder. Several brands of azathioprine tablets will disperse in water, in a closed system (see chapter 8); use of this method will reduce exposure. Gloves should be worn by staff handling azathioprine tablet suspension (the coating on the tablet would usually protect the handler).

Suggestions/recommendations

- Owing to risks of handling cytotoxic drugs, discontinue or use alternative drug where possible. However, in the majority of circumstances in which azathioprine is used it is likely that alternatives will also be cytotoxic.
- The preferred method is to disperse azathioprine tablets in 10 mL of water in the barrel of a syringe, as this is a closed system. Gloves should be worn during this procedure in case of accidental spillage.
- An extemporaneous formulation with 60 days' shelf-life can be made,[6] but this must be made in an environment with suitable containment facilities to handle crushed cytotoxic tablets.

Intragastric administration

1. Stop the enteral feed.
2. Flush the enteral feeding tube with the recommended volume of water.
3. Place the tablet in the barrel of an appropriate size and type of syringe.
4. Draw 10 mL of water into the syringe and allow the tablet to disperse, shaking if necessary.
5. Flush the medication dose down the feeding tube.
6. Draw another 10 mL of water into the oral syringe and also flush this via the feeding tube (this will rinse the syringe and ensure that the total dose is administered). Dispose of the syringe as cytotoxic waste.
7. Finally, flush with the recommended volume of water.
8. Re-start the feed, unless a prolonged break is required.

Intrajejunal administration

Jejunal administration would not be expected to affect bioavailability. Administer using the above method.

References

1. *BNF* 50, September 2005.
2. Imuran Tablets 25 mg, Summary of Product Characteristics; 23 December 2005.
3. BPNG data on file, 2004.
4. Personal Communication, GlaxoSmithKline; 22 January 2003.
5. Imuran Injection, Summary of Product Characteristics; 23 December 2005.
6. Allen LV, Erickson MA. Stability of acetazolamide, allopurinol, azathioprine, clonazepam, and flucytosine in extemporaneously compounded oral liquids. *Am J Health Syst Pharm.* 1996; 53: 1944–1949.
7. Personal communication, Nova Labs; 24 March 2005.

Baclofen

Formulations available[1]

Brand name (Manufacturer)	Formulation and strength	Product information/Administration information
Lioresal (Cephalon)	Tablets 10 mg	No specific data on enteral tube administration are available for this formulation.
Lioresal (Cephalon)	Liquid 5 mg/5 mL	Sugar-free liquid. Contains sorbitol, 2.75 g/5 mL dose.[7] May be diluted with water without affecting the formulation.[4]
Lyflex (Chemidex)	Oral solution 5 mg/5 mL	Sugar-free liquid. Contains sorbitol. May be further diluted with water.[8]
Baclofen (Alpharma, APS, Hillcross, IVAX, Sandoz)	Tablets 10 mg	Alpharma brand tablets can be crushed.[3] APS brand tablets disperse within 2 minutes when placed in 10 mL of water to produce a very fine white dispersion that flushes easily via an 8Fr NG tube.[6]
Baclospas (Ashbourne)	Tablets 10 mg	No specific data on enteral tube administration are available for this formulation.
Lioresal (Novartis)	Intrathecal injection 50 microgram/mL, 500 microgram/mL, 2 mg/mL	Not appropriate as a routine alternative to oral route.

Site of absorption (oral administration)

Baclofen is rapidly and completely absorbed from the GI tract, although the specific site of absorption is not documented. Liquid and tablet formulations are bioequivalent. Peak plasma concentration occurs 0.5–1.5 hours following oral dose.[2]

Alternative routes available

Intrathecal route is available but not an appropriate alternative to oral therapy. Diazepam is available in rectal and parenteral formulations if clinically indicated.

Interactions

Food does not affect the bioavailability of baclofen, but administration after food may reduce GI side-effects.[5]

Health and safety

Standard precautions apply.

Suggestions/recommendations

- Use liquid formulation for small doses. Consider dispersing tablets in water for higher doses owing to the sorbitol content of the liquid formulation.
- A prolonged break in feeding is not required.

Intragastric administration

Liquid formulation

1. Stop the enteral feed.
2. Flush the enteral feeding tube with the recommended volume of water.
3. Draw the medication solution into an appropriate size and type of syringe.
4. Flush the medication dose down the feeding tube.
5. Finally, flush with the recommended volume of water.
6. Re-start the feed, unless a prolonged break is required.

Alternatively, at step (3) measure the medicine in a suitable container and then draw into an appropriate syringe. Ensure that the measure is rinsed and that this rinsing water is administered also to ensure that the total dose is given. **Do not** measure liquid medicines using a catheter-tipped syringe as this results in excessive dosing owing to the volume of the tip.

Intrajejunal administration

Tablet formulation

1. Stop the enteral feed.
2. Flush the enteral feeding tube with the recommended volume of water.
3. Place the tablet in the barrel of an appropriate size and type of syringe.
4. Draw 10 mL of water into the syringe and allow the tablet to disperse, shaking if necessary.
5. Flush the medication dose down the feeding tube.
6. Draw another 10 mL of water into the syringe and also flush this via the feeding tube (this will rinse the syringe and ensure that the total dose is administered).
7. Finally, flush with the recommended volume of water.
8. Re-start the feed, unless a prolonged break is required.

Alternatively, at step (3) place the tablet into a medicine pot, add 10 mL of water and allow the tablet to disperse. Draw this into an appropriate syringe. Ensure that the measure is rinsed and that this rinsing water is administered also to ensure that the total dose is given.

References

1. *BNF 50*, September 2005.
2. Lioresal Tablets (Novartis), Summary of Product Characteristics; 22 February 2005.
3. Personal Communication, Alpharma Ltd; 21January 2003.
4. Lioresal Liquid (Novartis), Summary of Product Characteristics; 22 February 2005.
5. Dollery C. *Therapeutic Drugs*, 2nd edn. London: Churchill Livingstone; 1998.
6. BPNG data on file 2004.
7. Personal communication, Cephalon; July 2005.
8. Lyflex (Chemidex), Summary of Product Characteristics; 10 June 2004.

Balsalazide

Formulations available[1]

Brand name (Manufacturer)	Formulation and strength	Product information/Administration information
Colazide (Shire)	Capsules 750 mg	The capsules can be opened and the powder can be mixed with water; however, the company strongly discourage this as the azo dye will stain skin.[2]

Site of absorption (oral administration)

Balsalazide is not absorbed; the azo bond is cleaved in the colon, releasing mesalazine as the active component.[3]

Alternative routes available

Topical therapy using a rectal 5-ASA formulation should be used first line in local rectal disease.

Interactions

There is no documented interaction with food.[3]

Health and safety

Standard precautions apply. Capsule contents will stain.

Suggestions/recommendations

- Use topical preparations where clinically appropriate.
- Consider changing to sulfasalazine liquid preparation or using alternative therapy such as steroids.

References

1. *BNF* 50, September 2005.
2. Personal communication, Shire Pharmaceuticals; 17 February 2003.
3. Colozide (Shire), Summary of Product Characteristics; September 2005.

Bendroflumethiazide

Formulations available[1]

Brand name (Manufacturer)	Formulation and strength	Product information/Administration information
Bendroflumethiazide (Alpharma, APS, CP, Generics, Hillcross, IVAX)	Tablets 2.5 mg, 5 mg	Bendroflumethiazide is insoluble in water.[2] CP, APS and Alpharma brands of bendroflumethiazide all disperse within 2 minutes when placed in 10 mL of water. CP and APS give a very fine dispersion, Alpharma brand has slightly larger particles, but all flush down an 8Fr NG tube without blockage.[3]
Neo-NaClex (Goldshield)	Tablets 5 mg	No specific data on enteral tube administration are available for this formulation.
Aprinox (Sovereign)	Tablets 2.5 mg, 5 mg	No specific data on enteral tube administration are available for this formulation.

Site of absorption (oral administration)

Specific site of absorption is not documented. Bendroflumethiazide is completely absorbed from the GI tract; onset of diuretic action occurs within 2 hours, with a peak effect between 3 and 6 hours.[4]

Alternative routes available

None available for bendroflumethiazide. Other diuretics such as frusemide and bumetanide are available as injection.

Interactions

No interactions with food are documented.

Health and safety

Standard precautions apply.

Suggestions/recommendations

- Disperse tablets in water.
- A prolonged break in feeding is not required.

Intragastric administration

1. Stop the enteral feed.
2. Flush the enteral feeding tube with the recommended volume of water.
3. Place the tablet in the barrel of an appropriate size and type of syringe.
4. Draw 10 mL of water into the syringe and allow the tablet to disperse, shaking if necessary.
5. Flush the medication dose down the feeding tube.
6. Draw another 10 mL of water into the syringe and also flush this via the feeding tube (this will rinse the syringe and ensure that the total dose is administered).
7. Finally, flush with the recommended volume of water.
8. Re-start the feed, unless a prolonged break is required.

Alternatively, at step (3) place the tablet into a medicine pot, add 10 mL of water and allow the tablet to disperse. Draw this into an appropriate syringe. Ensure that the measure is rinsed and that this rinsing water is administered also to ensure that the total dose is given.

Intrajejunal administration

No specific data on jejunal administration. Administer using the above method.

References

1. *BNF* 50, September 2005.
2. Personal Communication, Alpharma Pharmaceuticals; 21 January 2003.
3. BPNG data on file, 2004.
4. Aprinox Tablets (Sovereign), Summary of Product Characteristics; March 2003.

Betahistine

Formulations available[1]

Brand name (Manufacturer)	Formulation and strength	Product information/Administration information
Serc (Solvay)	Tablets 8 mg, 16 mg	Betahistine is very soluble. The tablets can be crushed.[3]
Betahistine (Alpharma)	Tablets 8 mg, 16 mg	The tablets can be crushed.[4]
Betahistine (Kent)	Tablets 8 mg	Tablets do not disperse easily in water and require crushing to mix with water. When crushed finely the powder mixes easily with water and flushes down an 8Fr NG tube.[5]

Site of absorption (oral administration)

Specific site is not documented. Peak plasma concentration occurs within 1 hour of oral administration.[6]

Alternative routes available

No alternative is available.

Interactions

No specific interaction with food is documented.[6] Betahistine is recommended to be taken after food.[2]

Health and safety

Standard precautions apply.

Suggestions/recommendations

- Crush the tablets and disperse in water immediately prior to administration.
- A prolonged break in feeding is not required.
- Where possible, administer after feed.

Intragastric administration

1. Stop the enteral feed.
2. Flush the enteral feeding tube with the recommended volume of water.
3. Place the tablet in mortar and crush to a fine powder using the pestle.
4. Add a few millilitres of water and mix to form a paste.
5. Add up to 15 mL of water and mix thoroughly, ensuring that there are no large particles of tablet.
6. Draw this into an appropriate size and type of syringe.
7. Flush the medication dose down the feeding tube.
8. Add another 15 mL of water to the mortar and stir to ensure that any remaining drug is rinsed from the container. Draw this water into the syringe and also flush this via the feeding tube (this will rinse the mortar and syringe and ensure total dose is administered).
9. Finally, flush the enteral feeding tube with the recommended volume of water.
10. Re-start the feed, unless a prolonged break in feeding is required.

Intrajejunal administration

There is no specific information on jejunal administration of betahistine. Administer using the above method. Monitor for increased side-effects or loss of efficacy.

References

1. *BNF 50*, September 2005.
2. Serc (Solvay), Summary of Product Characteristics; April 2003.
3. Personal communication, Solvay Healthcare; 19 February 2003.
4. Personal communication, Alpharma Pharmaceuticals; 21 January 2003.
5. BPNG data on file, 2004.
6. Dollery C. *Therapeutic Drugs*, 2nd edn. London: Churchill Livingstone; 1998.

Betaine

Formulations available

Brand name (Manufacturer)	Formulation and strength	Product information/Administration information
Betaine Oral Liquid (Special Products Ltd)	Oral liquid 500 mg/mL	Manufactured 'special'. The oral liquid can be administered undiluted via an enteral feeding tube. [1] Liquid pH is 7–8.

Site of absorption (oral administration)

Specific site is not documented.

Alternative routes available

None available for betaine.

Interactions

No documented interactions with food.

Health and safety

Standard precautions apply.

Suggestions/recommendations

- Use liquid preparation.
- Titrate dose to response based on plasma-homocysteine concentrations. [2]

Intragastric administration

1. Stop the enteral feed.
2. Flush the enteral feeding tube with the recommended volume of water.
3. Draw the medication solution into an appropriate size and type of syringe.
4. Flush the medication dose down the feeding tube.
5. Finally, flush with the recommended volume of water.
6. Re-start the feed, unless a prolonged break is required.

Alternatively, at step (3) measure the medicine in a suitable container and then draw into an appropriate syringe. Ensure that the measure is rinsed and that this rinsing water is administered also to ensure that the total dose is given. **Do not** measure liquid medicines using a catheter-tipped syringe as this results in excessive dosing owing to the volume of the tip.

Intrajejunal administration

No specific data on administration via jejunostomy. Administer using the above method. Titrate dose to response.

References

1. Personal Communication, Special Products Ltd; 20 January 2003.
2. Sweetman SC, ed. *Martindale*, 34th edn. London: Pharmaceutical Press; 2005.

Betamethasone

Formulations available[1]

Brand name (Manufacturer)	Formulation and strength	Product information/Administration information
Betnelan (Celltech)	Tablet 500 microgram	Betamethasone PhEur.[2] No specific data on enteral tube administration are available for this formulation.
Betnesol (Celltech)	Soluble tablet 500 microgram	Betamethasone sodium phosphate equivalent to 500 microgram betamethasone.[3] Betnesol tablets dissolve completely in 10 mL of water to give a clear pink solution that flushes down an 8Fr NG tube without blockage.[5]
Betnesol (Celltech)	Injection 4 mg/mL	5.3 mg of betamethasone sodium phosphate equivalent to 4 mg betamethasone.[4] No specific data on enteral tube administration are available for this formulation.

Site of absorption (oral administration)

Betamethasone, like all steroids, is rapidly absorbed from the GI tract,[6] specific pharmacokinetics are not documented.[7]

Alternative routes available

The parenteral formulation can be given by i.v. injection or infusion or as a deep i.m. injection.[4]

Interactions

Should be taken after food.[1]

Health and safety

Standard precautions apply.

Suggestions/recommendations

- Use the dispersible tablets for administration via the feeding tubes.
- A prolonged break in feeding is not required.

Intragastric administration

1. Stop the enteral feed.
2. Flush the enteral feeding tube with the recommended volume of water.
3. Place the tablet in the barrel of an appropriate size and type of syringe.
4. Draw 10 mL of water into the syringe and allow the tablet to dissolve.
5. Flush the medication dose down the feeding tube.
6. Draw an equal volume of water into the syringe and also flush this via the feeding tube (this will rinse the syringe and ensure that the total dose is administered).
7. Finally, flush with the recommended volume of water.
8. Re-start the feed, unless a prolonged break is required.

Alternatively, at step (3) place the tablet into a medicine pot, add 10 mL of water and allow the tablet to dissolve. Draw this into an appropriate syringe. Ensure that the measure is rinsed and that this rinsing water is administered also to ensure that the total dose is given.

Intrajejunal administration

There are no specific data on the jejunal administration of betamethasone. Administer using the above method.

References

1. *BNF* 50, September 2005.
2. Betnelan Tablets, Summary of Product Characteristics; June 2005.
3. Betnesol Tablets, Summary of Product Characteristics; June 2005.
4. Betnesol Injection, Summary of Product Characteristics; June 2005.
5. BPNG data on file, 2004.
6. Personal communication, Celltech; 31 March 2003.
7. Sweetman SC, ed. *Martindale*, 34th edn. London: Pharmaceutical Press; 2005.

Bethanechol

Formulations available[1]

Brand name (Manufacturer)	Formulation and strength	Product information/Administration information
Myotonine (Greenwood)	Tablets 10 mg, 25 mg	Take half an hour before food.[2] Extemporaneous preparation can be made.[3] *Bethanechol suspension 5 mg/mL (60-day expiry):* Bethanechol 10 mg tablets 50 tablets Cherry syrup to 100 mL

Site of absorption (oral administration)

Therapeutic effect seen within 1 hour of oral administration.[2] Bethanechol is poorly absorbed from the GI tract.[4]

Alternative routes available

None available in the UK. An injection is licensed in the USA.[4]

Interactions

There is no documented interaction with food; however, bethanechol was discovered before pharmacokinetic studies were routinely completed and there are very few data on pharmacokinetics in general.[4]

Health and safety

Standard precautions apply.

Suggestions/recommendations

- Crush tablets and disperse in water immediately prior to administration.
- Alternatively, make an extemporaneous preparation.

Intragastric administration

1. Stop the enteral feed.
2. Flush the enteral feeding tube with the recommended volume of water.
3. Place the tablet in mortar and crush to a fine powder using the pestle.
4. Add a few millilitres of water and mix to form a paste.
5. Add up to 15 mL of water and mix thoroughly ensuring that there are no large particles of tablet.
6. Draw this into an appropriate size and type of syringe.
7. Flush the medication dose down the feeding tube.
8. Add another 15 mL of water to the mortar and stir to ensure that any remaining drug is rinsed from the container. Draw this water into the syringe and also flush this via the feeding tube (this will rinse the mortar and syringe and ensure total dose is administered).
9. Finally, flush the enteral feeding tube with the recommended volume of water.
10. Re-start the feed, unless a prolonged break is required.

Intrajejunal administration

There are no specific data relating to the jejunal administration of bethanechol. Administer using the above method. If using the extemporaneous suspension, dilute with an equal volume of water immediately prior to administration. Monitor for increased side-effects or loss of efficacy.

References

1. *BNF 50*, September 2005.
2. Myotonine (Glenwood), Summary of Product Characteristics; February 2000.
3. Allen LV, Erickson MA. Stability of bethanechol chloride, pyrazinamide, quinidine sulphate, rifampicin, and tetracycline hydrochloride in extemporaneously compounded oral liquids. *Am J Health Syst Pharm*. 1998; 55: 1804–1809.
4. Dollery C. *Therapeutic Drugs*, 2nd edn. London: Churchill Livingston; 1998.

Bexarotene

Formulations available[1]

Brand name (Manufacturer)	Formulation and strength	Product information/Administration information
Targretin (Zeneus)	Capsules 75 mg	Soft gelatin capsule. One of the ingredients inside the capsule is an irritant to the eyes, skin and mucous membranes and therefore the capsules must be swallowed whole and not chewed or broken open.[2]

Site of absorption (oral administration)

Specific site of absorption is unknown.

Alternative routes available

None.

Interactions

Although there are no documented interactions with food, absorption may be enhanced by food and all clinical trials were conducted in fed patients.[3]

Health and safety

Bexarotene is an antineoplastic drug and should be handled as a cytotoxic.

Suggestions/recommendations

- Do not attempt to withdraw contents from capsule.
- Seek specialist advice for alternative therapy.

References

1. *BNF* 50, September 2005.
2. Personal Communication, Elan Pharma Ltd; 16 January 2003.
3. Targretin Capsules (Zeneus), Summary of Product Characteristics; 14 June 2004.

Bezafibrate

Formulations available[1]

Brand name (Manufacturer)	Formulation and strength	Product information/Administration information
Bezalip (Roche)	Tablet 200 mg	Film-coated tablet.[2] The tablet swells and the coating splits when placed in 10 mL of water; this gives a coarse dispersion. The coating does not disperse and there is a high risk of tube blockage.[3]
Bezalip Mono (Roche)	M/R tablet 400 mg	Film-coated modified release tablet. Should not be crushed.[4] Not suitable for enteral tube administration.
Bezafibrate (Generics, PLIVA, Ratiopharm)	Tablet 200 mg	Ratiopharm brand tablets disperse in 10 mL of water if shaken for 5 minutes to form a coarse dispersion that may block fine-bore tubes but can be flushed through an 8Fr NG tube without blockage.[3]

Site of absorption (oral administration)

Specific site of absorption is not documented. Peak plasma concentration occurs 2 hours after oral administration.[2]

Alternative routes available

None.

Interactions

No specific documented interaction with food. Recommended to be taken after food.[2]

Health and safety

Standard precautions apply.

Suggestions/recommendations

- Bezafibrate requires three times a day dosing. Consider changing to a once daily fibrate or statin if clinically appropriate. See relevant monographs.
- If bezafibrate therapy is indicated, disperse the tablet in water and administer via the feeding tube; see notes above.

Intragastric administration

1. Stop the enteral feed.
2. Flush the enteral feeding tube with the recommended volume of water.
3. Place the tablet in the barrel of an appropriate size and type of syringe.
4. Draw 10 mL of water into the syringe and allow the tablet to disperse, shaking if necessary.
5. Flush the medication dose down the feeding tube.
6. Draw another 10 mL of water into the syringe and also flush this via the feeding tube (this will rinse the syringe and ensure that the total dose is administered).
7. Finally, flush with the recommended volume of water.
8. Re-start the feed, unless a prolonged break is required.

Alternatively, at step (4) place the tablet into a medicine pot, add 10 mL of water and allow the tablet to disperse. Draw this into an appropriate syringe. Ensure that the measure is rinsed and that this rinsing water is administered also to ensure that the total dose is given.

Intrajejunal administration

There are no specific data on jejunal administration. Administer using the above method. Monitor for increased side-effects or loss of efficacy.

References

1. *BNF* 50, September 2005.
2. Bezalip (Roche), Summary of Product Characteristics; 8 November 2005.
3. BPNG data on file 2005.
4. Bezalip Mono (Roche), Summary of Product Characteristics; 8 November 2005.

Bicalutamide

Formulations available[1]

Brand name (Manufacturer)	Formulation and strength	Product information/Administration information
Casodex (AstraZeneca)	Tablets 50 mg, 150 mg	Film-coated tablets. [2, 3] The tablets do not disperse even when agitated for more than 5 minutes in 10 mL of water; the tablets do crush and mix well with water to form a milky suspension. [4]

Site of absorption (oral administration)

Specific site of absorption unknown. Bicalutamide is well absorbed following oral administration. [2]

Alternative routes available

None available for bicalutamide. Other antiandrogens such as buserelin, goserelin, leuprorelin and triptorelin are available as injections or implants. [1]

Interactions

There is no evidence of any clinically relevant effect of food on bioavailability. [2]

Health and safety

Protective clothing should be worn when crushing bicalutamide tablets to minimise exposure to dry powder and reduce risk of inhalation. Bicalutamide is a potent anti-androgen. Tablets should not be crushed and handled by pregnant women.

Suggestions/recommendations

- Where possible change to different drug, available in an injectable/implantable formulation. If this is not possible and continuation of bicalutamide therapy is considered appropriate, the tablets should be crushed and mixed with water using a closed system where possible (e.g. crushing syringe).
- A prolonged break in the enteral feeding regimen is not necessary.

Intragastric administration

1. Stop the enteral feed.
2. Flush the enteral feeding tube with the recommended volume of water.
3. Place the tablet in a mortar and crush to a fine powder using the pestle; wear protective clothing and avoid inhalation.
4. Add a few millilitres of water and mix to form a paste.
5. Add up to 15 mL of water and mix thoroughly, ensuring that there are no large particles of tablet.
6. Draw this into an appropriate size and type of syringe.
7. Flush the medication dose down the feeding tube.
8. Add another 15 mL of water to the mortar and stir to ensure that any remaining drug is rinsed from the container. Draw this water into the syringe and also flush this via the feeding tube (this will rinse the mortar and syringe and ensure total dose is administered).
9. Finally, flush the enteral feeding tube with the recommended volume of water.
10. Re-start the feed, unless a prolonged break in feeding is required.

Intrajejunal administration

There are no specific data relating to the jejunal administration of bicalutamide. Administer using the above method. Monitor for increased side-effects or loss of efficacy.

References

1. *BNF* 50, September 2005.
2. Casodex Tablets 50 mg, Summary of Product Characteristics; 27 January 2004.
3. Casodex Tablets 150 mg, Summary of Product Characteristics; 5 December 2005.
4. BPNG data on file, 2004.

Bisacodyl

Formulations available[1]

Brand name (Manufacturer)	Formulation and strength	Product information/Administration information
Dulco-lax (Boehringer Ingelheim)	Enteric coated tablets 5 mg	Enteric coated tablets, do not crush.[2] The tablets are designed so that minimal drug is released in the small bowel; the active form is released in the colon by bacterial cleavage.[2]
Dulco-lax (Boehringer Ingelheim)	Suppositories 10 mg	For rectal administration only.
Dulco-lax (Boehringer Ingelheim)	Paediatric suppositories 5 mg	For rectal administration only.

Site of absorption (oral administration)

There is minimal systemic absorption. Bisacodyl exerts a topical effect in the colon.[3]

Alternative routes available

Rectal route.

Interactions

Not applicable.

Health and safety

Standard precautions apply.

Suggestions/recommendations

- Use the suppositories, 10 mg, in the morning.
- If not appropriate consider changing to docusate sodium liquid preparation (see monograph).

References

1. *BNF* 50, September 2005.
2. Dulco-lax Tablets 5 mg, Summary of Product Characteristics; March 2005.
3. Dulco-lax Suppositories, Summary of Product Characteristics; October 2003.

Bisoprolol fumarate

Formulations available[1]

Brand name (Manufacturer)	Formulation and strength	Product information/Administration information
Cardicor (Merck)	Tablets 1.25 mg, 2.5 mg, 3.75 mg, 5 mg, 7.5 mg, 10 mg	Film-coated tablet. PIL states do not crush or chew tablets.[2] Cardicor tablets are film-coated and scored but can be crushed if necessary.[3] Tablets disintegrate rapidly in 10 mL of water to form a fine suspension that flushes down an 8Fr NG tube without blockage.[5]
Emcor (Merck)	Tablets 5 mg, 10 mg	Film-coated tablet. Emcor tablets are film-coated and scored but can be crushed if necessary.[3]
Monocor (Lederle)	Tablets 5 mg, 10 mg	Film-coated tablet Tablet disperses rapidly in 10 mL of water to give fine white dispersion that settles quickly but flushes via 8Fr NG tube without blockage.[5]
Bisoprolol (Alpharma, APS, Ashbourne, Generics, Goldshield, Lexon, Niche, PLIVA)	Tablets 5 mg, 10 mg	APS brand tablets do not disperse readily in water but will disperse if shaken in 10 mL of water for 5 minutes, the resulting dispersion flushes via 8Fr NG tube without blockage.[5]

Site of absorption (oral administration)

Specific site of absorption is not documented. Peak plasma concentration occurs 3 hours after oral dosing.[4]

Alternative routes available

None for bisoprolol, other beta-blockers available in parenteral formulation are labetalol, metoprolol, propranolol and atenolol.

Interactions

Absorption is unaffected by food intake.[4]

Health and safety

Standard precautions apply.

Suggestions/recommendations

- Disperse tablets in water (preferably Merck or Lederle brand) immediately prior to administration.
- A prolonged break in feeding is not required.

Intragastric administration

1. Stop the enteral feed.
2. Flush the enteral feeding tube with the recommended volume of water.
3. Place the tablet in the barrel of an appropriate size and type of syringe.
4. Draw 10 mL of water into the syringe and allow the tablet to disperse, shaking if necessary.
5. Flush the medication dose down the feeding tube.
6. Draw another 10 mL of water into the syringe and also flush this via the feeding tube (this will rinse the syringe and ensure that the total dose is administered).
7. Finally, flush with the recommended volume of water.
8. Re-start the feed, unless a prolonged break is required.

Alternatively, at step (3) place the tablet into a medicine pot, add 10 mL of water and allow the tablet to disperse. Draw this into an appropriate syringe. Ensure that the measure is rinsed and that this rinsing water is administered also to ensure that the total dose is given.

Intrajejunal administration

There are no specific data relating to the jejunal administration of bisoprolol. Administer using the above method. Monitor for increased side-effects or loss of efficacy.

References

1. *BNF* 50, September 2005.
2. Patient Information Leaflet, Cardicor, September 1999.
3. Personal communication, Merck Pharmaceuticals Ltd; 23 January 2003.
4. Dollery C. *Therapeutic Drugs*, 2nd edn. London: Churchill Livingstone; 1998.
5. BPNG data on file 2004/05.

Bromocriptine mesilate

Formulations available[1]

Brand name (Manufacturer)	Formulation and strength	Product information/Administration information
Parlodel (Novartis)	Tablets 1 mg, 2.5 mg	Scored tablets No specific data on enteral tube administration are available for this formulation.
Parlodel (Novartis)	Capsules 5 mg, 10 mg	Hard gelatin capsules Capsules open easily, contents pour freely. Contents mix with water when powder is wetted; powder forms a fine dispersion that flushes easily via 8Fr NG tube without blockage.[2]
Bromocriptine (non-proprietary)	Tablets 2.5 mg	No specific data on enteral tube administration are available for this formulation.

Site of absorption (oral administration)

Specific site of absorption is not documented. Peak plasma concentration occurs 1–3 hours post dose.[3, 4]

Alternative routes available

None.

Interactions

Bromocriptine should be taken after food to minimise the rapid onset of adverse effects such as nausea, vomiting and postural hypotension.[5]

Health and safety

Standard precautions apply.

Suggestions/recommendations

- Disperse tablets in water or open capsules and disperse contents in water immediately prior to administration.
- Administer after feed.

Intragastric administration

Capsule administration

1. Stop the enteral feed.
2. Flush the enteral feeding tube with the recommended volume of water.
3. Avoid a prolonged break in feeding.
4. Open the capsule and pour the contents into a medicine pot.
5. Add 15 mL of water.
6. Stir to disperse the powder.
7. Draw into an appropriate size and type of syringe and administer via the feeding tube.
8. Add a further 15 mL of water to the medicine pot; stir to ensure that any powder remaining in the pot is mixed with water.
9. Draw up this dispersion and flush down the tube. This will ensure that the whole dose is given.
10. Flush the tube with water.
11. Restart the feed.

Tablet administration

1. Stop the enteral feed.
2. Flush the enteral feeding tube with the recommended volume of water.
3. Avoid a prolonged break in feeding.
4. Place the tablet in the barrel of an appropriate size and type of syringe.
5. Draw 10 mL of water into the syringe and allow the tablet to disperse, shaking if necessary.
6. Flush the medication dose down the feeding tube.
7. Draw another 10 mL of water into the syringe and also flush this via the feeding tube (this will rinse the syringe and ensure that the total dose is administered).
8. Finally, flush with the recommended volume of water.
9. Re-start the feed, unless a prolonged break is required.

Alternatively, at step (4) place the tablet into a medicine pot, add 10 mL of water and allow the tablet to disperse. Draw this into an appropriate syringe. Ensure that the measure is rinsed and that this rinsing water is administered also to ensure that the total dose is given.

Intrajejunal administration

There are no specific data relating to jejunal administration of bromocriptine. It is possible that absorption will be faster if the drug is delivered directly into the small bowel. Administer as above. Monitor for increased side-effects.

References

1. *BNF 50*, September 2005.
2. BPNG data on file 2005.
3. Parlodel Tablets, Summary of Product Characteristics; July 2004.
4. Parlodel Capsules, Summary of Product Characteristics; July 2004.
5. Dollery C. *Therapeutic Drugs*, 2nd edn. London: Churchill Livingstone; 1998.

Budesonide

Formulations available[1]

Brand name (Manufacturer)	Formulation and strength	Product information/Administration information
Budenofalk (Provalis)	Capsule 3 mg	Hard gelatin capsule containing enteric coated granules.[2] 'The capsules can be opened as long as the granules are not chewed or damaged. It may be difficult to try and wash the granules down an enteral feeding tube, as they may stick to the sides.'[4]
Entocort (AstraZeneca)	CR capsules 3 mg	Hard gelatin capsule containing enteric coated, modified release granules.[3] No specific data on enteral administration are available for this formulation.
Entocort (AstraZeneca)	Enema 2 mg/100 mL	Not appropriate for enteral administration.

Site of absorption (oral administration)

Budenofalk capsules, owing to their enteric coating, release the drug in the terminal ileum and caecum, giving a peak plasma concentration at 5 hours.[2] The peak plasma concentration of budesonide occurs at 3–5 hours post dose for Entocort capsules.[3]

Alternative routes available

Topical therapy using enema is licensed for colitis only.[1]

Interactions

Budenofalk and Entocort preparations are advised to be taken before food to reduce the effect on the coating of the enclosed granules and ensure delivery of drug to the desired area of the intestine.

Health and safety

Standard precautions apply.

Suggestions/recommendations

- Both Budenofalk and Entocort are formulated to release budesonide in the terminal ileum and ascending colon for the topical treatment of disease in this area. Alteration of this formulation will cause the drug to be released elsewhere and absorbed systemically.
- Patients should be converted to a therapeutically equivalent dose of prednisolone and the soluble tablets used (see prednisolone monograph).

References

1. *BNF* 50, September 2005.
2. Budenofalk 3 mg, Summary of Product Characteristics; April 2004.
3. Entocort 3 mg CR capsules, Summary of Product Characteristics; September 2004.
4. Personal Communication, Provalis Healthcare; 5 February 2003

Bumetanide

Formulations available

Brand name (Manufacturer)	Formulation and strength	Product information/Administration information
Bumetanide (Leo)	Liquid 1 mg/5 mL	Contains sorbitol.[2]
Bumetanide (Leo)	Injection 500 microgram/mL 4 mL ampoule	Can be given by i.v. or i.m. injection or i.v. infusion. Can be administered orally or enterally.[5]
Bumetanide (Alpharma, APS, CP, Generics, Hillcross, IVAX, Norton)	Tablets 1 mg, 5 mg	APS brand 1 mg tablet disperses in 10 mL of water when agitated for 5 minutes to give a fine dispersion that flushes down an 8Fr NG tube without blockage.[3] Norton brand 1 mg disperses in 10 mL of water when agitated for 5 minutes to give a fine dispersion that flushes down an 8Fr NG tube without blockage.[3] Alpharma brand: 'Tablets can be crushed.'[4]
Burinex (Leo)	Tablets 1 mg, 5 mg	Film-coated tablets, Leo do not recommend crushing tablets as a liquid preparation is available.[5]

Site of absorption (oral administration)

Specific site of absorption is not documented. Peak plasma concentration occurs between 0.5 and 2.2 hours following oral dosing.[6]

Alternative routes available

Parenteral route is available.

Interactions

Bioavailability is unaffected by food.[6]

Health and safety

Standard precautions apply.

Suggestions/recommendations

- Use a liquid preparation.
- A prolonged break in feeding is not required.

Intragastric administration

1. Stop the enteral feed.
2. Flush the enteral feeding tube with the recommended volume of water.
3. Draw the medication suspension into an appropriate size and type of syringe.
4. Flush the medication dose down the feeding tube.
5. Finally, flush with the recommended volume of water.
6. Re-start the feed, unless a prolonged break is required.

Alternatively, at step (3) measure the medicine in a suitable container. Draw this into an appropriate syringe. Ensure that the measure is rinsed and that this rinsing water is administered also to ensure that the total dose is given. **Do not** measure liquid medicines using a catheter-tipped syringe as this results in excessive dosing owing to the volume of the tip.

Intrajejunal administration

No specific information is available relating to jejunal administration of bumetanide. Administer using the above method. Consider dilution of the liquid formulation immediately prior to administration to reduce osmolarity. Monitor for side-effects or loss of efficacy.

References

1. *BNF* 50, September 2005.
2. Bumetanide liquid 0.2 mg/mL oral solution (Leo), Summary of Product Characteristics; January 2004.
3. BPNG data on file 2004.
4. Personal communication, Alpharma Ltd; 21 January 2003.
5. Personal communication, Leo Pharmaceuticals; 7 February 2003.
6. Dollery C. *Therapeutic Drugs*, 2nd edn. London: Churchill Livingstone; 1998.

Busulfan

Formulations available[1]

Brand name (Manufacturer)	Formulation and strength	Product information/Administration information
Myleran (GSK)	Film-coated tablet 2 mg	Cytotoxic – film coating protects the handler from exposure. GSK recommends that tablets should not be crushed or broken.[2] Extemporaneous preparation can be made: *Busulfan suspension 2 mg/mL:* Busulfan 2 mg tablets 30 tablets Simple syrup to 30 mL Expiry 30 days, stored in a refrigerator.[3] Any cytotoxic extemporaneous preparation should be made in facilities with suitable containment equipment.
Busulfan (Nova Labs)	Suspension 5–20 mg/5 mL	Manufactured 'special'. Eight-day expiry. Viscosity is suitable for administration via feeding tube.[4]

Formulations available[1] (continued)

Brand name (Manufacturer)	Formulation and strength	Product information/Administration information
Busilvex (Fabre)	Concentrate for infusion 6 mg/mL 10 mL vial	No specific data on enteral tube administration are available for this formulation.

Site of absorption (oral administration)

Specific site of absorption is not documented.[5]

Alternative routes available

Parenteral route available.

Interactions

No specific interaction with food are documented.[5]

Health and safety

Cytotoxic. Protective clothing should be worn. Dispose of contaminated disposable equipment as cytotoxic waste.

Suggestions/recommendations

- Use the manufactured special suspension when possible or prepare the extemporaneous suspension if suitable containment facilities are available.
- A prolonged break in feeding is not required.

Intragastric administration

1. Stop the enteral feed.
2. Flush the enteral feeding tube with the recommended volume of water.
3. Shake the medication bottle thoroughly to ensure adequate mixing.
4. Draw the medication suspension into an appropriate size and type of syringe.
5. Flush the medication dose down the feeding tube.
6. Finally, flush with the recommended volume of water.
7. Re-start the feed, unless a prolonged break is required.

Alternatively, at step (4) measure the medicine in a suitable container. Draw this into an appropriate syringe. Ensure that the measure is rinsed and that this rinsing water is administered also to ensure that the total dose is given. **Do not** measure liquid medicines using a catheter-tipped syringe as this results in excessive dosing owing to the volume of the tip.

Intrajejunal administration

There are no specific data relating to jejunal administration of busulfan. Seek specialist advice regarding alternative therapy. Administer using the above method. Monitor for loss of efficacy.

References

1. *BNF 50*, September 2005.
2. Personal Communication, GSK; 22 January 2003.
3. Allen LV. Busulfan oral suspension. *US Pharmacist*. 1990; 15: 94–95.
4. Personal communication, Nova Labs; 24 March 2005.
5. Dollery C. *Therapeutic Drugs*, 2nd edn. London: Churchill Livingstone; 1998.

Cabergoline

Formulations available[1]

Brand name (Manufacturer)	Formulation and strength	Product information/Administration information
Cabaser (Pharmacia)	Tablets 1 mg, 2 mg, 4 mg	Tablets can be crushed and mixed with tap water to prepare an oral solution.[2] Data available indicate that bioavailability is unaffected by formulation as a solution.[3] Tablets do not disperse readily in water, but will disperse completely to give a clear solution if shaken in 10 mL of water for 5 minutes, this solution flushes via an 8Fr NG tube without blockage.[4]

Site of absorption (oral administration)

Specific site of absorption is not documented. Peak plasma concentrations occur 0.5–4 hours post oral dosing.[5]

Alternative routes available

No alternative route is available for cabergoline. Selegiline is available as oral lyophilisate tablets, Zelapar (Athena).

Interactions

Food does not appear to affect absorption and disposition of cabergoline;[5] however, taking it with food improves tolerability.[6]

Health and safety

Standard precautions apply.

Suggestions/recommendations

- Disperse tablets in water immediately prior to dosing.
- Administer after feed.

Intragastric administration

1. Stop the enteral feed.
2. Flush the enteral feeding tube with the recommended volume of water.
3. Place the tablet in the barrel of an appropriate size and type of syringe.
4. Draw 10 mL of water into the syringe and allow the tablet to dissolve, shaking if necessary.
5. Flush the medication dose down the feeding tube.
6. Draw another 10 mL of water into the syringe and also flush this via the feeding tube (this will rinse the syringe and ensure that the total dose is administered).
7. Finally, flush with the recommended volume of water.
8. Re-start the feed, unless a prolonged break is required.

Intrajejunal administration

There are no specific data relating to jejunal administration of cabergoline. Administer using the above method. Monitor for increased side-effects or loss of efficacy.

References

1. *BNF* 50, September 2005.
2. Personal Communication, Pharmacia Ltd; 11 March 2003.
3. Persiani S, Sassolas G, Piscitelli G, *et al.* Pharmacodynamics and relative bioavailability of cabergoline tablets vs solution in healthy volunteers. *J Pharm Sci.* 1994; 83(10): 1421–1424.
4. BPNG data on file, 2005.
5. Cabaser Tablets 1 mg (Pharmacia), Summary of Product Characteristics; January 2005.
6. Dollery C. Therapeutic Drugs, 2nd edn. London: Churchill Livingstone; 1998.

Calcium folinate (Leucovorin)

Formulations available[1]

Brand name (Manufacturer)	Formulation and strength	Product information/Administration information
Calcium folinate (APS, Goldshield, Hillcross, Mayne, Pharmacia)	Tablets 15 mg	APS brand tablets will disperse in 10 mL of water within 5 minutes to give a fine white dispersion that flushes easily via an 8Fr NG tube without blockage.[2]
Folinic acid (CP, Lederle, Mayne, Pharmacia)	Injection 3 mg/mL, 7.5 mg/mL, 10 mg/mL	Pharmacia and Mayne brands of injection can be administered orally.[3, 4] (As calcium salt.)
Folinic acid (Goldshield)	Powder for reconstitution For injection 15 mg, 30 mg	No specific data on enteral tube administration are available for this formulation. (As calcium salt.)

Site of absorption (oral administration)

Specific site of absorption is not documented. Folinic acid is well absorbed following oral administration;[5] peak plasma concentration of folate occurs 1 hour following an oral dose.[6]

Alternative routes available

Injection can be given parenterally and orally.[3, 4]

Interactions

No specific interactions with food affecting the absorption of folinic acid are documented. However, many drugs owe their pharmacological activity or side-effect profile to their inhibition of dihydrofolate reductase; folinic acid is used to treat these side-effects or as rescue therapy, for example in chemotherapy regimens containing methotrexate. Folic acid is ineffective in these instances.[7]

Health and safety

Standard precautions apply.

Suggestions/recommendations

- Disperse tablets in water immediately prior to dosing.
- A prolonged break in feeding is not required.

Intragastric administration

1. Stop the enteral feed.
2. Flush the enteral feeding tube with the recommended volume of water.
3. Place the tablet in the barrel of an appropriate size and type of syringe.
4. Draw 10 mL of water into the syringe and allow the tablet to disperse, shaking if necessary.
5. Flush the medication dose down the feeding tube.
6. Draw another 10 mL of water into the syringe and also flush this via the feeding tube (this will rinse the syringe and ensure that the total dose is administered).
7. Finally, flush with the recommended volume of water.
8. Re-start the feed, unless a prolonged break is required.

Alternatively, at step (3) place the tablet into a medicine pot, add 10 mL of water and allow the tablet to disperse. Draw this into an appropriate syringe. Ensure that the measure is rinsed and that this rinsing water is administered also to ensure that the total dose is given.

Intrajejunal administration

Administer using the above method.

References

1. *BNF 50*, September 2005.
2. BPNG data on file, 2004.
3. Personal Communication, Pharmacia Ltd; 11 March 2003.
4. Personal communication, Mayne Pharma plc; 29 January 2003.
5. Sweetman SC, ed. *Martindale*, 34th edn. London: Pharmaceutical Press; 2005.
6. Calcium leucovorin tablets (Wyeth), Summary of Product Characteristics; March 2004.
7. White R, Ashworth A. How drug therapy can affect, threaten and compromise nutritional status. *J Hum Nutr Diet.* 2000; 13: 119–129.

Calcium resonium (Polystyrene sulphonate resins)

Formulations available[1]

Brand name (Manufacturer)	Formulation and strength	Product information/Administration information
Calcium Resonium (Sanofi-Synthelabo)	Powder Calcium polystyrene sulphonate	Oral adult dose 15 g three times daily. Rectal adult dose 30 g.[2]
Resonium A (Sanofi-Synthelabo)	Powder Sodium polystyrene sulphonate	No specific data on enteral tube administration are available for this formulation.

Site of absorption (oral administration)

These products are ion exchange resins and are not absorbed.[2]

Alternative routes available

Use the rectal route.

Interactions

Designed to reduce intestinal absorption of potassium; no other documented interaction with food.

Health and safety

Standard precautions apply.

Suggestions/recommendations

- When mixed with water, the resulting pastes are too thick to administer via a feeding tube.
- The rectal route should be used.

References

1. *BNF 50*, September 2005.
2. Calcium Resonium (Sanofi-Synthelabo), Summary of Product Characteristics; February 2005.

Calcium salts

Formulations available[1]

Brand name (Manufacturer)	Formulation and strength	Product information/Administration information
Calcium carbonate Cacit (Procter & Gamble)	Effervescent tablets 1.25 g	Providing 500 mg (12.6 mmol) as calcium citrate Tablet effervesces and dissolves in 10 mL of water. Flushes down an 8Fr NG tube without blockage.[3] This must be allowed to dissolve completely before administration but should not be stored as a solution once dissolved.[4]
Adcal (Straken)	Chewable tablet 1.5 g	Providing 600 mg calcium carbonate. No specific data on enteral tube administration are available for this formulation.
Calcichew (Shire)	Chewable tablet 1.25 g	Providing 500 mg (12.6 mmol) as calcium carbonate.
Calcichew Forte (Shire)	Chewable tablet 2.5 g	Providing 1 g (25 mmol) as calcium carbonate. Can crush tablets and dissolve in water.[6]
Calcium chloride Calcium chloride (Aurum, Celltech)	Injection 10% 0.68 mmol/mL	No specific data on enteral tube administration are available for this formulation.

Formulations available[1] (continued)

Brand name (Manufacturer)	Formulation and strength	Product information/Administration information
Calcium glubionate Calcium-Sandoz (Alliance)	Calcium glubionate 1.09 g and calcium lactobionate USP 0.727 g per 5 mL	1.85 mL Calcium-Sandoz syrup = 1 mmol calcium. The manufacturer has no data to support the administration of Calcium-Sandoz syrup via a PEG or NG tube.[2] pH = 6.7, Osmolarity = 2130 mosmol/kg.[2]
Calcium gluconate Calcium gluconate tablets 600 mg (Alpharma)	Tablets 600 mg	Contains 53.4 mg (1.35 mmol calcium)
Effervescent tablets 1 g (Alpharma)	Effervescent tablets 1 g	Contains 89 mg calcium (2.25 mmol), also contains 4.46 mmol sodium. Can be administered via a feeding tube, once dissolved.[5]
Injection (Phoenix)	Injection 10% 0.22 mmol/mL	
Calcium lactate Calcium lactate tablets (Alpharma)	300 mg	Tablets can be crushed.[5] Contain 1 mmol calcium
Sandocal-400 (Novartis)	400 mg	Effervescent tablets. Contain 10 mmol calcium
Sandocal-1000 (Novartis)	1000 mg	Effervescent tablets. Contain 25 mmol calcium

Site of absorption (oral administration)

Calcium salts are absorbed in the jejunum.

Alternative routes available

The parenteral route can be used in acute deficiency states, in medical emergencies or when GI absorption is compromised.

Interactions

Calcium may bind to phosphate in the enteral feed.

Health and safety

Standard precautions apply.

Suggestions/recommendations

- Use effervescent tablets dissolved in 30–50 mL of water.
- A prolonged break in feeding is not required, but the tube should be adequately flushed to ensure that the calcium supplement does not come into contact with the feed.

Intragastric administration

Effervescent tablets

1. Stop the enteral feed.
2. Flush the enteral feeding tube with the recommended volume of water.
3. Measure 30–50 mL of water into a measuring pot.
4. Add the effervescent tablet and allow to dissolve.
5. Draw into an appropriate size and type of syringe.
6. Flush the medication dose down the feeding tube.
7. Rinse the measure and administer this also to ensure that the total dose is given.
8. Finally, flush with the recommended volume of water.
9. Re-start the feed, unless a prolonged break is required.

Liquid formulation

1. Stop the enteral feed.
2. Flush the enteral feeding tube with the recommended volume of water.
3. Draw the medication liquid into an appropriate size and type of syringe.
4. Flush the medication dose down the feeding tube.
5. Finally, flush with the recommended volume of water.
6. Re-start the feed, unless a prolonged break is required.

Alternatively, at step (3) measure the medicine in a suitable container. Draw this into an appropriate syringe. Ensure that the measure is rinsed and that this rinsing water is administered also to ensure that the total dose is given. **Do not** measure liquid medicines using a catheter-tipped syringe as this results in excessive dosing owing to the volume of the tip.

Intrajejunal administration

Calcium salts are absorbed in the jejunum. Jejunal administration of the above products should not affect the bioavailability. Effervescent tablets are the preferred formulation for this route owing to the lower osmolarity.

References

1. *BNF* 50, September 2005.
2. Personal communication, Alliance Pharmaceuticals Ltd; January 2003.
3. BPNG data on file, 2004.
4. Personal communication, Procter & Gamble Pharmaceuticals; 22 January 2003.
5. Personal communication, Alpharma Ltd; 21 January 2003.
6. Personal communication, Shire Pharmaceuticals; 17 February 2003.

Calcium salts with vitamin D

Formulations available[1]

Brand name (Manufacturer)	Formulation and strength	Product information/Administration information
Adcal D3 (Strakan)	Chewable tablet 600 mg/400 IU	No specific data on enteral tube administration are available for this formulation.

Formulations available[1] (continued)

Brand name (Manufacturer)	Formulation and strength	Product information/Administration information
Cacit D3 (Procter & Gamble)	Effervescent granules	Possible to administer via an enteral feeding tube.[2] 4 g sachet provides 500 mg calcium, 440 IU cholecalciferol, also contains 0.22 mmol sodium.[5]
Calceos (Provalis)	Chewable tablet 500 mg/400 IU	No specific data on enteral tube administration are available for this formulation.
Calcichew D3 (Shire)	Chewable tablet 500 mg/200 IU	Tablets disperse in 10 mL water if agitated for 2 minutes.[6]
Calcichew D3 Forte (Shire)	Chewable tablet 500 mg/400 IU	Tablets can be crushed and dispersed in water.[4] Tablets disperse in 10 mL water if agitated for 5 minutes.[6]
Calcium and ergocalciferol (Alpharma)	Tablet 300 mg/400 IU	Tablets can be crushed.[3] 300 mg calcium lactate = 2.4 mmol calcium.

Site of absorption (oral administration)

Calcium salts are absorbed in the jejunum.

Alternative routes available

The parenteral route can be used in acute deficiency states, in medical emergencies or when GI absorption is compromised.

Interactions

Calcium will potentially bind to phosphate in the feed.[5]

Health and safety

Standard precautions apply.

Suggestions/recommendations

- Use the effervescent granules; dissolve in 30–50 mL of water.
- A prolonged break in feeding is not required.

Intragastric administration

1. Stop the enteral feed.
2. Flush the enteral feeding tube with the recommended volume of water.
3. Measure 30–50 mL of water into a measuring pot.
4. Add the granules and allow to dissolve.
5. Draw into an appropriate size and type of syringe.
6. Flush the medication dose down the feeding tube.
7. Rinse the measure and administer this also to ensure that the total dose is given.
8. Finally, flush with the recommended volume of water.
9. Re-start the feed, unless a prolonged break is required.

Intrajejunal administration

Calcium salts and vitamin D are absorbed in the small bowel; therefore jejunal administration is not expected to affect bioavailability. Administer using the above method.

References

1. *BNF 50*, September 2005.
2. Personal communication, Procter & Gamble Pharmaceuticals; 22 January 2003.
3. Personal communication, Alpharma Ltd; 21 January 2003.
4. Personal communication, Shire Pharmaceuticals; 17 February 2003.
5. Cacit D3 (Procter & Gamble), Summary of Product Characteristics; October 2002.
6. BPNG data on file, 2004.

Candesartan cilexetil

Formulations available[1]

Brand name (Manufacturer)	Formulation and strength	Product information/Administration information
Amias (Takeda)	Tablets 2 mg, 4 mg, 8 mg, 16 mg, 32 mg	16 mg tablets (other strengths not tested) do not disperse readily in water but crush easily and mix well with water to form fine suspension that flushes down an 8Fr NG tube without blockage.[3]

Site of absorption (oral administration)

Specific site of absorption is not documented. Peak plasma concentration is reached 3–4 hours after oral dosing.[2]

Alternative routes available

No other routes of administration are available for any of the angiotensin II receptor antagonists.

Interactions

The bioavailability of candesartan is not significantly affected by food.[2]

Health and safety

Standard precautions apply.

Suggestions/recommendations

- As tablets do not readily disperse, consider changing to irbesartan (see monograph).
- A prolonged break in feeding in not required.

References

1. *BNF 50*, September 2005.
2. Amias (Takeda), Summary of Product Characteristics; December 2004.
3. BPNG data on file, 2004

Captopril

Formulations available[1]

Brand name (Manufacturer)	Formulation and strength	Product information/Administration information
Capoten (Squibb)	Tablets 12.5 mg, 25 mg, 50 mg	Captopril is freely soluble in cold water (160 mg/mL).[2, 3] Tablets disperse in 10 mL of water within 2 minutes to give a fine dispersion that draws into a syringe easily and flushes down an 8Fr NG tube without blockage.[4]
Captopril (Alpharma)	Tablets 12.5 mg, 25 mg, 50 mg	Tablets can be crushed.[5]
Kaplon (Berk)	Tablets 12.5 mg, 25 mg, 50 mg	No specific data on enteral tube administration are available for this formulation.
Captopril (CP, Generics, Hillcross, Sandoz, Sovereign, Sterwin)	Tablets 12.5 mg, 25 mg, 50 mg	No specific data on enteral tube administration are available for this formulation.
Ecopace (Goldshield)	Tablets 12.5 mg, 25 mg, 50 mg	No specific data on enteral tube administration are available for this formulation.
Tensopril (IVAX)	Tablets 12.5 mg, 25 mg, 50 mg	No specific data on enteral tube administration are available for this formulation.
Captopril (Tillomed)	Tablets 12.5 mg, 25 mg, 50 mg	Disintegrates in 10 mL of water within 2 minutes, to give small particles. These tend to stick to the syringe, and one has to flush the syringe well to give the full dose, but do not block an 8Fr NG tube.[3]
Captopril unlicensed special (Martindale)	Suspension 5 mg/5 mL	Clear slightly viscous liquid. Some resistance on flushing. Nonaqueous suspension does not mix with water.[4]
Captopril extemporaneous preparation	Suspension	*Extemporaneous captopril solution 1 mg/mL:* Captopril 12.5 mg tablet 8 tablets Sodium ascorbate injection 500 mg Sterile water for irrigation to 100 mL Refrigerate; 56 days' stability.[7]

Site of absorption (oral administration)

Captopril is absorbed in the proximal small bowel.[2] Peak plasma concentrations are reached within 60–90 minutes.[5]

Alternative routes available

None available.

Interactions

The presence of food in the GI tract reduces absorption by 30–40%;[5] however, there is no recommendation to take before food.[6]

Health and safety

Standard precautions apply.

Suggestions/recommendations

- Captopril tablets can be dispersed in water immediately prior to dosing – a prolonged break in feed is not required – or alternatively the liquid preparation can be used.
- However, it may be more convenient to change to a once-daily dosed ACE inhibitor available as a liquid preparation, e.g. lisinopril (see monograph).

Intragastric administration

1. Stop the enteral feed.
2. Flush the enteral feeding tube with the recommended volume of water.
3. Place the tablet in the barrel of an appropriate size and type of syringe.
4. Draw 10 mL of water into the syringe and allow the tablet to disperse, shaking if necessary.
5. Flush the medication dose down the feeding tube.
6. Draw another 10 mL of water into the oral syringe and also flush this via the feeding tube (this will rinse the syringe and ensure that the total dose is administered).
7. Finally, flush with the recommended volume of water.
8. Re-start the feed, unless a prolonged break is required.

Alternatively, at step (3) place the tablet into a medicine pot, add 10 mL of water and allow the tablet to disperse. Draw this into an appropriate syringe. Ensure that the measure is rinsed and that this rinsing water is administered also to ensure that the total dose is given.

Intrajejunal administration

There is no specific information on jejunal administration of captopril. Administer using the above method. Monitor for loss of efficacy or increased side-effects.

References

1. *BNF 50*, September 2005.
2. Personal communication, Bristol-Myers Squibb; 24 January 2004.
3. Dollery C. *Therapeutic Drugs*, 2nd edn. London: Churchill Livingstone; 1998.
4. BPNG data on file, 2004/5.
5. Personal communication, Alpharma Ltd; 21 January 2004.
6. Capoten (Squibb), Summary of Product Characteristics; June 2005.
7. Nahata M, Morosco R, Hipple T. Stability of captopril in three liquid dosage forms. *Am J Hosp Pharm*. 1994; 51: 95–96.

Carbamazepine

Formulations available[1]

Brand name (Manufacturer)	Formulation and strength	Product information/Administration information
Tegretol (Cephalon)	Tablets 100 mg, 200 mg, 400 mg	Tablets disintegrate rapidly when placed in 10 mL of water to give a coarse dispersion; this draws up easily into a syringe but the risk of blocking a fine-bore tube is high unless care is taken to keep the granules suspended.[2]
Tegretol (Cephalon)	Chewtabs 100 mg, 200 mg	No specific data on enteral tube administration are available for this formulation.
Tegretol (Cephalon)	Liquid 100 mg/5 ml	Sugar-free liquid Contains sorbitol,[3] 1.25 g/5 mL dose.[6] There are data to suggest that the liquid preparation may adsorb onto the tube and reduce the dose administered. Diluting with an equal volume of water immediately prior to administration appears to prevent this.[5]
Tegretol (Cephalon)	Suppositories 125 mg, 250 mg	Rectal administration only. Licensed for short-term use (7 days). 125 mg suppository is equivalent to 100 mg tablets.[1]
Tegretol Retard (Cephalon)	M/R tablets 200 mg, 400 mg	Modified-release preparation – do not crush. Convert to the liquid preparation. Divide the total daily dose by 4 to give the liquid dose, e.g. 400 mg b.d. M/R tablets = 200 mg q.d.s. liquid
Carbamazepine (Alpharma, APS, Generics, Hillcross, IVAX)	Tablets 100 mg, 200 mg, 400 mg	No specific data on enteral tube administration are available for this formulation.
Teril Retard (Taro)	M/R tablets 200 mg, 400 mg	Modified-release preparation – do not crush. See notes above for Tegretol Retard.
Timonil Retard (CP)	M/R tablets 200 mg, 400 mg	Modified-release preparation – do not crush. See notes above for Tegretol Retard.
Carbagen (Generics)	M/R tablets 200 mg, 400 mg	Modified-release preparation – do not crush. See notes above for Tegretol Retard.

Site of absorption (oral administration)

Specific site is not documented; however, peak plasma concentration occurs up to 12 hours post oral dose with the tablet formulation; the liquid formulation produces higher and earlier peak plasma concentrations[7] which may be associated with an increase in side-effects.[3]

Alternative routes available

Suppositories are available (see notes above).

Interactions

Food has no significant effect on absorption from all the dosage forms of carbamazepine;[3] however, enteral feeding may slightly delay and reduce absorption of the liquid preparation, which may help to reduce side-effects such as mild drowsiness and lightheadedness.[4]

Health and safety

Standard precautions apply.

Suggestions/recommendations

- Use the liquid preparation. Dilute with an equal volume of water immediately prior to administration. If giving doses higher than 400 mg/day, divide into 4 equal doses. Doses above 800 mg/day may cause bloating due to the sorbitol content of the liquid.
- A prolonged break in feeding is not necessary.
- Plasma concentrations can be monitored if subtherapeutic or toxic concentrations are suspected. Dosage should be titrated to effect.

Intragastric administration

1. Stop the enteral feed.
2. Flush the enteral feeding tube with the recommended volume of water.
3. Shake the medication bottle thoroughly to ensure adequate mixing.
4. Draw the medication liquid into an appropriate size and type of syringe.
5. Draw an equal volume of water and a little air into the syringe and shake to mix thoroughly.
6. Flush the medication dose down the feeding tube.
7. Finally, flush with the recommended volume of water.
8. Re-start the feed, unless a prolonged break is required.

Alternatively, at step (4) measure the medicine in a suitable container and then add an equal volume of water and mix thoroughly. Draw this into an appropriate syringe. Ensure that the measure is rinsed and that this rinsing water is administered also to ensure that the total dose is given. **Do not** measure liquid medicines using a catheter-tipped syringe as this results in excessive dosing owing to the volume of the tip.

Intrajejunal administration

There are no specific data relating to jejunal administration of carbamazepine. Administer using the above method. An increase in side-effects such as dizziness is possible owing to the rapid delivery into the small bowel. Monitor for increased side-effects or loss of efficacy. Consider decreasing the dose and increasing the dosing frequency if side-effects are problematic.

References

1. *BNF 50*, September 2005.
2. BPNG data on file, 2004.
3. Tegretol liquid (Novartis), Summary of Product Characteristics; January 2003.
4. Bass J, Miles MV, Tennison MB, Holcombe BJ, Thorn MD. Effects of enteral tube feeding on the absorption and pharmacokinetic profile of carbamazepine suspension. *Epilepsia*. 1989; 30(3): 364–369.
5. Clark-Schmidt AL, Garnett WR, Lowe DR, Karnes HT. Loss of carbamazepine suspension through nasogastric feeding tubes. *Am J Hosp Pharm*. 1990; 47(9): 2034–2037.
6. Greenwood J. Sugar content of liquid prescription medicines. *Pharm J.* 1989(Oct.): 553–557.
7. Dollery C. *Therapeutic Drugs*, 2nd edn. London: Churchill Livingstone; 1998.

Carbimazole

Formulations available[1]

Brand name (Manufacturer)	Formulation and strength	Product information/Administration information
Neo-Mercazole (Roche)	Tablets 5 mg, 20 mg	The active component is contained in the central white core of the tablet; the coloured compression coat is inert. The tablets can be crushed and dispersed in a suitable suspending agent, e.g. methylcellulose. A short expiry should be allocated (3 days, refrigerated) owing to the rapid hydrolysis of the drug.[2] Tablets will disperse in 10 mL of water if shaken vigorously for 5 minutes; the resulting fine dispersion flushes via an 8Fr NG tube without blockage.[3]

Site of absorption (oral administration)

Specific site is not documented. Peak plasma concentrations of the active metabolite, methimazole, occur 1–2 hours following oral dosing of carbimazole.[4]

Alternative routes available

None available for carbimazole.

Interactions

No specified effect of food.[2]

Health and safety

Standard precautions apply.

Suggestions/recommendations

- Disperse tablets in water immediately prior to use.
- A prolonged break in feeding is not required.

Intragastric administration

1. Stop the enteral feed.
2. Flush the enteral feeding tube with the recommended volume of water.
3. Place the tablet in the barrel of an appropriate size and type of syringe.
4. Draw 10 mL of water into the syringe and allow the tablet to disperse, shaking if necessary.
5. Flush the medication dose down the feeding tube.
6. Draw another 10 mL of water into the syringe and also flush this via the feeding tube (this will rinse the syringe and ensure that the total dose is administered).
7. Finally, flush with the recommended volume of water.
8. Re-start the feed, unless a prolonged break is required.

Alternatively, at step (3) place the tablet into a medicine pot, add 10 mL of water and allow the tablet to disperse. Draw this into an appropriate syringe. Ensure that the measure is rinsed and that this rinsing water is administered also to ensure that the total dose is given.

Intrajejunal administration

There are no specific data relating to this route of administration. Administer using the above method. Monitor for increased side-effects or loss of efficacy.

References

1. *BNF 50*, September 2005.
2. Personal communication, Roche; 6 February 2003.
3. BPNG data on file, 2005.
4. Dollery C. *Therapeutic Drugs*, 2nd edn. London: Churchill Livingstone; 1998.

Carvedilol

Formulations available[1]

Brand name (Manufacturer)	Formulation and strength	Product information/Administration information
Eucardic (Roche)	Tablets 3.125 mg, 6.25 mg, 12.5 mg, 25 mg	Eucardic tablets may be crushed for patients having difficulty swallowing. The tablets will not dissolve in water but will form a suspension of small particle size. There are no stability data on crushing tablets, so it is recommended that the tablets be crushed immediately before administration.[2] The tablets will disperse in 10 mL of water if shaken for 5 minutes; the higher strength may take longer to disperse. The resulting dispersion will flush down an 8Fr NG tube without blockage.[5]
Carvedilol (APS)	Tablets 12.5 mg, 25 mg	The tablets will disperse in 10 mL of water if shaken for 5 minutes; the resulting dispersion has visible particles but these do not block an 8Fr NG feeding
tube.[5]	Carvedilol (Alpharma)	Tablets 12.5 mg, 25 mg

Site of absorption (oral administration)

Maximum plasma concentration occurs 1–2 hours post oral dose.[3] The absorption rate decreases progressively from the jejunum to the ileum through to the colon, and the absorption is delayed by bile and some mucoadhesive agents.[4]

Alternative routes available

None available for carvedilol; other beta-blockers are available as parenteral formulations.

Interactions

The absolute bioavailability of carvedilol is not affected by food, but absorption is delayed. For this reason it is recommended that carvedilol be taken after food as this reduces the incidence of rapid vasodilation, rapid hypotension and flushing.[2]

Health and safety

Standard precautions apply.

Suggestions/recommendations

- Disperse tablets in water immediately prior to administration.
- Administer after feed.
- If administering during feeding, a prolonged break is not necessary.

Intragastric administration

1. Stop the enteral feed.
2. Flush the enteral feeding tube with the recommended volume of water.
3. Avoid a prolonged break to reduce incidence of profound hypotension.
4. Place the tablet in the barrel of an appropriate size and type of syringe.
5. Draw 10 mL of water into the syringe and allow the tablet to disperse, shaking if necessary.
6. Flush the medication dose down the feeding tube.
7. Draw an equal volume of water into the syringe and also flush this via the feeding tube (this will rinse the syringe and ensure that the total dose is administered).
8. Finally, flush with the recommended volume of water.
9. Re-start the feed, unless a prolonged break is required.

Alternatively, at step (4) place the tablet into a medicine pot, add 10 mL of water and allow the tablet to disperse. Draw this into an appropriate syringe. Ensure that the measure is rinsed and that this rinsing water is administered also to ensure that the total dose is given.

Intrajejunal administration

Jejunal administration is unlikely to affect absorption. Administer using the above method.

References

1. *BNF 50*, September 2005.
2. Personal communication, Roche Pharmaceuticals Ltd; 6 February 2003.
3. Dollery C. *Therapeutic Drugs*, 2nd edn. London: Churchill Livingstone; 1998.
4. Cheng J, Kamiya K, Kodama I. Carvedilol: molecular and cellular basis for its multifaceted therapeutic potential. *Cardiovasc Drug Rev.* 2001; 19(2): 152–171.
5. BPNG data on file, 2004/5.

Cefalexin (Cephalexin)

Formulations available[1]

Brand name (Manufacturer)	Formulation and strength	Product information/Administration information
Cefalexin (Alpharma, APS, Arrow, Generics, Hillcross, IVAX, Kent, Ranbaxy)	Capsules 250 mg, 500 mg	See safety information below.

Formulations available[1] (*continued*)

Brand name (Manufacturer)	Formulation and strength	Product information/Administration information
Cefalexin (Alpharma, APS, Arrow, Hillcross, IVAX, Kent)	Tablets 250 mg, 500 mg	See safety information below.
Cefalexin (Alpharma, APS, Arrow, Hillcross, IVAX, Kent)	Oral suspension 125 mg/5 mL, 250 mg/5 mL	No specific data on enteral tube administration are available for this formulation.
Ceporex (Galen)	Capsules 250 mg, 500 mg	See safety information below.
Ceporex (Galen)	Tablets 250 mg, 500 mg	See safety information below.
Ceporex (Galen)	Syrup 125 mg/5 mL, 250 mg/5 mL, 500 mg/5 mL	Orange suspension when reconstituted. Flushes with some resistance. Mixes easily with an equal volume of water; this reduces resistance to flushing.[2]
Keflex (Lilly)	Capsules 250 mg, 500 mg	See safety information below.
Keflex (Lilly)	Tablets 250 mg, 500 mg	See safety information below.
Keflex (Lilly)	Suspension 125 mg/5 mL, 250 mg/5 mL	Powder for reconstitution contains active drug, sucrose, flavouring and colour only.[3]

Site of absorption (oral administration)

Peak plasma concentration occurs 1 hour following oral administration.[3] Cefalexin is thought to be absorbed from the duodenum and therefore absorption may be reduced by jejunal administration.[4]

Alternative routes available

None available for cefalexin. Cefradine (alternative first-generation cephalosporin) is available in parenteral formulation.

Interactions

Absorption is slightly reduced by co-administration with food.[3] This is unlikely to be clinically relevant.

Health and safety

Avoid crushing tablets or opening capsules owing to the risk of sensitisation to cephalosporins.

Suggestions/recommendations

- Use liquid preparation. Give as twice daily dose if clinically appropriate.
- A prolonged break in feeding is not required.

Intragastric administration

1. Stop the enteral feed.
2. Flush the enteral feeding tube with the recommended volume of water.
3. Shake the medication bottle thoroughly to ensure adequate mixing.
4. Draw the medication suspension into an appropriate size and type of syringe.
5. Draw an equal volume of water and a little air into the syringe and shake to mix thoroughly.
6. Flush the medication dose down the feeding tube.
7. Finally, flush with the recommended volume of water.
8. Re-start the feed, unless a prolonged break is required.

Alternatively, at step (4) measure the medicine in a suitable container and then add an equal volume of water and mix thoroughly. Draw this into an appropriate syringe. Ensure that the measure is rinsed and that this rinsing water is administered also to ensure that the total dose is given. **Do not** measure liquid medicines using a catheter-tipped syringe as this results in excessive dosing owing to the volume of the tip.

Intrajejunal administration

See notes above; absorption may be reduced. Use the higher end of the dose range. Administer using the above method.

References

1. *BNF 50*, September 2005.
2. BPNG data on file, 2005.
3. Keflex (Lilly), Summary of Product Characteristics; September 2005.
4. Adams D. Administration of drugs through a jejunostomy tube. *Br J Intensive Care.* 1994; 4(1): 10–17.

Cefixime

Formulations available[1]

Brand name (Manufacturer)	Formulation and strength	Product information/Administration information
Suprax (Rhône-Poulenc Rorer)	Tablets 200 mg	Film-coated. No specific data on enteral tube administration are available for this formulation.
Suprax (Rhône-Poulenc Rorer)	Suspension 100 mg/5 mL	Dilution not recommended. Absorption is better from suspension than tablets.[2] Contains 2.5 g sucrose/5 mL. Does not contain sorbitol.[3]

Site of absorption (oral administration)

Specific site of absorption is not documented.

Alternative routes available

No alternative routes are available for cefixime. Other cephalosporins are available as parenteral formulations.

Interactions

Absorption of cefixime is not significantly modified by food. Peak concentration may be delayed.[2]

Health and safety

Standard precautions apply.

Suggestions/recommendations

- Use liquid preparation. Flush well before and after dose. Do not dilute suspension.
- A prolonged break in feeding is not required.

Intragastric administration

1. Stop the enteral feed.
2. Flush the enteral feeding tube with the recommended volume of water.
3. Draw the medication solution into an appropriate size and type of syringe.
4. Flush the medication dose down the feeding tube.
5. Finally, flush with the recommended volume of water.
6. Re-start the feed.

Alternatively, at step (3) measure the medicine in a suitable container and then draw into an appropriate syringe. Ensure that the measure is rinsed and that this rinsing water is administered also to ensure that the total dose is given. **Do not** measure liquid medicines using a catheter-tipped syringe as this results in excessive dosing owing to the volume of the tip.

Intrajejunal administration

There are no specific data relating to jejunal administration of cefixime. Administer using the above method. Flush well before and after dosing to reduce the osmolarity of the suspension. Monitor for lack of effect.

References

1. *BNF* 50, September 2005.
2. Personal communication, Aventis; 13 February 2003.
3. Suprax (Sanofi-Aventis), Summary of Product Characteristics; April 2004.

Cefradine (Cephradine)

Formulations available[1]

Brand name (Manufacturer)	Formulation and strength	Product information/Administration information
Cefradine (APS, Galen, Generics, IVAX)	Capsules 250 mg, 500 mg	See safety information below.
Velosef (Squibb)	Capsules 250 mg, 500 mg	Squibb recommend using liquid preparation in preference to opening the capsules, although this is outside the product license.[2] See safety information below.

Formulations available[1] (*continued*)

Brand name (Manufacturer)	Formulation and strength	Product information/Administration information
Velosef (Squibb)	Syrup 250 mg/5 ml	Sucrose-based oral powder for reconstitution.[3]
Velosef (Squibb)	Injection 500 mg, 1 g	No specific data on enteral tube administration are available for this formulation.

Site of absorption (oral administration)

Specific site is not documented. Peak plasma concentration occurs within 1 hour of oral dosing.[3]

Alternative routes available

Parenteral route available.

Interactions

Food delays the absorption but does not affect total bioavailability.[3, 4]

Health and safety

Standard precautions apply. Do not open capsules. Avoid inhalation of capsule contents owing to risk of cephalosporin sensitisation.

Suggestions/recommendations

- Use liquid preparation. Change to twice-daily dosing, if clinically appropriate, to simplify the regimen.
- A prolonged break in feeding is not required.

Intragastric administration

1. Stop the enteral feed.
2. Flush the enteral feeding tube with the recommended volume of water.
3. Shake the medication bottle thoroughly to ensure adequate mixing.
4. Draw the medication suspension into an appropriate size and type of syringe.
5. Finally, flush with the recommended volume of water.
6. Re-start the feed, unless a prolonged break is required.

Alternatively, at step (4) measure the medicine in a suitable container. Draw this into an appropriate syringe. Ensure that the measure is rinsed and that this rinsing water is administered also to ensure that the total dose is given. **Do not** measure liquid medicines using a catheter-tipped syringe as this results in excessive dosing owing to the volume of the tip.

Intrajejunal administration

There are no specific data relating to the jejunal administration of cefradine. Administer using the above method.

References

1. *BNF 50*, September 2005.
2. Personal communication, Squibb; 24 January 2003.
3. Velosef (Squibb), Summary of Product Characteristics; June 2005.
4. Dollery C. *Therapeutic Drugs*, 2nd edn. London: Churchill Livingstone; 1998.

Cefuroxime

Formulations available[1]

Brand name (Manufacturer)	Formulation and strength	Product information/Administration information
Zinnat (GSK)	Tablet 125 mg, 250 mg	Film-coated tablet.[1] Cefuroxime axetil. Tablets may be easily dispersed in water; this may be easier than the suspension to administer via nasogastric tube.[2]
Zinnat (GSK)	Suspension 125 mg/5 mL	Cefuroxime axetil. The suspension may be too viscous to administer via fine bore feeding tubes.[2] Granules for reconstitution.[3]
Zinnat (GSK)	Sachets 125 mg per sachet	Cefuroxime axetil. Same formulation as suspension. Each sachet should be mixed with 10 mL of water immediately prior to administration.[3]
Cefuroxime (Lilly) Zinacef (GSK)	Injection 750 mg, 1.5 g	Cefuroxime sodium. No specific data on enteral tube administration are available for this formulation.

Site of absorption (oral administration)

Specific site is not documented. Cefuroxime axetil is hydrolysed in the intestine to cefuroxime.[4] Peak plasma concentration occurs 2–3 hours following oral dosing.[3]

Alternative routes available

The parenteral route is available.

Interactions

Food increased the peak plasma concentration and total bioavailability of oral cefuroxime axetil; the peak was delayed slightly.[5,6] The data are inconsistent, with a few studies demonstrating reduced peak levels; however, antimicrobial activity is unaffected.[7]

Health and safety

Crushing tablets should be avoided owing to risks of cephalosporin sensitisation.

Suggestions/recommendations

- For a wider bore tube > 10Fr, use suspension formulation. For finer bore tube, consider using tablets dispersed in 10 mL of water.
- For intrajejunal tubes, use the tablets dispersed in water; this may be preferable owing to the lower osmolarity.
- A prolonged break in feeding is not required.

Intragastric administration

See notes above.

Suspension

1. Stop the enteral feed.
2. Flush the enteral feeding tube with the recommended volume of water.
3. Shake the medication bottle thoroughly to ensure adequate mixing.
4. Draw the medication into an appropriate size and type of syringe.
5. Flush the medication dose down the feeding tube.
6. Finally, flush with the recommended volume of water.
7. Re-start the feed, unless a prolonged break is required.

Alternatively, at step (4) measure the medicine in a suitable container and then draw into an appropriate syringe. Ensure that the measure is rinsed and that this rinsing water is administered also to ensure that the total dose is given. **Do not** measure liquid medicines using a catheter-tipped syringe as this results in excessive dosing owing to the volume of the tip.

Intrajejunal administration

There are no specific data relating to jejunal administration of cefuroxime axetil; however, as conversion to cefuroxime occurs in the small bowel, it is unlikely that bioavailability will be affected. Administer using the above method, also see below.

Tablet administration

1. Stop the enteral feed.
2. Flush the enteral feeding tube with the recommended volume of water.
3. Place the tablet in the barrel of an appropriate size and type of syringe.
4. Draw 10 mL of water into the syringe and allow the tablet to disperse, shaking if necessary.
5. Flush the medication dose down the feeding tube.
6. Draw another 10 mL of water into the oral syringe and also flush this via the feeding tube (this will rinse the syringe and ensure that the total dose is administered).
7. Finally, flush with the recommended volume of water.
8. Re-start the feed, unless a prolonged break is required.

Alternatively, at step (3) place the tablet into a medicine pot, add 10 mL of water and allow the tablet to disperse. Draw this into an appropriate syringe. Ensure that the measure is rinsed and that this rinsing water is administered also to ensure that the total dose is given.

References

1. *BNF 50*, September 2005.
2. Personal communication, GSK; 22 January 2003.
3. Zinnat Suspension (GSK), Summary of Product Characteristics; 28 June 2005.
4. Dollery C. *Therapeutic Drugs*, 2nd edn. London: Churchill Livingstone; 1998.
5. Williams PE, Harding SM. The absolute bioavailability of oral cefuroxime axetil in male and female volunteers after fasting and after food. *J Antimicrob Chemother*. 1984; 13: 191–196.
6. Finn A, Straughb A, Meyer M, *et al*. Effect of dose and food on the bioavailability of cefuroxime axetil. *Biopharm Drug Dispos*. 1987; 8(5): 519–526.
7. Garraffo R, Drugeon HB, Chiche D. Pharmacokinetics and pharmacodynamics of two oral forms of cefuroxime axetil. *Fundam Clin Pharmacol*. 1997; 11: 90–95.

Celecoxib

Formulations available[1]

Brand name (Manufacturer)	Formulation and strength	Product information/Administration information
Celebrex (Pharmacia)	Capsules 100 mg, 200 mg	The contents of the capsules pour easily from an opened capsule and mix easily with 10 mL of water to form a milky suspension that flushes down an 8Fr NG tube without blockage.[2] However, this requires a degree of manual dexterity owing to the small size of the capsules. Pharmacia do not recommend that the capsules be opened and mixed with water, but state that the contents of the capsule can be mixed with pudding or apple sauce immediately prior to administration.[3]

Site of absorption (oral administration)

Specific site of absorption is not documented. Peak plasma concentration occurs 2–3 hours after oral dosing.[4]

Alternative routes available

Meloxicam (COX II-selective) is available as suppositories. Rectal, topical and parenteral routes are available for other NSAIDs.

Interactions

A high-fat meal delays peak concentrations by approximately 1 hour. Celecoxib can be taken before or after food.[4]

Health and safety

Standard precautions apply.

Suggestions/recommendations

- Change to an alternative COX II-selective NSAID such as meloxicam, etoricoxib or valdecoxib (see monographs).

References

1. *BNF 50*, September 2005.
2. BPNG data on file, 2005.
3. Personal communication, Pharmacia; 11 March 2003.
4. Celebrex (Pharmacia), Summary of Product Characteristics; 28 November 2005.

Celiprolol hydrochloride

Formulations available[1]

Brand name (Manufacturer)	Formulation and strength	Product information/Administration information
Celectol (Sanofi-Aventis)	Tablets 200 mg, 400 mg	Solubility in water 151 g/L.[2] Film-coated tablets.[1] No specific data on enteral tube administration are available for this formulation.
Celiprolol (APS, Generics, IVAX, Ranbaxy, Sovereign)	Tablets 200 mg, 400 mg	Ranbaxy 200 mg tablets disperse in 10 mL of water within 5 minutes and flush via an 8Fr NG tube without blockage.[3]

Site of absorption (oral administration)

Specific site of absorption is not documented. Peak plasma concentration occurs between 2 and 3 hours after oral dosing.[2]

Alternative routes available

None available for celiprolol; other beta-blockers are available as parenteral formulations.

Interactions

Celiprolol absorption is significantly affected by food but it is not thought to be clinically relevant.[2]

Health and safety

Standard precautions apply.

Suggestions/recommendations

- Owing to limited data, consider changing to alternative beta-blocker such as atenolol or propranolol (see monographs).

References

1. *BNF 50*, September 2005.
2. Dollery C. *Therapeutic Drugs*, 2nd edn. London: Churchill Livingstone; 1998.
3. BPNG data on file, 2005.

Cetirizine hydrochloride

Formulations available[1]

Brand name (Manufacturer)	Formulation and strength	Product information/Administration information
Cetirizine (Alpharma, APS, CP, Generics, Ratiopharm, Sandoz, Sterwin, Tillomed)	Tablets 10 mg	Alpharma does not recommend crushing tablets as the coating may not pulverise.[2] Tillomed brand tablets do not disperse readily in water but will disintegrate if shaken in 10 mL of water for 5 minutes; this forms a fine dispersion that flushes via an 8Fr tube without blockage.[3]
Cetirizine (Ratiopharm, Sandoz)	Oral solution 5 mg/5 mL	OTC oral solutions (Zirtec) available. Contains sorbitol.

Site of absorption (oral administration)

Specific site of absorption is not documented. Peak plasma concentration occurs 30–60 minutes following oral dosing.[4]

Alternative routes available

Parenteral formulation is available for chlorpheniramine.

Interactions

No specific interaction with food are documented.

Health and safety

Standard precautions apply.

Suggestions/recommendations

- Use the liquid preparation, unless sorbitol is contraindicated.
- A prolonged break in feeding is not required.

Intragastric administration

1. Stop the enteral feed.
2. Flush the enteral feeding tube with the recommended volume of water.
3. Draw the medication solution into an appropriate size and type of syringe.
4. Flush the medication dose down the feeding tube.
5. Finally, flush with the recommended volume of water.
6. Re-start the feed, unless a prolonged break is required.

Alternatively, at step (3) measure the medicine in a suitable container and then draw into an appropriate syringe. Ensure that the measure is rinsed and that this rinsing water is administered also to ensure that the total dose is given. **Do not** measure liquid medicines using a catheter-tipped syringe as this results in excessive dosing owing to the volume of the tip.

Intrajejunal administration

There are no specific data relating to jejunal administration of cetirizine. Monitor for reduced effect or increased side-effects. Administer as above.

References

1. *BNF* 50, September 2005.
2. Personal communication, Alpharma; 21 January 2003.
3. BPNG data on file, 2004.
4. Zirtec (UCB Pharma), Summary of Product Characteristics; January 2003.

Chloroquine

Formulations available[1]

Brand name (Manufacturer)	Formulation and strength	Product information/Administration information
Avoclor (AstraZeneca)	Tablets 250 mg	250 mg chloroquine phosphate = 155 mg chloroquine base. No specific data on enteral tube administration are available for this formulation.
Nivaquine (Beacon)	Tablets 200 mg	200 mg chloroquine sulfate = 150 mg chloroquine base. Tablets can be crushed, although chloroquine has a very bitter taste.[2]
Nivaquine (Beacon)	Syrup 68 mg/5 mL	Chloroquine base 50 mg/5 mL. Contains sugar base; does not contain sorbitol.[3]
Malarivon (Wallace Mfg)	Syrup 80 mg/5 mL	Chloroquine phosphate 80 mg/5 mL = chloroquine base 50 mg/5 mL.
Chloroquine sulphate (Beacon)	Injection 54.5 mg/mL	Chloroquine base 40 mg/mL. No specific data on enteral tube administration are available for this formulation.

Site of absorption (oral administration)

Specific site is not documented.

Alternative routes available

Parenteral route is available; usually reserved for treatment of malaria.

Interactions

Food does not affect the bioavailability of chloroquine. The SPC recommends taking with food or milk to minimise the possibility of gastrointestinal irritation.[2]

Health and safety

Standard precautions apply.

Suggestions/recommendations

- Use liquid preparation for intragastric administration.
- Owing to the likely high viscosity and volume of dose for adults (30 mL) of the liquid preparation, consider dilution with water immediately prior to administration.
- A prolonged break in feeding is not required.

Intragastric administration

1. Stop the enteral feed.
2. Flush the enteral feeding tube with the recommended volume of water.
3. Shake the medication bottle thoroughly to ensure adequate mixing.
4. Draw the medication suspension into an appropriate size and type of syringe.
5. Flush the medication dose down the feeding tube.
6. Finally, flush with the recommended volume of water.
7. Re-start the feed, unless a prolonged break is required.

Alternatively, at step (4) measure the medicine in a suitable container. Draw this into an appropriate syringe. Ensure that the measure is rinsed and that this rinsing water is administered also to ensure that the total dose is given. **Do not** measure liquid medicines using a catheter-tipped syringe as this results in excessive dosing owing to the volume of the tip.

Intrajejunal administration

See notes above. Use the above method; ensure tube is flushed well. High osmolarity may increase the incidence of GI side-effects.

References

1. *BNF* 50, September 2005.
2. Personal communication, Beacon; 24 February 2003.
3. Nivaquine Syrup (Sanofi-Aventis), Summary of Product Characteristics; January 2005.

Chlorphenamine (Chlorpheniramine) maleate

Formulations available[1]

Brand name (Manufacturer)	Formulation and strength	Product information/Administration information
Chlorphenamine (Various manufacturers)	Tablets 4 mg	Chlorphenamine is soluble 1 : 5 in water.[2] Tablets can be crushed and mixed with water.[3]
Chlorphenamine (Sandoz)	Oral solution 2 mg/5 mL	No specific data on enteral tube administration are available for this formulation.
Chlorphenamine (Link)	Injection 10 mg/mL (1 mL)	No specific data relating to enteral tube administration of the injection.

Formulations available[1] (*continued*)

Brand name (Manufacturer)	Formulation and strength	Product information/Administration information
Piriton (GSK Healthcare)	Tablets 4 mg	No specific data on enteral tube administration are available for this formulation.
Piriton (GSK Healthcare)	Syrup 2 mg/5 mL	Liquid flushes via fine-bore tube with some resistance, mixes easily with an equal volume of water.[4]

Site of absorption (oral administration)

Specific site is not documented. Peak plasma concentration occurs 2–3 hours following oral dosing.[2]

Alternative routes available

Parenteral formulation is available.

Interactions

Administration with food significantly reduces bioavailability;[2] however, no specific recommendations are made in the SPC.

Health and safety

Standard precautions apply.

Suggestions/recommendations

- Use liquid preparation.
- A prolonged break in feeding is not required.

Intragastric administration

1. Stop the enteral feed.
2. Flush the enteral feeding tube with the recommended volume of water.
3. Shake the medication bottle thoroughly to ensure adequate mixing.
4. Draw the medication syrup into an appropriate size and type of syringe.
5. Flush the medication dose down the feeding tube.
6. Finally, flush with the recommended volume of water.
7. Re-start the feed, unless a prolonged break is required.

Alternatively, at step (4) measure the medicine in a suitable container. Draw this into an appropriate syringe. Ensure that the measure is rinsed and that this rinsing water is administered also to ensure that the total dose is given. **Do not** measure liquid medicines using a catheter-tipped syringe as this results in excessive dosing owing to the volume of the tip.

Intrajejunal administration

There are no specific data relating to jejunal administration of chlorphenamine. Monitor for loss of effect or increased side-effects. Administer as above. Consider diluting the syrup immediately prior to administration to reduce osmolarity.

References

1. *BNF 50*, September 2005.
2. Dollery C. *Therapeutic Drugs*, 2nd edn. London: Churchill Livingstone; 1998.
3. Personal communication, Alpharma; 21 January 2003.
4. BPNG data on file, 2004.

Chlorpromazine hydrochloride

Formulations available[1]

Brand name (Manufacturer)	Formulation and strength	Product information/Administration information
Chlorpromazine (various manufacturers)	Tablets 10 mg, 25 mg, 50 mg, 100 mg	Coated tablets. Do not crush, see below.
Chlorpromazine (Hillcross, Rosemont)	Oral solution 25 mg/5 mL, 100 mg/5 mL	Rosemont preparation contains 0.45 g sorbitol/5 mL.[2]
Chlorpromazine (Antigen)	Injection 25 mg/mL (1.2 mL)	Licensed for i.m. administration. No specific data on enteral tube administration are available for this formulation.
Chlorpromazine (Martindale)	Suppositories 100 mg	'Special order' product only. *For equivalent therapeutic effect:* 100 mg rectal = 20–25 mg i.m. = 40–50 mg orally.[1]
Largactil (Hawgreen)	Tablets 10 mg, 25 mg, 50 mg, 100 mg	Coated tablets. Do not crush, see below.
Largactil (Hawgreen)	Syrup 25 mg/5 mL	Sucrose-based syrup; does not contain sorbitol.[3]
Largactil (Hawgreen)	Suspension forte 100 mg/5 mL	Contains sorbitol.[3]
Largactil (Hawgreen)	Injection 25 mg/mL (2 mL)	No specific data on enteral tube administration are available for this formulation.

Site of absorption (oral administration)

Specific site is not documented. Peak plasma concentration occurs 2–4 hours following oral administration.[4]

Alternative routes available

Parenteral route is available. Suppositories are available by special order only.

Interactions

No specific documented interaction with food.[4]

Health and safety

Owing to the risks of contact sensitisation, tablets should not be crushed and solutions should be handled with care.[1]

Suggestions/recommendations

- Use oral solution where possible.
- A prolonged break in feeding is not required.

Intragastric administration

1. Stop the enteral feed.
2. Flush the enteral feeding tube with the recommended volume of water.
3. Draw the medication solution into an appropriate size and type of syringe.
4. Flush the medication dose down the feeding tube.
5. Finally, flush with the recommended volume of water.
6. Re-start the feed, unless a prolonged break is required.

Alternatively, at step (3) measure the medicine in a suitable container and then draw into an appropriate syringe. Ensure that the measure is rinsed and that this rinsing water is administered also to ensure that the total dose is given. **Do not** measure liquid medicines using a catheter-tipped syringe as this results in excessive dosing owing to the volume of the tip.

Intrajejunal administration

There are no specific data relating to jejunal administration of chlorpromazine. Administer using the above method. Monitor for increased side-effects.

References

1. *BNF* 50, September 2005.
2. Personal communication, Rosemont; 20 January 2005.
3. Largactil (Hawgreen), Summary of Product Characteristics; March 2004.
4. Dollery C. *Therapeutic Drugs*, 2nd edn. London: Churchill Livingstone; 1998.

Chlortalidone (Chlorthalidone)

Formulations available[1]

Brand name (Manufacturer)	Formulation and strength	Product information/Administration information
Hygroton (Alliance)	Tablet 50 mg	Scored tablets. Tablet disintegrates within 2 minutes when placed in 10 mL of water; the pale yellow dispersion flushes via an 8Fr NG tube without blockage.[2]

Site of absorption (oral administration)

Specific site is not documented. Peak plasma concentration occurs 8–12 hours following oral administration.[3]

Alternative routes available

None for chlortalidone. Other diuretics are available in parenteral formulations.

Interactions

No specific interaction with food is documented.[3, 4]

Health and safety

Standard precautions apply.

Suggestions/recommendations

- Disperse the tablet in immediately prior to administration.
- A prolonged break in feeding is not required.

Intragastric administration

1. Stop the enteral feed.
2. Flush the enteral feeding tube with the recommended volume of water.
3. Place the tablet in the barrel of an appropriate size and type of syringe.
4. Draw 10 mL of water into the syringe and allow the tablet to disperse, shaking if necessary.
5. Flush the medication dose down the feeding tube.
6. Draw another 10 mL of water into the syringe and also flush this via the feeding tube (this will rinse the syringe and ensure that the total dose is administered).
7. Finally, flush with the recommended volume of water.
8. Re-start the feed, unless a prolonged break is required.

Alternatively, at step (3) place the tablet into a medicine pot, add 10 mL of water and allow the tablet to disperse. Draw this into an appropriate syringe. Ensure that the measure is rinsed and that this rinsing water is administered also to ensure that the total dose is given.

Intrajejunal administration

There are no specific data on jejunal administration of chlortalidone. Administer using the above method. Monitor for increased side-effects or loss of efficacy.

References

1. *BNF* 50, September 2005.
2. BPNG data on file, 2005.
3. Hygroton (Alliance), Summary of Product Characteristics; February 2004.
4. Dollery C. *Therapeutic Drugs*, 2nd edn. London: Churchill Livingstone; 1998.

Cilazapril

Formulations available[1]

Brand name (Manufacturer)	Formulation and strength	Product information/Administration information
Vascace (Roche)	Tablets 500 microgram, 1 mg, 2.5 mg, 5 mg	Film-coated tablets.[2] Solubility 1 : 200 in water.[3] No specific data on enteral tube administration are available for this formulation.

Site of absorption (oral administration)

Specific site of absorption is unknown. Peak plasma concentration is reached within 2 hours of oral administration.[2]

Alternative routes available

None available.

Interactions

Food delays and reduces absorption of cilazapril, but this is therapeutically irrelevant.[2]

Health and safety

Standard precautions apply.

Suggestions/recommendations

- Limited data are available.
- Consider changing to alternative once daily dosed ACE inhibitor, for example ramipril or lisinopril (see monographs).

References

1. *BNF* 50, September 2005.
2. Vascace (Roche), Summary of Product Characteristics; September 2005.
3. Dollery C. *Therapeutic Drugs*, 2nd edn. London: Churchill Livingstone; 1998.

Cimetidine

Formulations available[1]

Brand name (Manufacturer)	Formulation and strength	Product information/Administration information
Tagamet (GSK)	Tablets 200 mg, 400 mg, 800 mg Effervescent tablet 400 mg	Effervescent tablets contain 18 mmol sodium/tablet.[2]
Tagamet (GSK)	Syrup 200 mg/5 mL	Contains insignificant quantity of sorbitol.[2]
Tagamet (GSK)	Injection 100 mg/mL	Injection can be administered enterally.[3]
Dyspamet (Goldshield)	Suspension 200 mg/5 mL	Contains sorbitol 2.79 g/5 mL.[1]
Cimetidine (Rosemont)	Oral solution 200 mg/5 mL	No specific data.
Cimetidine (Alpharma, APS, Ashbourne, Berk, BHR, CP, Dexcel, Eastern, Hillcross, IVAX, Kent, Opus, Sovereign)	Tablets 200 mg, 400 mg, 800 mg	Alpharma brand tablets can be crushed but the manufacturer advises against this.[5]

Site of absorption (oral administration)

Absorption is from the proximal small bowel. Peak plasma concentration occurs 60–90 minutes after oral dosing.[4]

Alternative routes available

Parenteral formulation is available.

Interactions

Peak concentrations are reduced by food, but overall absorption is unaffected.[4]

Health and safety

Standard precautions apply.

Suggestions/recommendations

- Use liquid preparation or effervescent tablets.
- Caution is needed when using high doses owing to the sorbitol content of the sugar-free liquids and the sodium content of the effervescent tablets.
- A prolonged break in feeding is not required.

Intragastric administration

Liquid preparation (see below for effervescent tablets).

1. Stop the enteral feed.
2. Flush the enteral feeding tube with the recommended volume of water.
3. Shake the medication bottle thoroughly to ensure adequate mixing.
4. Draw the medication dose into an appropriate size and type of syringe.
5. Flush the medication dose down the feeding tube.
6. Finally, flush with the recommended volume of water.
7. Re-start the feed, unless a prolonged break is required.

Alternatively, at step (4) measure the medicine in a suitable container. Draw this into an appropriate syringe. Ensure that the measure is rinsed and that this rinsing water is administered also to ensure that the total dose is given. **Do not** measure liquid medicines using a catheter-tipped syringe as this results in excessive dosing owing to the volume of the tip.

Intrajejunal administration

Cimetidine can be administered into the jejunum; for this route the effervescent tablets, dissolved in at least 30 mL of water, or the injection should be used.[3]

1. Stop the enteral feed.
2. Flush the enteral feeding tube with the recommended volume of water.
3. Measure 30 mL of water into a measuring pot.
4. Add the effervescent tablet and allow to dissolve.
5. Draw into an appropriate size and type of syringe.
6. Flush the medication dose down the feeding tube.
7. Rinse the measure and administer this also to ensure that the total dose is given.
8. Finally, flush with the recommended volume of water.
9. Re-start the feed, unless a prolonged break is required.

References

1. *BNF 50*, September 2005.
2. Tagamet (Chemidex), Summary of Product Characteristics; June 2004.
3. Adams D. Administration of drugs through a jejunostomy tube. *Br J Intensive Care*, 1994; 4(1): 10–17.
4. Dollery C. *Therapeutic Drugs*, 2nd edn. London: Churchill Livingstone; 1998.
5. Personal communication, Alpharma Ltd; 21 January 2003.

Cinnarizine

Formulations available[1]

Brand name (Manufacturer)	Formulation and strength	Product information/Administration information
Cinnarizine (Alpharma, APS, Ashbourne, Generics, Hillcross, IVAX, Norton)	Tablets 15 mg	Norton brand tablets disperse in 10 mL of water within 5 minutes to give a fine dispersion that flushes easily via an 8Fr NG tube without blockage.[2]
Stugeron (Janssen-Cilag)	Tablets 15 mg	Tablets may be chewed, sucked or swallowed whole.[3]
Stugeron Forte (Janssen-Cilag)	Capsules 75 mg	Indicated for peripheral vascular disease and Raynaud syndrome. No specific data on enteral tube administration are available for this formulation.

Site of absorption (oral administration)

No specific information on site on absorption. Peak plasma concentration occurs 1–4 hours following oral administration in fasted subjects.[4]

Alternative routes available

None available for cinnarizine; parenteral and rectal formulations are available for other antiemetics and antihistamines.

Interactions

No specific interaction with food is documented; the dose should be taken after meals.[5]

Health and safety

Standard precautions apply.

Suggestions/recommendations

- Disperse the tablets in water immediately prior to administration.
- A prolonged break in feeding is not necessary.
- The dose should be administered after feed if practicable.

Intragastric administration

1. Stop the enteral feed.
2. Flush the enteral feeding tube with the recommended volume of water.
3. Place the tablet in the barrel of an appropriate size and type of syringe.
4. Draw 10 mL of water into the syringe and allow the tablet to disperse, shaking if necessary.
5. Flush the medication dose down the feeding tube.
6. Draw another 10 mL of water into the syringe and also flush this via the feeding tube (this will rinse the syringe and ensure that the total dose is administered).
7. Finally, flush with the recommended volume of water.
8. Re-start the feed, unless a prolonged break in feeding is required.

Alternatively, at step (4) place the tablet into a medicine pot, add 10 mL of water and allow the tablet to disperse. Draw this into an appropriate syringe. Ensure that the measure is rinsed and that this rinsing water is administered also to ensure that the total dose is given.

Intrajejunal administration

There are no specific data relating to jejunal administration of cinnarizine. Administer as above. Monitor for loss of efficacy or increase side-effects.

References

1. *BNF 50*, September 2005.
2. BPNG data on file, 2005.
3. Personal communication, Janssen-Cilag; 22 January 2003.
4. Dollery C. *Therapeutic Drugs*, 2nd edn. London: Churchill Livingstone; 1998.
5. Stugeron (Janssen-Cilag), Summary of Product Characteristics; 20 February 2006.

Ciprofloxacin

Formulations available[1]

Brand name (Manufacturer)	Formulation and strength	Product information/Administration information
Ciprofloxacin (Alpharma, APS, Arrow, Chemidex, Generics, PLIVA, Sandoz, Sterwin, Tillomed)	Tablets 100 mg, 250 mg, 500 mg, 750 mg	Ciprofloxacin hydrochloride. Generics and Ranbaxy brand of tablets disperse in water within 2–5 minutes. Owing to the tablet's bulk, it is quite difficult to see the particles, but the dispersion flushes via an 8Fr NG tube without blockage.[2] Alpharma brand tablets can be crushed.[3]
Ciproxin (Bayer)	Tablets 100 mg, 250 mg, 500 mg, 750 mg	Ciprofloxacin hydrochloride. The 750 mg tablets have been crushed and mixed with 50 mL of water and delivered via gastric tube.[4]
Ciproxin (Bayer)	Suspension 250 mg/mL	Granules for suspension. Very thick nonaqueous granular suspension. High risk of tube blockage with fine-bore tubes.[2]
Ciproxin (Bayer)	I.v. infusion 2 mg/mL (100 mL, 200 mL)	Ciprofloxacin lactate. No specific data on enteral tube administration are available for this formulation.

Site of absorption (oral administration)

Specific site of absorption is unknown. Peak plasma concentration occurs 60–75 minutes following an oral dose.[5] There is case report evidence that ciprofloxacin is absorbed when delivered into the jejunum but that plasma concentrations may be lower; it is recommended that the higher end of the dose range be used.[6]

Alternative routes available

Parenteral route available.

Interactions

The interaction between ciprofloxacin and enteral feeds is well established. Ciprofloxacin binds to divalent ions in the feed. In a study using Pulmocare (high in calcium and magnesium compared to Osmolite and Ensure), the absorption of ciprofloxacin was significantly reduced when Pulmocare was administered immediately following a dose of ciprofloxacin; however, the plasma level achieved was still above the MIC for many important pathogenic bacteria.[4]

When ciprofloxacin, levofloxacin and ofloxacin were added directly to enteral feeds, a loss of dose was observed for all antibiotics; however, the losses were 83%, 61% and 46%, respectively.[7]

A reduction in absorption was also noted when the enteral feed was resumed immediately following dosing. The standard fibre feed contained less than half the electrolyte content of Pulmocare; the mean peak level was 44%.[8]

Health and safety

Standard precautions apply.

Suggestions/recommendations

- Disperse the tablets in water immediately prior to dosing.
- It is recommended that the upper end of the dose range be used.[9]
- Although there is no evidence that a break in feeding is beneficial, it would appear logical to administer the dose during a break in feeding where possible.
- The upper end of the dose range should be also be used for intrajejunal administration.
- The patient should be monitored closely for signs of treatment failure.[9]
- Alternatively, the patient could be transferred to an alternative quinolone as the scale of the interaction appears less, although there are fewer publications relating to these antibiotics.

Intragastric administration

1. Stop the enteral feed.
2. Flush the enteral feeding tube with the recommended volume of water.
3. Allow a break in feeding if possible.
4. Place the tablet in the barrel of an appropriate size and type of syringe.
5. Draw 20 mL of water into the syringe and allow the tablet to disperse, shaking if necessary.
6. Flush the medication dose down the feeding tube.
7. Draw another 10 mL of water into the oral syringe and also flush this via the feeding tube (this will rinse the syringe and ensure that the total dose is administered).
8. Finally, flush with the recommended volume of water.
9. Re-start the feed, unless a prolonged break is required.

Alternatively, at step (4) place the tablet into a medicine pot, add 20 mL of water and allow the tablet to disperse. Draw this into an appropriate syringe. Ensure that the measure is rinsed and that this rinsing water is administered also to ensure that the total dose is given.

Intrajejunal administration

Administer as above. See notes above.

References

1. *BNF 50*, September 2005.
2. BPNG data on file, 2004.
3. Personal communication, Alpharma; 21 January 2003.
4. Cohn SM, Sawyer MD, Burns GA, *et al.* Enteric absorption of ciprofloxacin during tube feeding in the critically ill. *J Antimicrob Chemother.* 1996; 38: 871–876.
5. Dollery C. *Therapeutic Drugs*, 2nd edn. London: Churchill Livingstone; 1998.
6. Adams D. Administration of drugs through a jejunostomy tube. *Br J Intensive Care*, 1994; 4(1): 10–17.
7. Wright DH, Pietz SL, Konstantinides FN, Rotschafer JC. Decreased in vitro fluoroquinolone concentrations after admixture with an enteral feeding formulation. *JPEN J Parenter Enteral Nutr.* 2000; 24: 42–48.
8. Mimoz O, Binter V, Jacolot A, *et al.* Pharmacokinetics and absolute bioavailability of ciprofloxacin administered through a nasogastric tube with continuous enteral feeding to critically ill patients. *Intensive Care Med.* 1998; 24: 1047–1051.
9. Stockley IH. *Drug Interactions*, 4th edn. London: Pharmaceutical Press, 1996.

Citalopram

Formulations available[1]

Brand name (Manufacturer)	Formulation and strength	Product information/Administration information
Citalopram (Generics, Niche, Sandoz, Sterwin)	Tablets 10 mg, 20 mg, 40 mg	Citalopram hydrobromide. Generic brand tablets are very slow to disperse but will disintegrate if shaken in 10 mL of water for 5 minutes to give a fine dispersion that flushes via an 8Fr NG tube without blockage.[2]
Cipramil (Lundbeck)	Tablets 10 mg, 20 mg, 40 mg	Citalopram hydrobromide. Film-coated tablets. No specific data on enteral tube administration are available for this formulation.
Cipramil (Lundbeck)	Oral drops 40 mg/mL	Citalopram hydrochloride. 8 mg citalopram hydrochloride = 10 mg citalopram hydrobromide. 8 mg = 4 drops Can be mixed with water, orange juice or apple juice.[3]

Site of absorption (oral administration)

Specific site of absorption is not documented. Peak plasma concentration occurs 2–4 hours following oral dosing.[4]

Alternative routes available

An intravenous infusion is available from Lundbeck on a named-patient basis. Contact the manufacturer for further details.[4]

Interactions

Absorption is unaffected by food.[5]

Health and safety

Standard precautions apply.

Suggestions/recommendations

- Use oral drops.
- A prolonged break in feeding is not required.

Intragastric administration

1. Stop the enteral feed.
2. Flush the enteral feeding tube with the recommended volume of water.
3. Add 4 drops of the oral solution for every 10 mg of the tablets to 10 mL of water.
4. Draw the medication solution into an appropriate size and type of syringe.
5. Flush the medication dose down the feeding tube.
6. Finally, flush with the recommended volume of water.
7. Re-start the feed, unless a prolonged break is required.

Intrajejunal administration

There are no specific data relating to the jejunal administration of citalopram. Administer using the above method. Monitor for increased side-effects or loss of efficacy.

References

1. *BNF 50*, September 2005.
2. BPNG data on file, 2004.
3. Cipramil Drops (Lundbeck), Summary of Product Characteristics; April 2003.
4. Personal communication, Lundbeck; January 2006.
5. Dollery C. *Therapeutic Drugs*, 2nd edn. London: Churchill Livingstone; 1998.

Clarithromycin

Formulations available[1]

Brand name (Manufacturer)	Formulation and strength	Product information/Administration information
Clarithromycin (nonproprietary)	Tablets 250 mg, 500 mg	No specific data on enteral tube administration are available for this formulation.
Klaricid (Abbott)	Tablets 250 mg, 500 mg	No specific data on enteral tube administration are available for this formulation.

Formulations available[1] (continued)

Brand name (Manufacturer)	Formulation and strength	Product information/Administration information
Klaricid (Abbott)	Paediatric suspension 125 mg/5 mL, 250 mg/5 mL	Very thick creamy, slightly granular/gritty suspension. Blocks fine NG tube (less than 9Fr) because of the presence of granules and viscosity. If the dose is diluted with an equal volume of water immediately prior to administration, the viscosity is reduced, but there is still a risk of tube blockage with very fine-bore tubes.[2]
Klaricid (Abbott)	Granules 250 mg/sachet	No specific data on enteral tube administration are available for this formulation.
Klaricid (Abbott)	I.v. infusion 500 mg	Not suitable for enteral use.
Klaricid XL (Abbott)	Tablets 500 mg	Modified-release tablets. Not suitable for administration via feeding tube.

Site of absorption (oral administration)

Specific site is not documented. Peak plasma concentration occurs at 2 hours following oral administration.[3]

Alternative routes available

Parenteral route is available.

Interactions

Food delays peak plasma concentrations slightly, but does not affect bioavailability.[3] There does not appear to be any interaction with enteral feed.

Health and safety

Standard precautions apply.

Suggestions/recommendations

- Clarithromycin suspension has been successfully administered via NG tube to 16 ICU patients.[4]
- For tubes 9Fr or larger, use the suspension formulation, diluted with an equal volume of water immediately prior to administration.
- A prolonged break in feeding is not required.
- Consider parenteral therapy or an alternative macrolide such as azithromycin.

Intragastric administration

1. Stop the enteral feed.
2. Flush the enteral feeding tube with the recommended volume of water.
3. Shake the medication bottle thoroughly to ensure adequate mixing.
4. Draw the medication suspension into an appropriate size and type of syringe.
5. Draw an equal volume of water and a little air into the syringe and shake to mix thoroughly.
6. Flush the medication dose down the feeding tube.
7. Finally, flush with the recommended volume of water.
8. Re-start the feed, unless a prolonged break is required.

Alternatively, at step (4) measure the medicine in a suitable container and then add an equal volume of water and mix thoroughly. Draw this into an appropriate syringe. Ensure that the measure is rinsed and that this rinsing water is administered also to ensure that the total dose is given. **Do not** measure liquid medicines using a catheter-tipped syringe as this results in excessive dosing owing to the volume of the tip.

Intrajejunal administration

There are no specific reports of jejunal administration. Administer using the above method. Monitor for loss of efficacy.

References

1. *BNF* 50, September 2005.
2. BPNG data on file, 2004.
3. Dollery C. *Therapeutic Drugs*, 2nd edn. London: Churchill Livingstone; 1998.
4. Fish DN, Abraham E. Pharmacokinetics of a clarithromycin suspension administered via nasogastric tube to seriously ill patients. *Antimicrob Agents Chemother.* 1999; 43(5): 1277–1280.

Clindamycin

Formulations available[1]

Brand name (Manufacturer)	Formulation and strength	Product information/Administration information
Clindamycin (Sandoz)	Capsules 150 mg	Clindamycin is soluble 1 : 2 in water.[2]
Dalacin C (Pharmacia)	Capsules 75 mg, 150 mg	Pharmacia have no data to support the administration of clindamycin via enteral feeding tubes.[3] The capsules open easily and the powder pours from the capsule when squeezed; care must be taken to ensure the entire contents of the capsule are emptied out. The powder mixes easily with water and flushes via an 8Fr NG tube without blockage.[4]
Dalacin C (Pharmacia)	Injection 150 mg/mL (2 mL, 4 mL)	For i.m. injection or i.v. infusion.[1]
Dalacin (Pharmacia)	Paediatric suspension	Discontinued in the UK. Still available via importers, e.g. IDIS.[3]

Site of absorption (oral administration)

Specific site is not documented. Peak plasma concentration occurs within 1 hour of oral administration.[5]

Alternative routes available

Parenteral route is available. Cream is available for topical treatment only.

Interactions

Standard precautions apply. Avoid inhalation of capsule contents.

Health and safety

Food delays the absorption of clindamycin but does not affect the peak concentration.[2, 5]

Suggestions/recommendations

- Where clinically appropriate, change to an alternative antibiotic available as a liquid or dispersible tablet.
- To administer clindamycin, open the capsules and disperse in water immediately prior to administration. Avoid inhalation of capsule contents.
- A prolonged break in feeding is not required.

Intragastric administration

1. Stop the enteral feed.
2. Flush the enteral feeding tube with the recommended volume of water.
3. Open the capsule and pour the contents into a medicine pot.
4. Add 15 mL of water.
5. Stir to disperse the powder.
6. Draw into an appropriate size and type of syringe and administer via the feeding tube.
7. Add a further 15 mL of water to the medicine pot; stir to ensure that any powder remaining in the pot is mixed with water.
8. Draw up this dispersion and flush down the tube. This will ensure that the whole dose is given.
9. Flush the tube with water.
10. Re-start the feed, unless a prolonged break in feeding is required.

Intrajejunal administration

There are no specific data relating to jejunal administration of clindamycin. Administer as above.

References

1. *BNF* 50, September 2005.
2. Dollery C. *Therapeutic Drugs*, 2nd edn. London: Churchill Livingstone; 1998.
3. Personal communication, Pharmacia; 11 March 2003.
4. BPNG data on file, 2004.
5. Dalacin C (Pharmacia), Summary of Product Characteristics; February 2004.

Clobazam

Formulations available[1]

Brand name (Manufacturer)	Formulation and strength	Product information/Administration information
Frisium (Aventis)	Tablets 10 mg	Not coated.[2] Tablets should disperse in water or be crushed.

Manufactured 'specials' are available in a variety of strengths, contact specials manufacturers for details.

Site of absorption (oral administration)

Specific site of absorption is not documented. Peak plasma concentration occurs 1–4 hours after oral dosing.[3]

Alternative routes available

None available for clobazam.

Interactions

Administration with food delays peak plasma concentrations but does not reduce overall bioavailability.[3]

Health and safety

Standard precautions apply.

Suggestions/recommendations

- Use an alternative drug where clinically appropriate. It should be possible to disperse the tablets and suspend them in water immediately prior to administration.
- Alternatively, a manufactured 'special' liquid preparation can be obtained.
- A prolonged break in feeding is not required.

Intragastric administration

1. Stop the enteral feed.
2. Flush the enteral feeding tube with the recommended volume of water.
3. Place the tablet in the barrel of an appropriate size and type of syringe.
4. Draw 10 mL of water into the syringe and allow the tablet to disperse, shaking if necessary.
5. Flush the medication dose down the feeding tube.
6. Draw another 10 mL of water into the oral syringe and also flush this via the feeding tube (this will rinse the syringe and ensure that the total dose is administered).
7. Finally, flush with the recommended volume of water.
8. Re-start the feed, unless a prolonged break is required.

Alternatively, at step (4) place the tablet into a medicine pot, add 10 mL of water and allow the tablet to disperse. Draw this into an appropriate syringe. Ensure that the measure is rinsed and that this rinsing water is administered also to ensure that the total dose is given.

Intrajejunal administration

There are no specific data on jejunal administration of clobazam. Administer using the above method. Monitor for increased side-effects or loss of efficacy.

References

1. *BNF* 50, September 2005.
2. Frisium (Aventis) Summary of Product Characteristics; January 2002.
3. Dollery C. *Therapeutic Drugs*, 2nd edn. London: Churchill Livingstone; 1998.

Clomipramine hydrochloride

Formulations available[1]

Brand name (Manufacturer)	Formulation and strength	Product information/Administration information
Clomipramine (Alpharma, APS, Generics, Hillcross, IVAX)	Capsules 10 mg, 25 mg, 50 mg	APS brand capsules – contents pour easily from capsules and disperse in 10 mL of water; this flushes via an 8Fr NG tube without blockage. Requires sufficient manual dexterity owing to the size of the capsules.[2]
Anafranil (Cephalon)	Capsules 10 mg, 25 mg, 50 mg	All size 4 capsules.[3] No specific data on enteral tube administration are available for this formulation.
Anafranil SR (Cephalon)	Tablets 75 mg	Modified release tablets. Cannot be crushed. Unsuitable for administration via the feeding tube.

Site of absorption (oral administration)

Specific site of absorption or time to peak plasma concentrations are not documented in the SPC.[3]

Alternative routes available

None available for clomipramine.[3]

Interactions

Food does not significantly affect bioavailability of clomipramine but the peak serum concentrations and therefore onset of action may be delayed.[3]

Health and safety

Standard precautions apply.

Suggestions/recommendations

- Capsules can be opened and the contents mixed with water immediately prior to administration.
- The capsules are very small and this may not be practical; consideration should therefore be given to changing to alternate therapy.
- A prolonged break in feeding is not required.

Intragastric administration

1. Stop the enteral feed.
2. Flush the enteral feeding tube with the recommended volume of water.
3. Open the capsule and pour the contents into a medicine pot.
4. Add 15 mL of water.
5. Stir to disperse the powder.
6. Draw into an appropriate size and type of syringe and administer via the feeding tube.
7. Add further 15 mL of water to the medicine pot; stir to ensure that any powder remaining in the pot is mixed with water.
8. Draw up this dispersion and flush down the tube. This will ensure that the whole dose is given.
9. Flush the tube with water.
10. Re-start the feed, unless a prolonged break is required.

Intrajejunal administration

There are no specific data relating to site of absorption of clomipramine. Administer using the above method. Monitor for loss of efficacy or increased side-effects.

References

1. *BNF* 50, September 2005.
2. BPNG data on file, 2004.
3. Anafranil (Novartis), Summary of Product Characteristics; 19 July 2004.

Clonazepam

Formulations available[1]

Brand name (Manufacturer)	Formulation and strength	Product information/Administration information
Rivotril (Roche)	Tablets 500 microgram, 2 mg	Scored. Tablets disperse in 10 mL of water within 5 minutes to form a coarse dispersion that breaks up when drawn into the syringe and flushes down an 8Fr NG tube without blockage.[3]
Clonazepam (Rosemont)	Oral solution 0.5 mg/5 mL, 2 mg/5 mL	Unlicensed special: 6 months shelf-life.[4]
Clonazepam (extemporaneous preparation)		*Extemporaneous preparation 200 microgram/5 mL:*[2] Clonazepam tablets 2 mg — 20 tablets Keltrol — 0.4% w/v Methylhydroxybenzoate — 0.1 g Propylhydroxybenzoate — 0.02 g Propylene glycol — 2 mL Syrup BP — 40 mL Purified water — to 1000 mL Three months' shelf-life at room temperature.
Rivotril (Roche)	Injection 1 mg/mL	No specific data on enteral tube administration of injection formulation.

Site of absorption (oral administration)

Specific site of absorption is not documented. Peak plasma concentration occurs 1–4 hours after an oral dose.[5]

Alternative routes available

The parenteral route is available and is licensed for the treatment of status epilepticus.

Interactions

No specific interaction with food is documented.[5]

Health and safety

Standard precautions apply.

Suggestions/recommendations

- Disperse the tablets in water immediately prior to administration.
- For very fine-bore tubes consider using a liquid preparation.
- A prolonged break in feeding is not necessary.

Intragastric administration

1. Stop the enteral feed.
2. Flush the enteral feeding tube with the recommended volume of water.
3. Place the tablet in the barrel of an appropriate size and type of syringe.
4. Draw 10 mL of water into the syringe and allow the tablet to disperse, shaking if necessary.
5. Flush the medication dose down the feeding tube.
6. Draw another 10 mL of water into the oral syringe and also flush this via the feeding tube (this will rinse the syringe and ensure that the total dose is administered).
7. Finally, flush with the recommended volume of water.
8. Re-start the feed, unless a prolonged break is required.

Alternatively, at step (3) place the tablet into a medicine pot, add 10 mL of water and allow the tablet to disperse. Draw this into an appropriate syringe. Ensure that the measure is rinsed and that this rinsing water is administered also to ensure that the total dose is given.

Intrajejunal administration

There are no specific data relating to jejunal administration. Administer using the above method. Monitor for loss of efficacy or increased side-effects.

References

1. *BNF* 50, September 2005.
2. Personal communication, Roche; 6 February 2003.
3. BPNG data on file, 2004.
4. Personal communication, Rosemont; July 2004.
5. Rivotril Tablets (Roche), Summary of Product Characteristics; September 2005.

Clonidine hydrochloride

Formulations available[1]

Brand name (Manufacturer)	Formulation and strength	Product information/Administration information
Catapres (Boehringer Ingelheim)	Tablets 100 microgram, 300 microgram	Scored tablets. Tablets can be crushed.[2] 100 microgram tablets disperse within 2 minutes when placed in 10 mL of water, to give a fine white dispersion that flushes via an 8Fr NG tube without blockage.[3]
Catapres (Boehringer Ingelheim)	Injection 150 microgram/mL (1 mL)	Injection can be given orally.[2] pH = 4–4.5.
Dixarit (Boehringer Ingelheim)	Tablets 25 microgram	Film-coated tablets. Tablets can be crushed.[2] Tablets do not disperse readily in water.

Formulations available[1] (continued)

Brand name (Manufacturer)	Formulation and strength	Product information/Administration information
Clonidine (Sandoz)	Tablets 25 microgram	No specific data on enteral tube administration are available for this formulation.
Clonidine (extemporaneous preparation)	Suspension	*Extemporaneous clonidine suspension 0.1 mg/mL:* Clonidine 300 microgram tablets 10 tablets Sterile water 1–2 mL Simple syrup to 30 mL Expiry 28 days in a refrigerator.[4]

Site of absorption (oral administration)

Specific absorption site is not documented. Clonidine is well absorbed when administered orally. Peak plasma concentration occurs 3–5 hours after administration.[5]

Alternative routes available

Parenteral is formulation available.

Interactions

No specific interaction with food is documented.[6, 7]

Health and safety

Standard precautions apply.

Suggestions/recommendations

- Use 100 microgram tablets, disperse in water immediately prior to administration.
- A prolonged break in feeding is not required.

Intragastric administration

1. Stop the enteral feed.
2. Flush the enteral feeding tube with the recommended volume of water.
3. Place the tablet in the barrel of an appropriate size and type of syringe.
4. Draw 10 mL of water into the syringe and allow the tablet to disperse, shaking if necessary.
5. Flush the medication dose down the feeding tube.
6. Draw another 10 mL of water into the syringe and also flush this via the feeding tube (this will rinse the syringe and ensure that the total dose is administered).
7. Finally, flush with the recommended volume of water.
8. Re-start the feed, unless a prolonged break is required.

Alternatively, at step (3) place the tablet into a medicine pot, add 10 mL of water and allow the tablet to disperse. Draw this into an appropriate syringe. Ensure that the measure is rinsed and that this rinsing water is administered also to ensure that the total dose is given.

Intrajejunal administration

Owing to the lack of data, administer using the above method. Monitor for increased side-effects or loss of efficacy.

References

1. *BNF* 50, September 2005.
2. Personal communication, Boehringer Ingelheim; 6 March 2003.
3. BPNG data on file, 2005.
4. Levinson ML, Johnson CE. Stability of an extemporaneously compounded clonidine hydrochloride oral liquid. *Am J Hosp Pharm*. 1992; 49: 122–125.
5. Catapres (Boehringer Ingelheim), Summary of Product Characteristics; November 2003.
6. Dollery C. *Therapeutic Drugs*, 2nd edn. London: Churchill Livingstone; 1998.
7. Sweetman SC, ed. *Martindale*, 34th edn. London: Pharmaceutical Press; 2005.

Clopidogrel

Formulations available[1]

Brand name (Manufacturer)	Formulation and strength	Product information/Administration information
Plavix (Bristol-Myers Squibb)	Tablets 75 mg	Film-coated. Although the manufacturer has no specific information on this route of administration, there are likely to be alteration in the pharmacokinetics if the tablets are crushed. However, this is unlikely to cause any adverse effects.[2] The tablets can be crushed and mixed with water and flushed down a feeding tube.[2] The tablets do not disperse readily in water. They can be crushed (although this is difficult owing to the coating) and then mixed with 10 mL water; the resulting suspension can then be flushed down an 8Fr NG feeding tube without blockage.[3]

Site of absorption (oral administration)

Specific site of absorption is not documented. The active metabolite cannot be detected in the plasma and therefore time to reach peak plasma concentration has not been defined.[4]

Alternative routes available

None.

Interactions

No specific interaction with food is documented.

Health and safety

Standard precautions apply.

Suggestions/recommendations

- Crush tablets and disperse in water immediately prior to administration.
- A prolonged break in feeding is not required.

Intragastric administration

1. Stop the enteral feed.
2. Flush the enteral feeding tube with the recommended volume of water.
3. Place the tablet in mortar and crush to a fine powder using the pestle.
4. Add a few millilitres of water and mix to form a paste.
5. Add up to 15 mL of water and mix thoroughly ensuring that there are no large particles of tablet.
6. Draw this into an appropriate size and type of syringe.
7. Flush the medication dose down the feeding tube.
8. Add another 15 mL of water to the mortar and stir to ensure that any remaining drug is rinsed from the container. Draw this water into the syringe and also flush this via the feeding tube (this will rinse the mortar and syringe and ensure that the total dose is administered).
9. Finally, flush the enteral feeding tube with the recommended volume of water.
10. Re-start the feed, unless a prolonged break is required.

Intrajejunal administration

There are no specific reports of jejunal administration of clopidogrel. Administer as above.

References

1. *BNF* 50, September 2005.
2. Personal communication, Bristol-Myers Squibb; 20 January 2003.
3. BPNG data on file, 2004.
4. Plavix (Bristol-Myers Squibb), Summary of Product Characteristics; January 2005.

Co-amilofruse

Formulations available[1]

Brand name (Manufacturer)	Formulation and strength	Product information/Administration information
Co-amilofruse (Alpharma, CP, Helios, Hillcross, Sandoz)	Tablets 2.5 mg/20 mg	Amiloride 2.5 mg/furosemide 20 mg All tablets are immediate-release and in theory can be crushed. Alpharma brand can be crushed.[2] CP brand tablets disperse in 10 mL of water within 2 minutes to give a fine dispersion that flushes via an 8Fr NG tube without blockage.[3]
Co-amilofruse (Alpharma, APS, Ashbourne, Borg, CP, Helios, Hillcross, IVAX, Sandoz, Sovereign)	Tablets 5 mg/40 mg	Amiloride 5 mg/furosemide 40 mg All tablets are immediate-release and in theory can be crushed. Alpharma brand can be crushed.[2] CP brand tablets disperse in 10 mL of water within 2–5 minutes to give a fine dispersion, with some visible particles, that flushes via an 8Fr NG tube without blockage; risk of blocking finer bore tubes.[3]
Co-amilofruse (CP, Helios)	Tablets 10 mg/80 mg	Amiloride 10 mg/furosemide 80 mg All tablets are immediate-release and in theory can be crushed.

Site of absorption (oral administration)

Amiloride and furosemide are absorbed in the proximal small bowel; see monographs on individual components.

Alternative routes available

Furosemide injection is available.

Interactions

No specific interaction with food is documented.

Health and safety

Standard precautions apply.

Suggestions/recommendations

- Tablets can be dispersed in water, or crushed and mixed with water immediately prior to administration.
- A break in feeding is not required.
- For very fine-bore tubes, consider using the individual components as liquid preparations (see monographs).

Intragastric administration

1. Stop the enteral feed.
2. Flush the enteral feeding tube with the recommended volume of water.
3. Place the tablet in the barrel of an appropriate size and type of syringe.
4. Draw 10 mL of water into the syringe and allow the tablet to disperse, shaking if necessary.
5. Flush the medication dose down the feeding tube.
6. Draw another 10 mL of water into the syringe and also flush this via the feeding tube (this will rinse the syringe and ensure that the total dose is administered).
7. Finally, flush with the recommended volume of water.
8. Re-start the feed, unless a prolonged break is required.

Alternatively, at step (3) place the tablet into a medicine pot, add 10 mL of water and allow the tablet to disperse. Draw this into an appropriate syringe. Ensure that the measure is rinsed and that this rinsing water is administered also to ensure that the total dose is given.

Intrajejunal administration

Bioavailability is unlikely to be affected by jejunal administration. Administer using the above method.

References

1. *BNF* 50, September 2005.
2. Personal communication, Alpharma; 21 January 2003.
3. BPNG data on file, 2004.

Co-amilozide

Formulations available[1]

Brand name (Manufacturer)	Formulation and strength	Product information/Administration information
Co-amilozide (CP, Bristol-Myers Squibb)	Tablets 2.5 mg/25 mg	Amiloride 2.5 mg/hydrochlorthiazide 25 mg. CP brand tablets disintegrate rapidly in 10 mL of water to form a coarse dispersion that settles quickly but flushes via an 8Fr NG tube without blockage.[2]
Co-amilozide (Alpharma, APS, CP, Bristol-Myers Squibb, Hillcross, IVAX)	Tablets 5 mg/50 mg	Amiloride 5 mg/hydrochlorthiazide 50 mg. Tablets can be crushed and dispersed in water.[3] APS brand tablets disperse in 10 mL of water if shaken vigorously for a few minutes; the resulting dispersion flushes via an 8Fr NG tube without blockage.[2]

Site of absorption (oral administration)

Both drugs are absorbed well from the small intestine. Onset of action of both drugs occurs within 2 hours of administration.[4]

Alternative routes available

None. Other diuretics are available in parenteral formulations.

Interactions

No specific interaction with food is documented.

Health and safety

Standard precautions apply.

Suggestions/recommendations

- Disperse the tablets in water immediately prior to administration.
- A prolonged break in feeding is not required.

Intragastric administration

1. Stop the enteral feed.
2. Flush the enteral feeding tube with the recommended volume of water.
3. Place the tablet in the barrel of an appropriate size and type of syringe.
4. Draw 10 mL of water into the syringe and allow the tablet to disperse, shaking if necessary.
5. Flush the medication dose down the feeding tube.
6. Draw another 10 mL of water into the syringe and also flush this via the feeding tube (this will rinse the syringe and ensure that the total dose is administered).
7. Finally, flush with the recommended volume of water.
8. Re-start the feed, unless a prolonged break is required.

Alternatively, at step (3) place the tablet into a medicine pot, add 10 mL of water and allow the tablet to disperse. Draw this into an appropriate syringe. Ensure that the measure is rinsed and that this rinsing water is administered also to ensure that the total dose is given.

Intrajejunal administration

Administer using the above method. Monitor for increased side-effects or loss of efficacy.

References

1. *BNF 50*, September 2005.
2. BPNG data on file, 2005.
3. Personal communication, Alpharma; 21 January 2003.
4. Moduretic (Bristol-Myers Squibb), Summary of Product Characteristics; October 2003.

Co-amoxiclav

Formulations available[1]

Brand name (Manufacturer)	Formulation and strength	Product information/Administration information
Co-amoxiclav (various manufacturers)	Tablets 250/125 mg, 500/125 mg	Tablets do not disperse readily in water.[2]
Co-amoxiclav (APS, Generics, IVAX, Sterwin)	Oral suspension 125/31 mg/5 mL, 260/62 mg/5 mL	No specific data on enteral tube administration are available for this formulation.
Augmentin (GSK)	Tablets 375 mg, 625 mg	No specific data on enteral tube administration are available for this formulation.
Augmentin (GSK)	Dispersible tablets 250/125 mg	Large tablet, disperses in 10 mL of water within 2 minutes to form a milky suspension that flushes easily with little resistance.[2]
Augmentin (GSK)	Suspension 125/31 mg/5 mL, 250/62 mg/5 mL	When reconstituted is an off-white, creamy suspension, very resistant to flushing. Mixes with an equal volume of water only if shaken.[2]
Augmentin (GSK)	Injection 600 mg, 1.2 g	No specific data on enteral tube administration are available for this formulation.
Augmentin Duo (GSK)	Suspension 400/57 mg/5 mL	No specific data on enteral tube administration are available for this formulation.

Site of absorption (oral administration)

Specific site is not documented. Peak plasma concentration occurs within 1 hour following oral administration.[3]

Alternative routes available

Co-amoxiclav injection is available for parenteral administration.

Interactions

No specific interaction with food is documented. Absorption of Augmentin is optimised at the start of a meal.[3]

Health and safety

Standard precautions apply.

Suggestions/recommendations

- Use dispersible tablets.
- Disperse in water immediately prior to administration.
- Administer at the start of feed if practicable.

Intragastric administration

1. Stop the enteral feed.
2. Flush the enteral feeding tube with the recommended volume of water.
3. Place the tablet in the barrel of an appropriate size and type of syringe.
4. Draw 10 mL of water into the syringe and allow the tablet to disperse.
5. Flush the medication dose down the feeding tube.
6. Draw an equal volume of water into the syringe and also flush this via the feeding tube (this will rinse the syringe and ensure that the total dose is administered).
7. Finally, flush with the recommended volume of water.
8. Re-start the feed, unless a prolonged break is required.

Alternatively, at step (3) place the tablet into a medicine pot, add 10 mL of water and allow the tablet to disperse. Draw this into an appropriate syringe. Ensure that the measure is rinsed and that this rinsing water is administered also to ensure that the total dose is given.

Intrajejunal administration

There are no specific data on jejunal administration. Administer using the above method.

References

1. *BNF* 50, September 2005.
2. BPNG data on file, 2005.
3. Augmentin (GSK), Summary of Product Characteristics; 16 November 2005.

Co-codamol

Formulations available

(Owing to the large number of formulations available, only those that might be considered suitable are included below.)[1]

Brand name (Manufacturer)	Formulation and strength	Product information/Administration information
Co-codamol 8/500 Co-codamol 8/500 (Generics, Roche Consumer Health, Sandoz, Sterwin)	Dispersible tablets 8 mg/500 mg	Roche brand contains 420 mg sodium (18 mmol) per tablet.[2] Sterwin brand contains 388 mg sodium (16.9 mmol) per tablet.[7] Generics and Lagap brand contains 438 mg sodium (19.1 mmol) per tablet.[8]

Formulations available (continued)

Brand name (Manufacturer)	Formulation and strength	Product information/Administration information
Co-codamol 30/500 Kapake (Galen)	Effervescent tablets 30 mg/500 mg	Each tablets contains 388 mg (16.9 mmol) sodium. [1]
Co-codamol (Sterwin)	Effervescent tablets 30 mg/500 mg	Each tablets contains 388 mg (16.9 mmol) sodium. [7]
Solpadol (Sanofi-Synthelabo)	Effervescent tablets 30 mg/500 mg	Each tablet contains 16.9 mmol sodium (388 mg) [3]. Tablet will disperse adequately in 10 mL of water with insignificant residue giving no risk of tube blockage. [6]
Tylex (Schwarz)	Effervescent tablets 30 mg/500 mg	Each tablet contains 312.9 mg Sodium (13.7 mmol). [4]
Co-codamol 60/1000 Kapake (Galen)	Sachets 60 mg/1000 mg	No specific data on enteral tube administration are available for this formulation.

Site of absorption (oral administration)

Paracetamol is absorbed rapidly following oral administration. Administration into the jejunum achieves similar plasma concentrations to oral administration. [5]

Alternative routes available

Rectal and parenteral routes are available for paracetamol; parenteral route is available for codeine.

Interactions

No interaction with food or enteral feed is documented.

Health and safety

Standard precautions apply.

Suggestions/recommendations

- Use tablets dispersed in 50 mL of water (for adults) for intragastric or intrajejunal administration. If the sodium content is problematical, use liquid preparations of individual components (see monographs).
- Suppositories or injection can be considered useful alternatives.

Intragastric administration

1. Stop the enteral feed.
2. Flush the enteral feeding tube with the recommended volume of water.
3. Measure 50 mL of water into a measuring pot.
4. Add the effervescent tablet and allow to dissolve.
5. Draw into an appropriate size and type of syringe.
6. Flush the medication dose down the feeding tube.
7. Rinse the measure with 10–20 mL of water and administer this also to ensure that the total dose is given.
8. Finally, flush with the recommended volume of water.
9. Re-start the feed, unless a prolonged break is required.

Intrajejunal administration

Administer using the above method. Bioavailability should be unaffected.

References

1. *BNF 50*, September 2005.
2. Co-codamol Effervescent (Roche), Summary of Product Characteristics; March 1999.
3. Solpadol (Sanofi), Summary of Product Characteristics; October 2004.
4. Tylex (Schwarz), Summary of Product Characteristics; May 2005.
5. Adams D. Administration of drugs through a jejunostomy tube. *Br J Intensive Care*, 1994; 4(1): 10–17.
6. BPNG data on file, 2004.
7. Personal communication, Sterwin; 26 July 2005.
8. *Nottingham Prescriber*. 2002; 7(3): 1.

Codeine phosphate

Formulations available[1]

Brand name (Manufacturer)	Formulation and strength	Product information/Administration information
Codeine (various manufacturers)	Tablets 15 mg, 30 mg, 60 mg	No specific data on enteral tube administration are available for this formulation.
Codeine (various manufacturers)	Syrup BPC 25 mg/5 mL	Syrup based formulation. Very viscous, difficult to flush via an 8Fr NG tube. Mixes with an equal volume of water, which reduces resistance to flushing.[2]
Codeine (various manufacturers)	Injection 60 mg/mL	No specific data on enteral tube administration are available for this formulation.

Site of absorption (oral administration)

Specific site is not documented. Peak plasma concentration occurs within 1 hour of oral dosing.[3]

Alternative routes available

Parenteral route is available.

Interactions

No interactions are documented.

Health and safety

Standard precautions apply.

Suggestions/recommendations

- Use a liquid preparation. Dilute immediately before use.
- A prolonged break in feeding is not required.

Intragastric administration

1. Stop the enteral feed.
2. Flush the enteral feeding tube with the recommended volume of water.
3. Draw the medication syrup into an appropriate size and type of syringe.
4. Draw an equal volume of water and a little air into the syringe and shake to mix thoroughly.
5. Flush the medication dose down the feeding tube.
6. Draw an equal volume of water into the syringe and also flush this via the feeding tube (this will rinse the syringe and ensure that the total dose is administered).
7. Finally, flush with the recommended volume of water.
8. Re-start the feed, unless a prolonged break is required.

Alternatively, at step (3) measure the medicine in a suitable container and then add an equal volume of water and mix thoroughly. Draw this into an appropriate syringe. Ensure that the measure is rinsed and that this rinsing water is administered also to ensure that the total dose is given. **Do not** measure liquid medicines using a catheter-tipped syringe as this results in excessive dosing owing to the volume of the tip.

Intrajejunal administration

Administer using the above method. Consider diluting liquid with 3–4 times the dose volume of water to reduce osmolarity.

References

1. *BNF* 50, September 2005.
2. BPNG data on file, 2005.
3. Dollery C. *Therapeutic Drugs*, 2nd edn. London: Churchill Livingstone; 1998.

Colchicine

Formulations available[1]

Brand name (Manufacturer)	Formulation and strength	Product information/Administration information
Colchicine (Celltech, CP, IVAX)	Tablets 500 microgram	Tablets can be crushed.[2] Celltech tablets disperse within 2 minutes when placed in 10 mL of water to give a coarse dispersion that breaks up further when drawn into the syringe. Flushes via an 8Fr NG tube without blockage.[3]

Site of absorption (oral administration)

Specific site of absorption is not documented. Peak plasma concentration occurs 2 hours following oral dosing.[4]

Alternative routes available

None available for colchicines. An intra-articular injection of steroids could be considered for acute monoarticular gout if clinically appropriate.

Interactions

No specific interaction with food documented.

Health and safety

Standard precautions apply.

Suggestions/recommendations

- Disperse the tablets in water immediately prior to administration.
- A prolonged break in feeding is not required.

Intragastric administration

1. Stop the enteral feed.
2. Flush the enteral feeding tube with the recommended volume of water.
3. Place the tablet in the barrel of an appropriate size and type of syringe.
4. Draw 10 mL of water into the syringe and allow the tablet to disperse, shaking if necessary.
5. Flush the medication dose down the feeding tube.
6. Draw another 10 mL of water into the syringe and also flush this via the feeding tube (this will rinse the syringe and ensure that the total dose is administered).
7. Finally, flush with the recommended volume of water.
8. Re-start the feed, unless a prolonged break is required.

Alternatively, at step (3) place the tablet into a medicine pot, add 10 mL of water and allow the tablet to disperse. Draw this into an appropriate syringe. Ensure that the measure is rinsed and that this rinsing water is administered also to ensure that the total dose is given.

Intrajejunal administration

There are no specific data on jejunal administration. Administer using the above method. Monitor for increased side-effects or loss of efficacy.

References

1. *BNF* 50, September 2005.
2. Personal communication, Celltech; 31 March 2003.
3. BPNG data on file, 2005.
4. Colchicine (Celltech), Summary of Product Characteristics; July 2001.

Co-phenotrope

Formulations available[1]

Brand name (Manufacturer)	Formulation and strength	Product information/Administration information
Lomotil (Goldshield)	Tablets 2.5 mg/25 microgram	Diphenoxylate hydrochloride 2.5 mg, atropine sulfate 25 microgram. Tablets disperse in 10 mL of water within 5 minutes when agitated to give very fine white dispersion that flushes down an 8Fr NG tube without blockage.[2]

Site of absorption (oral administration)

Specific site of absorption is not documented. Atropine is readily absorbed from the GI tract, mucous membranes, the eye and intact skin.[3] Diphenoxylate hydrochloride is well absorbed from the GI tract.

Alternative routes available

None.

Interactions

No specific interaction with food is documented.

Health and safety

Standard precautions apply.

Suggestions/recommendations

- Disperse tablets in water immediately prior to administration.
- Consider changing therapy to loperamide (see monograph).

Intragastric administration

1. Stop the enteral feed.
2. Flush the enteral feeding tube with the recommended volume of water.
3. Place the tablet in the barrel of an appropriate size and type of syringe.
4. Draw 10 mL of water into the syringe and allow the tablet to disperse, shaking if necessary.
5. Flush the medication dose down the feeding tube.
6. Draw another 10 mL of water into the syringe and also flush this via the feeding tube (this will rinse the syringe and ensure that the total dose is administered).
7. Finally, flush with the recommended volume of water.
8. Re-start the feed, unless a prolonged break is required.

Alternatively, at step (3) place the tablet into a medicine pot, add 10 mL of water and allow the tablet to disperse. Draw this into an appropriate syringe. Ensure that the measure is rinsed and that this rinsing water is administered also to ensure that the total dose is given.

Intrajejunal administration

There is no specific information on jejunal administration. Administer using the above method.

References

1. *BNF* 50, September 2005.
2. BPNG data on file, 2004.
3. Sweetman SC, ed. *Martindale*, 34th edn. London: Pharmaceutical Press; 2005.

Co-trimoxazole

Contains a mixture of trimethoprim and sulfamethoxazole in the proportions of 1 part to 5 parts.

Formulations available[1]

Brand name (Manufacturer)	Formulation and strength	Product information/Administration information
Co-trimoxazole (Alpharma, DDSA, Hillcross, IVAX)	Tablets 480 mg, 960 mg	Alpharma does not recommend crushing tablets as there are alternative formulations available.[2]
Co-trimoxazole (IVAX)	Paediatric oral suspension 240 mg/5 mL	No specific data on enteral tube administration are available for this formulation.
Co-trimoxazole (Kent)	Oral suspension 480 mg/5 mL	No specific data on enteral tube administration are available for this formulation.
Co-trimoxazole (Mayne)	Injection 96 mg/mL (5 mL, 10 mL)	No specific data on enteral tube administration are available for this formulation.

Formulations available (continued)

Brand name (Manufacturer)	Formulation and strength	Product information/Administration information
Septrin (GSK)	Tablets 480 mg, 960 mg	GSK has no information on the administration of Septrin products via NG or PEG tubes. [3]
Septrin (GSK)	Paediatric oral suspension 240 mg/5 mL	Extremely viscous creamy suspension. Very difficult to flush via a fine-bore tube. Does not mix readily with water owing to its viscosity; requires shaking. Mixing with 2–3 times the volume with water reduces the viscosity sufficiently to facilitate flushing via a fine-bore tube. [4] Contains sorbitol. [3]
Septrin (GSK)	Adult suspension 480 mg/5 mL	Creamy, very viscous suspension, very resistant to flushing. Mixes with an equal volume of water if shaken, this reduces resistance to flushing. Viscosity is less than that of paediatric liquid. [4]
Septrin (GSK)	Injection 96 mg/mL (5 mL)	No specific data on enteral tube administration.

Site of absorption (oral administration)

Specific site is not documented. Peak plasma concentration occurs 1–4 hours following oral administration. [5]

Alternative routes available

Parenteral route is available, no change in dose is required.

Interactions

The presence of food does not delay or reduce absorption. [5]

Health and safety

Standard precautions apply.

Suggestions/recommendations

- Use a liquid preparation. Dilute with 2–3 times volume of water (immediately before use) and shake well before administration.
- A prolonged break in feeding is not required.

Intragastric administration

1. Stop the enteral feed.
2. Flush the enteral feeding tube with the recommended volume of water.
3. Shake the medication bottle thoroughly to ensure adequate mixing.
4. Draw the medication suspension into an appropriate size and type of syringe.
5. Draw 2–3 times the dosage volume of water and a little air into the syringe and shake to mix thoroughly.
6. Flush the medication dose down the feeding tube.
7. Draw an equal volume of water into the syringe and also flush this via the feeding tube (this will rinse the syringe and ensure that the total dose is administered).
8. Finally, flush with the recommended volume of water.
9. Re-start the feed, unless a prolonged break is required.

Alternatively, at step (4) measure the medicine in a suitable container and then add 2–3 times the dose volume of water and mix thoroughly. Draw this into an appropriate syringe. Ensure that the measure is rinsed and that this rinsing water is administered also to ensure that the total dose is given. **Do not** measure liquid medicines using a catheter-tipped syringe as this results in excessive dosing owing to the volume of the tip.

Intrajejunal administration

There are no specific data relating to jejunal administration. Administer as above but dilute the dose with at least three times the volume of water to reduce osmolarity.

References

1. *BNF* 50, September 2005.
2. Personal communication, Alpharma; 21 January 2003.
3. Personal communication, GSK; 22 January 2003.
4. BPNG data on file, 2005.
5. Septrin Oral Products (GSK), Summary of Product Characteristics; 22 June 2005.

Cyclizine

Formulations available[1]

Brand name (Manufacturer)	Formulation and strength	Product information/Administration information
Valoid (Amdipharm)	Tablets 50 mg	Scored. Cyclizine hydrochloride. Tablets do not disintegrate readily in water, but will disperse if shaken in 10 mL of water for 5 minutes, resulting in a fine dispersion that flushes down an 8Fr NG tube without blockage.[2]
Valoid (Amdipharm)	Injection 50 mg/mL (1 mL)	Can be given i.m. or i.v. Cyclizine lactate. No specific data on enteral tube administration are available for this formulation.

Site of absorption (oral administration)

Oral cyclizine is absorbed via the GI tract, with an onset of action within 2 h.[3]

Alternative routes available

Parenteral route is available.

Interactions

No specific interaction with food is documented.[3]

Health and safety

Standard precautions apply.

Suggestions/recommendations

- As cyclizine tablets do not disperse readily in water, consider changing to an alternative antihistamine antiemetic such as promethazine (see monograph), or, if sedation is problematical, consider using a phenothiazine such as prochlorperazine (see monograph).
- Alternatively the tablets can be dispersed in water if shaken for 5 minutes; the resulting dispersion should be administered immediately.
- The injection could be used for short-term management.
- A prolonged break in feeding is not necessary.

Intragastric administration

1. Stop the enteral feed.
2. Flush the enteral feeding tube with the recommended volume of water.
3. Place the tablet in the barrel of an appropriate size and type of syringe.
4. Draw 10 mL of water into the syringe and allow the tablet to disperse, shaking as required.
5. Flush the medication dose down the feeding tube.
6. Draw another 10 mL of water into the syringe and also flush this via the feeding tube (this will rinse the syringe and ensure that the total dose is administered).
7. Finally, flush with the recommended volume of water.
8. Re-start the feed, unless a prolonged break is required.

Alternatively, at step (3) place the tablet into a medicine pot, add 10 mL of water and allow the tablet to disperse. Draw this into an appropriate syringe. Ensure that the measure is rinsed and that this rinsing water is administered also to ensure that the total dose is given.

Intrajejunal administration

There is no specific information relating to jejunal administration of cyclizine. Administer using the above method.

References

1. *BNF* 50, September 2005.
2. BPNG data on file, 2004.
3. Sweetman SC, ed. *Martindale*, 34th edn. London: Pharmaceutical Press; 2005.

Cyclophosphamide

Formulations available[1]

Brand name (Manufacturer)	Formulation and strength	Product information/Administration information
Cyclophosphamide (Pharmacia)	Tablets 50 mg	Tablet may be difficult to crush owing to small size. Possible health risk from dust exposure.[2]
Cyclophosphamide (Pharmacia)	Injection 500 mg, 1 g	The injection can be used to prepare a solution for oral use.[2]
Endoxana (Baxter Oncology)	Tablets 50 mg	No specific data on enteral tube administration are available for this formulation.
Endoxana (Baxter Oncology)	Injection 200 mg, 500 mg, 1 g	Can be administered enterally.[3]
Cyclophosphamide (Nova Labs)	Solution 25–100 mg/5 mL	Manufactured 'special'. 15 days shelf-life. Suitable for enteral tube administration.[4]

Site of absorption (oral administration)

Specific site of absorption is not documented. Peak plasma concentration occurs 1 hour after oral dosing.[5]

Alternative routes available

Parenteral route available.

Interactions

No specific interaction with food is documented.

Health and safety

Cytotoxic. Avoid crushing tablets. Handle as cytotoxic. Treat all contaminated waste, e.g. syringes, as cytotoxic waste.

Suggestions/recommendations

- Do not crush the tablets.
- Use the injection to prepare an oral solution. This should be undertaken in appropriate facilities.

Intragastric administration

1. Stop the enteral feed.
2. Flush the enteral feeding tube with the recommended volume of water.
3. Draw the medication solution into an appropriate size and type of syringe.
4. Flush the medication dose down the feeding tube.
5. Draw an equal volume of water into the syringe and also flush this via the feeding tube (this will rinse the syringe and ensure that the total dose is administered).
6. Finally, flush with the recommended volume of water.
7. Re-start the feed, unless a prolonged break is required.

Do not measure liquid medicines using a catheter-tipped syringe as this results in excessive dosing owing to the volume of the tip.

Intrajejunal administration

There are no specific data relating to jejunal administration of cyclophosphamide. Consideration should be given to using the parenteral route. Seek specialist advice. If clinically appropriate Administer using the above method.

References

1. *BNF 50*, September 2005.
2. Personal communication, Pharmacia; 11 March 2003.
3. Brooke D, Davis RE, Bequette RJ. Chemical stability of cyclophosphamide in aromatic elixir USP. *Am J Hosp Pharm*. 1973; 30: 618–620.
4. Personal communication, Nova Labs; 24 March 2005.
5. Cyclophosphamide Tablets (Pharmacia), Summary of Product Characteristics; 25 June 2005.

Dantron (Danthron)

Formulations available[1]

Brand name (Manufacturer)	Formulation and strength	Product information/Administration information
Co-danthramer (Napp)	Capsules 25 mg/200 mg, 37.5 mg/500 mg	Dantron 25 mg + poloxamer '188' 200 mg Dantron 37.5 mg + poloxamer '188' 500 mg No specific data on enteral administration are available for this formulation.
Co-danthramer (Hillcross, Napp, Sovereign, Pinewood)	Suspension 25 mg/200 mg in 5 mL, 75 mg/1000 mg in 5 mL	25 mg/200 mg in 5 mL liquid – quite viscous liquid but flushes down a fine bore tube with little resistance but requires flushing well.[2]

Formulations available[1] (continued)

Brand name (Manufacturer)	Formulation and strength	Product information/Administration information
Co-danthrusate (APS, Celltech, Galen, Hillcross, IVAX, Sterwin)	Capsules 50 mg/60 mg	Dantron 50 mg + docusate 60 mg No specific data on enteral tube administration are available for this formulation.
Co-danthrusate (Celltech)	Suspension 50 mg/60 mg	Dantron 50 mg + docusate 60 mg per 5 mL dose No specific data on enteral tube administration are available for this formulation.

Site of absorption (oral administration)

Dantron is partially absorbed in the small intestine.[3] The other constituents of the combination products – poloxamer and docusate – are both wetting agents and are not absorbed.

Alternative routes available

Not applicable.

Interactions

No significant interaction with food.

Health and safety

Standard precautions apply.

Suggestions/recommendations

- Use a liquid preparation. Flush well after dosing.
- A prolonged break in feeding is not required.

Intragastric administration

1. Stop the enteral feed.
2. Flush the enteral feeding tube with the recommended volume of water.
3. Draw the medication solution into an appropriate size and type of syringe.
4. Flush the medication dose down the feeding tube.
5. Finally, flush with the recommended volume of water.
6. Re-start the feed, unless a prolonged break is required.

Alternatively, at step (3) measure the medicine in a suitable container and then draw into an appropriate syringe. Ensure that the measure is rinsed and that this rinsing water is administered also to ensure that the total dose is given. **Do not** measure liquid medicines using a catheter-tipped syringe as this results in excessive dosing owing to the volume of the tip.

Intrajejunal administration

Administration into the jejunum is unlikely to affect pharmacological response. Administer using the above method.

References

1. *BNF 50*, September 2005.
2. BPNG data on file, 2004.
3. Co-danthramer (Napp), Summary of Product Characteristics; July 2002.

Deflazacort

Formulations available[1]

Brand name (Manufacturer)	Formulation and strength	Product information/Administration information
Calcort (Shire)	Tablets 1 mg, 6 mg, 30 mg	Tablets can be crushed.[2] Tablets disintegrate rapidly when placed in 10 mL of water, to produce a fine white dispersion that flushes down an 8Fr NG tube without blockage.[3]

Site of absorption (oral administration)

Deflazacort is rapidly absorbed following oral administration. Peak plasma concentration of the active metabolite is found in the plasma after 1.5–2 hours.[4]

Alternative routes available

None available for deflazacort, other steroids available in parenteral and rectal formulations.

Interactions

No specific interaction with food is documented.

Health and safety

Standard precautions apply.

Suggestions/recommendations

- Disperse the tablets in water immediately prior to administration.
- A prolonged break in feeding is not required.

Intragastric administration

1. Stop the enteral feed.
2. Flush the enteral feeding tube with the recommended volume of water.
3. Place the tablet in the barrel of an appropriate size and type of syringe.
4. Draw 10 mL of water into the syringe and allow the tablet to disperse, shaking if necessary.
5. Flush the medication dose down the feeding tube.
6. Draw another 10 mL of water into the syringe and also flush this via the feeding tube (this will rinse the syringe and ensure that the total dose is administered).
7. Finally, flush with the recommended volume of water.
8. Re-start the feed, unless a prolonged break is required.

Alternatively, at step (4) place the tablet into a medicine pot, add 10 mL of water and allow the tablet to disperse. Draw this into an appropriate syringe. Ensure that the measure is rinsed and that this rinsing water is administered also to ensure that the total dose is given.

Intrajejunal administration

There are no specific data relating to the jejunal administration of deflazacort. Administer using the above method; monitor for increased side-effects or loss of efficacy.

References

1. *BNF* 50, September 2005.
2. Personal communication, Shire; 17 February 2003.
3. BPNG data on file, 2004.
4. Calcort (Shire), Summary of Product Characteristics; August 2002.

Desmopressin acetate

Formulations available[1]

Brand name (Manufacturer)	Formulation and strength	Product information/Administration information
DDAVP (Ferring)	Tablets 100 microgram, 200 microgram	Tablets can be crushed and dispersed in water;[2] this does not affect oral bioavailability.[3] Tablet disintegrates within 5 minutes when placed in 10 mL of water, the resulting dispersion flushes via an 8Fr NG tube without blockage.[4]
Desmotabs (Ferring)	Tablets 200 microgram	As above.
Desmopressin acetate (PLIVA)	Nasal spray 10 microgram/spray	Intranasal use only.
DDAVP Melt (Ferring)	Oral lyophilisate 60 microgram, 120 microgram	Oral lyophilisate, for sublingual use only;[6] not suitable for administration via enteral feeding tube.
DDAVP (Ferring)	Nasal solution 100 microgram/mL	Used for paediatric doses less than 10 microgram.
Desmospray (Ferring)	Nasal spray 10 microgram/spray	Intranasal use only.
Nocutil (Norgine)	Nasal spray 10 microgram/spray	Intranasal use only.
DDAVP (Ferring)	Injection 4 microgram/mL	Primarily for diagnostic use. Licensed for diabetes insipidus treatment.

Site of absorption (oral administration)

Following oral administration, absorption occurs primarily in the duodenum and proximal jejunum.[2] Desmopressin is also absorbed sublingually.[6]

Alternative routes available

Nasal, sublingual and parenteral route are available; indications for parenteral route are limited (consult SPC).

Interactions

A standardised 27% fat meal significantly reduced the absorption of oral desmopressin; however, the pharmacodynamic effect was unaffected.[5]

Health and safety

Standard precautions apply.

Suggestions/recommendations

- Convert to sublingual tablets or to intranasal administration where possible for long-term therapy. If necessary the conventional tablets can be dispersed in water immediately prior to administration, see below.
- A prolonged break in feeding is not required.

Intragastric administration

1. Stop the enteral feed.
2. Flush the enteral feeding tube with the recommended volume of water.
3. Place the tablet in the barrel of an appropriate size and type of syringe.
4. Draw 10 mL of water into the syringe and allow the tablet to disperse, shaking if necessary.
5. Flush the medication dose down the feeding tube.
6. Draw another 10 mL of water into the syringe and also flush this via the feeding tube (this will rinse the syringe and ensure that the total dose is administered).
7. Finally, flush with the recommended volume of water.
8. Re-start the feed, unless prolonged break required.

Alternatively, at step (3) place the tablet into a medicine pot, add 10 mL of water and allow the tablet to disperse. Draw this into an appropriate syringe. Ensure that the measure is rinsed and that this rinsing water is administered also to ensure that the total dose is given.

Intrajejunal administration

There are no data to support administration via this route; owing to the site of absorption it is possible that the bioavailability may be reduced. If indicated, use the method detailed above and monitor for loss of efficacy.

References

1. *BNF 50*, September 2005.
2. Personal communication, Ferring Pharmaceuticals; 20 January 2003.
3. Argenti D, Ireland D, Heald DL. A pharmacokinetic and pharmacodynamic comparison of desmopressin administered whole, chewed and crushed tablets, and as an oral solution. *J Urol.* 2001; 165(5): 1446–1451.
4. BPNG data on file, 2005.
5. DDAVP Tablets (Ferring), Summary of Product Characteristics; May 2003.
6. DDAVP Melt (Ferring), Summary of Product Characteristics; 19 January 2006.

Dexamethasone

Formulations available[1]

Brand name (Manufacturer)	Formulation and strength	Product information/Administration information
Dexamethasone (Organon)	Tablets 500 microgram, 2 mg	Tablets disperse quickly when placed in 10 mL of water; the dispersion settles quite quickly but flushes down an 8Fr NG tube without blockage.[2]
Dexamethasone (Rosemont)	Oral solution 2 mg/5 mL	Dexamethasone sodium phosphate. Contains sorbitol 0.49 g/5 mL.[3]
Dexamethasone (Mayne)	Injection 4 mg/mL, 24 mg/mL	Dexamethasone phosphate. No specific data on enteral tube administration are available for this formulation.
Dexamethasone (Organon)	Injection 5 mg/mL	Dexamethasone sodium phosphate. No specific data on enteral tube administration are available for this formulation.
Decadron (MSD)	Tablets 500 microgram	No specific data on enteral tube administration are available for this formulation.

Site of absorption (oral administration)

Dexamethasone is readily absorbed from the GI tract, peak plasma concentration occurs 1–2 hours following oral dosing.[4]

Alternative routes available

Parenteral formulation is available, can be administered via i.v, i.m. or s.c. routes and rectal drip.

Interactions

No specific interaction with food is documented.

Health and safety

Standard precautions apply.

Suggestions/recommendations

- Use oral solution. Alternatively, the tablets can be dispersed in water immediately prior to administration.
- A prolonged break in feeding is not required.

Intragastric administration

1. Stop the enteral feed.
2. Flush the enteral feeding tube with the recommended volume of water.
3. Draw the medication liquid into an appropriate size and type of syringe.
4. Flush the medication dose down the feeding tube.
5. Draw an equal volume of water into the syringe and also flush this via the feeding tube (this will rinse the syringe and ensure that the total dose is administered).
6. Finally, flush with the recommended volume of water.
7. Re-start the feed, unless a prolonged break is required.

Alternatively, at step (3) measure the medicine in a suitable container and then add an equal volume of water and mix thoroughly. Draw this into an appropriate syringe. Ensure that the measure is rinsed and that this rinsing water is administered also to ensure that the total dose is given. **Do not** measure liquid medicines using a catheter-tipped syringe as this results in excessive dosing owing to the volume of the tip.

Intrajejunal administration

The liquid can be administered using the above method. Alternatively, administer tablets using the method below.

1. Stop the enteral feed.
2. Flush the enteral feeding tube with the recommended volume of water.
3. Place the tablet in the barrel of an appropriate size and type of syringe.
4. Draw 10 mL of water into the syringe and allow the tablet to disperse, shaking if necessary.
5. Flush the medication dose down the feeding tube.
6. Draw another 10 mL of water into the syringe and also flush this via the feeding tube (this will rinse the syringe and ensure that the total dose is administered).
7. Finally, flush with the recommended volume of water.
8. Re-start the feed, unless a prolonged break is required.

Alternatively, at step (3) place the tablet into a medicine pot, add 10 mL of water and allow the tablet to disperse. Draw this into an appropriate syringe. Ensure that the measure is rinsed and that this rinsing water is administered also to ensure that the total dose is given.

References

1. *BNF* 50, September 2005.
2. BPNG data on file, 2004.
3. Personal communication, Rosemont; 20 January 2005.
4. Dexsol (Rosemont), Summary of Product Characteristics; September 2000.

Diazepam

Formulations available[1]

Brand name (Manufacturer)	Formulation and strength	Product information/Administration information
Diazepam (Alpharma, APS, Arrow, DDSA, Generics, IVAX, Ranbaxy)	Tablets 2 mg, 5 mg, 10 mg	Tablets can be crushed and dispersed in water.[2] APS brand tablets disperse in water within 2 minutes to give fine dispersion that does not block an 8Fr NG tube.[3]
Diazepam (Alpharma, Sandoz)	Oral solution 2 mg/5 mL	Slightly viscous liquid. Some resistance on flushing. Mixes with an equal volume of water to reduce resistance.[3]
Diazepam (Sandoz)	Strong oral solution 5 mg/5 mL	No specific data on enteral tube administration are available for this formulation.
Diazepam (CP, Phoenix)	Injection (solution) 5 mg/mL (2 mL)	For i.m. injection. No specific data on enteral tube administration are available for this formulation.
Diazepam (Alpharma)	Injection (emulsion) 5 mg/mL (2 mL)	For i.v. injection for infusion. Diazemuls.
Diazepam (Alpharma, CP, Sandoz)	Rectal tubes 2.5 mg, 5 mg, 10 mg	For rectal administration. No specific data on enteral tube administration are available for this formulation.
Diazepam (Durbin)	Suppositories 10 mg	For rectal administration.
Diazepam (Rosemont)	Suspension 2.5 mg/5 mL, 10 mg/5 mL	Manufactured 'special'. Contains 0.68 g sorbitol/5 mL dose.[4]

Site of absorption (oral administration)

Specific site is not documented. Peak plasma concentration occurs 15–90 minutes following oral administration.[5] The pharmacokinetics of the liquid preparation are similar to the tablet formulation.

Alternative routes available

Rectal and parenteral routes available.

Interactions

Specific interaction with food is not documented.

Health and safety

Standard precautions apply.

Suggestions/recommendations

- For intragastric use, use liquid preparation.
- For intrajejunal use consider using tablets dispersed in water to reduce osmolarity.
- A prolonged break in feeding is not required.
- The rectal or parenteral route can be used if GI absorption is compromised.

Intragastric administration

Liquid administration

1. Stop the enteral feed.
2. Flush the enteral feeding tube with the recommended volume of water.
3. Shake the medication bottle thoroughly to ensure adequate mixing.
4. Draw the medication suspension into an appropriate size and type of syringe.
5. Flush the medication dose down the feeding tube.
6. Finally, flush with the recommended volume of water.
7. Re-start the feed, unless a prolonged break is required.

Alternatively, at step (4) measure the medicine in a suitable container. Draw this into an appropriate syringe. Ensure that the measure is rinsed and that this rinsing water is administered also to ensure that the total dose is given. **Do not** measure liquid medicines using a catheter-tipped syringe as this results in excessive dosing owing to the volume of the tip.

Intrajejunal administration

Tablet administration

1. Stop the enteral feed.
2. Flush the enteral feeding tube with the recommended volume of water.
3. Place the tablet in the barrel of an appropriate size and type of syringe.
4. Draw 10 mL of water into the syringe and allow the tablet to disperse, shaking if necessary.
5. Flush the medication dose down the feeding tube.
6. Draw another 10 mL of water into the syringe and also flush this via the feeding tube (this will rinse the syringe and ensure that the total dose is administered).
7. Finally, flush with the recommended volume of water.
8. Re-start the feed, unless a prolonged break is required.

Alternatively, at step (3) place the tablet into a medicine pot, add 10 mL of water and allow the tablet to disperse. Draw this into an appropriate syringe. Ensure that the measure is rinsed and that this rinsing water is administered also to ensure that the total dose is given.

References

1. *BNF* 50, September 2005.
2. Personal communication, Alpharma; 21 January 2003.
3. BPNG data on file, 2004.
4. Personal communication, Rosemont; 20 January 2005.
5. Dollery C. *Therapeutic Drugs*, 2nd edn. London: Churchill Livingstone; 1998.

Diclofenac sodium

Formulations available[1]

Brand name (Manufacturer)	Formulation and strength	Product information/Administration information
Voltarol (Novartis)	Tablets 25 mg, 50 mg	Enteric coated – do not crush.
Voltarol (Novartis)	Dispersible tablet 50 mg	Tablet swells and disperses to give bright pink, cherry-flavoured dispersion. Flushes easily via an 8Fr NG tube.[2]
Voltarol (Novartis)	Injection 25 mg/mL (3 mL)	Licensed for i.m. and i.v. use. Maximum of 2 days' therapy recommended.[7]
Voltarol (Novartis)	Suppositories 12.5 mg, 25 mg, 50 mg, 100 mg	Rate of absorption is slower than enteric coated tablets; peak plasma concentrations are reached after 1 hour. Bioavailability is two-thirds that of equivalent oral dose.[8]
Diclofenac sodium (various manufacturers)	Tablets 25 mg, 50 mg	Enteric coated – do not crush.
Diclofenac sodium (Goldshield)	Suppositories 100 mg	Rectal administration.
Diclofenac sodium (Antigen)	Injection 25 mg/mL (3 mL)	Licensed for i.m. use only. No specific data on enteral tube administration are available for this formulation.
Voltarol Rapid (Novartis)	Tablets 25 mg, 50 mg	Sugar coated. Diclofenac potassium.
Diclofenac M/R (various manufacturers)	M/R tablets and M/R capsules 75 mg, 100 mg	Modified-release preparations – not suitable for administration via feeding tube.
Diclofenac (Rosemont)	Oral suspension 50 mg/5 mL	Unlicensed special product (12 month shelf life)[3]. Sugar-free oral liquid.
Diclofenac (Special Products Ltd)	Dispersible tablets 10 mg	Unlicensed special product. Tablets should be stirred in 10 mL of water for 2 minutes to dissolve the active drug. The suspension should be allowed to settle for 1 minute, then the clear solution can be drawn up and flushed down the feeding tube using a syringe.[4]

Formulations available [1] (continued)

Brand name (Manufacturer)	Formulation and strength	Product information/Administration information
Arthrotec (Pharmacia)	Tablets '50', '75'	'50' tablets contain 50 mg diclofenac + misoprostil 200 microgram. '75' tablets contain 75 mg diclofenac + misoprostil 200 microgram. Tablets contain diclofenac in an enteric coated core surrounded by misoprostil, and therefore should not be crushed. [5]

Site of absorption (oral administration)

Specific site of absorption is unknown. Time to peak plasma concentration varies depending on formulation used. [6] As enteric coated preparations are available it is unlikely that jejunal administration will affect bioavailability.

Alternative routes available

Rectal and parenteral routes are available, route does not affect dosing.

Interactions

No specific interaction with food is documented.

Health and safety

Standard precautions apply.

Suggestions/recommendations

- Use dispersible tablets. Disperse tablets in water immediately prior to administration. There should be no reduction in bioavailability from jejunal administration.
- For mild localised pain, consider topical NSAIDs; see BNF for further details.
- A prolonged break in feeding is not required.

Intragastric administration

1. Stop the enteral feed.
2. Flush the enteral feeding tube with the recommended volume of water.
3. Place the tablet in the barrel of an appropriate size and type of syringe.
4. Draw 10 mL of water into the syringe and allow the tablet to disperse, shaking if necessary.
5. Flush the medication dose down the feeding tube.
6. Draw an equal volume of water into the syringe and also flush this via the feeding tube (this will rinse the syringe and ensure that the total dose is administered).
7. Finally, flush with the recommended volume of water.
8. Re-start the feed, unless a prolonged break is required.

Alternatively, at step (3) place the tablet into a medicine pot, add 10 mL of water and allow the tablet to disperse. Draw this into an appropriate syringe. Ensure that the measure is rinsed and that this rinsing water is administered also to ensure that the total dose is given.

Intrajejunal administration

Administer as above.

References

1. *BNF* 50, September 2005.
2. BPNG data on file, 2004.
3. Personal communication, Rosemont; July 2004.
4. Personal communication, Special Products Ltd; 20 January 2003.
5. Personal communication, Pharmacia; 11 March 2003.
6. Dollery C. *Therapeutic Drugs*, 2nd edn. London: Churchill Livingstone; 1998.
7. Voltarol Ampoules (Novartis), Summary of Product Characteristics; December 2000.
8. Voltarol Suppositories (Novartis), Summary of Product Characteristics; June 2005.

Dicycloverine (Dicyclomine) hydrochloride

Formulations available[1]

Brand name (Manufacturer)	Formulation and strength	Product information/Administration information
Merbentyl (Florizel)	Tablets 10 mg, 20 mg	No specific data on enteral tube administration are available for this formulation.
Merbentyl (Florizel)	Syrup 10 mg/5 mL	Merbentyl syrup can be diluted with water immediately prior to administration.[2]

Site of absorption (oral administration)

Specific site of absorption is not documented. Peak plasma concentration occurs 1–1.5 hours post dose.[3]

Alternative routes available

None.

Interactions

There is no documented interaction with food.

Health and safety

Standard precautions apply.

Suggestions/recommendations

- Use the syrup, dilute with an equal volume of water immediately prior to administration to reduce viscosity; flush after administration.
- A prolonged break in feeding is not necessary.

Intragastric administration

1. Stop the enteral feed.
2. Flush the enteral feeding tube with the recommended volume of water.
3. Shake the medication bottle thoroughly to ensure adequate mixing.
4. Draw the medication suspension into an appropriate size and type of syringe.
5. Draw an equal volume of water and a little air into the syringe and shake to mix thoroughly.
6. Flush the medication dose down the feeding tube.
7. Draw an equal volume of water into the syringe and also flush this via the feeding tube (this will rinse the syringe and ensure that the total dose is administered).
8. Finally, flush with the recommended volume of water.
9. Re-start the feed, unless a prolonged break is required.

Alternatively, at step (4) measure the medicine in a suitable container and then add an equal volume of water and mix thoroughly. Draw this into an appropriate syringe. Ensure that the measure is rinsed and that this rinsing water is administered also to ensure that the total dose is given. **Do not** measure liquid medicines using a catheter-tipped syringe as this results in excessive dosing owing to the volume of the tip.

Intrajejunal administration

There are no specific data relating to the jejunal administration of dicycloverine. Administer using the above method.

References

1. *BNF 50*, September 2005.
2. Merbentyl Syrup (Florizel), Summary of Product Characteristics; February 2001.
3. Merbentyl Tablets (Florizel), Summary of Product Characteristics; December 2000.

Digitoxin

Formulations available[1]

Brand name (Manufacturer)	Formulation and strength	Product information/Administration information
Digitoxin (various manufacturers)	Tablets 100 microgram	The tablets are uncoated, so can be crushed. There are no bioavailability data from the use of crushed tablets.[2] Tablets disperse in water within 2 minutes to give a fine dispersion that flushes via an 8Fr NG tube without blockage.[3]

Site of absorption (oral administration)

Absorption is from the small intestine. Peak plasma concentration occurs 1.5–2.5 hours following an oral dose.[4]

Alternative routes available

Digoxin is available for parenteral administration.

Interactions

There is no specific documented interaction with food.[4]

Health and safety

Standard precautions apply.

Suggestions/recommendations

- Disperse the tablets in water immediately prior to administration.
- A prolonged break in feeding is not required.
- Consider changing to digoxin liquid.

Intragastric administration

1. Stop the enteral feed.
2. Flush the enteral feeding tube with the recommended volume of water.
3. Place the tablet in the barrel of an appropriate size and type of syringe.
4. Draw 10 mL of water into the syringe and allow the tablet to disperse, shaking if necessary.
5. Flush the medication dose down the feeding tube.
6. Draw another 10 mL of water into the syringe and also flush this via the feeding tube (this will rinse the syringe and ensure that the total dose is administered).
7. Finally, flush with the recommended volume of water.
8. Re-start the feed, unless a prolonged break is required.

Alternatively, at step (3) place the tablet into a medicine pot, add 10 mL of water and allow the tablet to disperse. Draw this into an appropriate syringe. Ensure that the measure is rinsed and that this rinsing water is administered also to ensure that the total dose is given.

Intrajejunal administration

There are no specific data relating to the jejunal administration of digitoxin. Administer using the above method. Monitor for increased side-effects or loss of efficacy. Digitoxin plasma concentrations can be monitored.

References

1. *BNF* 50, September 2005.
2. Personal communication, Celltech; 31 March 2003.
3. BPNG data on file, 2005.
4. Digitoxin (Celltech), Summary of Product Characteristics; July 2001.

Digoxin

Formulations available[1]

Brand name (Manufacturer)	Formulation and strength	Product information/Administration information
Digoxin (various manufacturers)	Tablets 62.5 microgram, 125 microgram, 150 microgram	No specific data on enteral tube administration are available for this formulation.

Formulations available[1] (continued)

Brand name (Manufacturer)	Formulation and strength	Product information/Administration information
Digoxin (Antigen)	Injection 250 microgram/mL	No specific data on enteral tube administration are available for this formulation.
Digoxin (BCM specials)	Paediatric injection 100 microgram/mL	No specific data on enteral tube administration are available for this formulation.
Lanoxin (GSK)	Tablets 125 microgram, 250 microgram	Bioavailability approximately 63%.[2] No specific data on enteral tube administration are available for this formulation.
Lanoxin (GSK)	Injections 250 microgram/mL	No specific data on enteral tube administration are available for this formulation.
Lanoxin-PG (GSK)	Tablets 62.5 microgram	No specific data on enteral tube administration are available for this formulation.
Lanoxin-PG (GSK)	Elixir 50 microgram/mL	Do not dilute.[2] Bioavailability is approximately 75%.[2] Does not contain sorbitol.[2] Bright yellow liquid, slightly viscous, flushes via an 8Fr NG tube with very little resistance.[3]

Site of absorption (oral administration)

Absorption of digoxin is mainly from the proximal small intestine. Gastric absorption is minimal. Absorption is not affected by gastrectomy or jejunoileal bypass.[4] Case reports have suggested that absorption of digoxin is not compromised when administered via jejunostomy tube.[5] However, owing to the difference in pharmacokinetics properties between the tablets and liquid formulation, plasma concentrations should be monitored following any administration changes. Absorption may be reduced in malabsorption syndromes and following reconstructive surgery; increased doses may be necessary.[2]

Alternative routes available

Parenteral route is available. The SPC recommends dose reduction of 33% when changing from oral to i.v. route.

Interactions

Absorption of digoxin is slowed and reduced by concurrent intake of high-fibre (high-hemicellulose) meals. Although this is thought to be clinically insignificant, plasma concentrations should be checked when using a high-fibre feed (e.g. Jevity).

Health and safety

Standard precautions apply.

Suggestions/recommendations

- Use liquid preparation. Although in theory a dose reduction is indicated, in practice it is unlikely to be clinically important. If the patient is on a high-fibre feed, administer during a break in the regimen if possible. If on a standard feed, a prolonged break in feeding is not required.
- The liquid formulation has a high osmolarity, but dose volumes are small; therefore, flushing well with water immediately post dose should reduce any possibility of related side-effects.

Intragastric administration

1. Stop the enteral feed.
2. Flush the enteral feeding tube with the recommended volume of water.
3. Draw the medication solution into an appropriate size and type of syringe.
4. Flush the medication dose down the feeding tube.
5. Finally, flush with the recommended volume of water.
6. Re-start the feed, unless a prolonged break is required.

Alternatively, at step (3) measure the medicine in a suitable container and then draw into the syringe with an appropriate adapter for the tube connector. Ensure that the measure is rinsed and that this rinsing water is administered also to ensure that the total dose is given. **Do not** measure liquid medicines using a catheter-tipped syringe as this results in excessive dosing owing to the volume of the tip.

Intrajejunal administration

Administer using the above method. Plasma concentration can be monitored.

References

1. *BNF* 50, September 2005.
2. Lanoxin PG Elixir (GSK), Summary of Product Characteristics; 21 May 2003.
3. BPNG data on file, 2005.
4. Personal communication, GSK; 22 January 2003.
5. Adams D. Administration of drugs through a jejunostomy tube. *Br J Intensive Care*. 1994; 4(1): 10–17.

Dihydrocodeine tartrate

Formulations available[1]

Brand name (Manufacturer)	Formulation and strength	Product information/Administration information
Dihydrocodeine (various manufacturers)	Tablets 30 mg	Tablets can be crushed, but liquid preparation is available.[2]
Dihydrocodeine (Martindale)	Oral solution 10 mg/5 mL	Cola coloured and flavoured slightly viscous liquid. Some resistance to flushing via fine-bore NG tube. Mixes easily with an equal volume of water to reduce viscosity.[3]

Formulations available[1] (continued)

Brand name (Manufacturer)	Formulation and strength	Product information/Administration information
Dihydrocodeine (Aurum)	Injection 50 mg/mL (1 mL)	Licensed for s.c. or i.m. injection. No specific data on enteral tube administration are available for this formulation.
DF118 Forte (Martindale)	Tablets 40 mg	No specific data on enteral tube administration are available for this formulation.
DHC Continuous (Napp)	60 mg, 90 mg, 120 mg	Modified-release tablets. **Do not** crush. Not suitable for enteral feeding tube administration. Convert to liquid preparation; divide total daily dose into 6–4 doses given every 4–6 hours.

Site of absorption (oral administration)

Specific site of absorption is not documented. Peak plasma concentration occurs 1.2–1.8 hours after oral dosing.[4, 5]

Alternative routes available

Parenteral route is available.

Interactions

No specific interaction with food is documented.

Health and safety

Standard precautions apply.

Suggestions/recommendations

- Use a liquid preparation.
- A prolonged break in feeding is not required.

Intragastric administration

1. Stop the enteral feed.
2. Flush the enteral feeding tube with the recommended volume of water.
3. Draw medication liquid into appropriate size and type of syringe.
4. Draw an equal volume of water and a little air into the syringe and shake to mix thoroughly.
5. Flush the medication dose down the feeding tube.
6. Finally, flush with the recommended volume of water.
7. Re-start the feed, unless a prolonged break is required.

Alternatively, at step (3) measure the medicine in a suitable container and then add an equal volume of water and mix thoroughly. Draw this into an appropriate syringe. Ensure that the measure is rinsed and that this rinsing water is administered also to ensure that the total dose is given. **Do not** measure liquid medicines using a catheter-tipped syringe as this results in excessive dosing owing to the volume of the tip.

Intrajejunal administration

Administer using the above method.

References

1. *BNF* 50, September 2005.
2. Personal communication, Alpharma; 21 January 2003.
3. BPNG data on file, 2005.
4. Dollery C. *Therapeutic Drugs*, 2nd edn. London: Churchill Livingstone; 1998.
5. Sweetman SC, ed. *Martindale*, 34th edn. London: Pharmaceutical Press; 2005.

Diltiazem

Formulations available[1]

Brand name (Manufacturer)	Formulation and strength	Product information/Administration information
Tildiem (Sanofi-Synthelabo)	Tablets 60 mg	Tablets may be crushed; although this is likely to affect the pharmacokinetics, it is unlikely to cause adverse effects.[2]
Diltiazem (Alpharma, APS, Ashbourne, Hillcross, IVAX, Niche, Opus, Sterwin)	Tablets 60 mg	Alpharma does not recommend crushing tablets.[3] Sterwin brand tablets do not disperse readily in water but do crush and mix with 10 mL of water to form fine suspension that flushes via an 8Fr NG tube without blockage.[7]
Adizem SR (Napp)	M/R capsules 90 mg, 120 mg, 180 mg M/R Tablets 120 mg	Twice daily dosing. In-house studies conducted by Napp conclude that there is significant risk of blockage if the spheroids in the capsules are administered via an enteral feeding tube. The company does not recommend this method of administration.[4]
Adizem XL (Napp)	M/R capsules 120 mg, 180 mg, 200 mg, 240 mg, 300 mg	Once daily dosing. In-house studies conducted by Napp conclude that there is significant risk of blockage if the spheroids in the capsules are administered via an enteral feeding tube. The company does not recommend this method of administration.[4]
Angitil SR (Trinity)	M/R capsules 90 mg, 120 mg, 180 mg	No specific data on enteral tube administration are available for this formulation.
Angitil XL (Trinity)	M/R capsules 240 mg, 300 mg	No specific data on enteral tube administration are available for this formulation.
Calcicard CR (IVAX)	M/R tablets 90 mg, 120 mg	Modified-release tablets; not suitable for enteral tube administration.
Dilcardia SR (Generics)	M/R capsules 60 mg, 90 mg, 120 mg	No specific data on enteral tube administration are available for this formulation.

Formulations available[1] (continued)

Brand name (Manufacturer)	Formulation and strength	Product information/Administration information
Dilzem SR (Zeneus)	M/R capsules 60 mg, 90 mg, 120 mg	The capsules contain modified-release granules. The capsules can be opened to facilitate administration providing the contents are not crushed.[5] No information available on size of granules or risk of blockage. Bioavailability is similar to that of conventional tablets.[13]
Dilzem XL (Zeneus)	M/R capsules 120 mg, 180 mg, 240 mg	The capsules contain modified-release granules. The capsules can be opened to facilitate administration providing the contents are not crushed.[5] No information available on size of granules or risk of blockage. Bioavailability is similar to that of conventional tablets.[14]
Slozem (Merck)	M/R capsules 120 mg, 180 mg, 240 mg, 300 mg	Sustained-release pellets must not be crushed. Capsules can be opened and pellets administered via feeding tube. Pellets may get stuck within the tube, especially smaller-sized tubes.[6] The bioavailability of the capsules is equivalent to the same dose given as conventional tablets[11].
Tildiem LA (Sanofi-Synthelabo)	M/R capsules 200 mg, 300 mg	Pellets can be removed from the capsule but should not be crushed,[2] no information available on tube administration. Bioavailability is 80% of the conventional tablets[10].
Tildiem Retard (Sanofi-Synthelabo)	M/R tablets 90 mg, 120 mg	These tablets should not be crushed.[2] Bioavailability is 90% of the conventional tablets.[9]
Viazem XL (Genus)	M/R capsules 120 mg, 180 mg, 240 mg, 300 mg, 360 mg	No specific data on enteral tube administration are available for this formulation.
Zemzard (Galen)	M/R capsules 120 mg, 180 mg, 240 mg, 300 mg	No specific data on enteral tube administration are available for this formulation.
Extemporaneous preparation	Suspension	*Extemporaneous diltiazem suspension 12 mg/mL:* Diltiazem 60 mg tablets 20 tablets Cherry syrup to 100 mL Room temperature storage; 60-day expiry. (Adapted from ref. 12.)

Site of absorption (oral administration)

Diltiazem is well absorbed from immediate-release preparations (90%). Peak plasma concentration occurs 3–4 hours after an oral dose.[8] First-pass effect reduces bioavailability to 40%.

Alternative routes available

None.

Interactions

There is no documented interaction with food.

Health and safety

Standard precautions apply.

Suggestions/recommendations

- Where clinically appropriate, consider changing to an alternative once daily calcium-channel blocker such as amlodipine (see monograph).
- Bioavailability varies among the sustained-release diltiazem preparations. Therefore, despite the theoretical dose being administered, if changing to crushed 60 mg tablets it would be prudent to start at 60 mg three times a day. Owing to the unknown effect on pharmacokinetics of crushing the 60 mg tablets, if the dose is to be increased, increase the frequency to four times daily.

Intragastric administration

1. Stop the enteral feed.
2. Flush the enteral feeding tube with the recommended volume of water.
3. Place the tablet in a mortar and crush to a fine powder using the pestle.
4. Add a few millilitres of water and mix to form a paste.
5. Add up to 15 mL of water and mix thoroughly, ensuring that there are no large particles of tablet.
6. Draw this into an appropriate size and type of syringe.
7. Flush the medication dose down the feeding tube.
8. Add another 15 mL of water to the mortar and stir to ensure that any remaining drug is rinsed from the container. Draw this water into the syringe and also flush this via the feeding tube (this will rinse the mortar and syringe and ensure that the total dose is administered).
9. Finally, flush the enteral feeding tube with the recommended volume of water.
10. Re-start the feed, unless prolonged break required.

Intrajejunal administration

There are no specific data on jejunal administration of diltiazem. Consider changing therapy. If administering as above, monitor for lack of efficacy or increased side-effects.

References

1. *BNF 50*, September 2005.
2. Personal communication, Sanofi-Synthelabo; 3 February 2003.
3. Personal communication, Alpharma; 21 January 2003.
4. Personal communication, Napp Pharmaceuticals; 29 January 2003.
5. Personal communication, Elan Pharma; 16 January 2003.
6. Personal communication, Merck Pharmaceuticals; 23 January 2003.
7. BPNG data on file, 2004.
8. Tildiem (Sanofi-Synthelabo), Summary of Product Characteristics; July 2002.
9. Tildiem Retard (Sanofi-Synthelabo), Summary of Product Characteristics; August 2003.
10. Tildiem LA (Sanofi-Synthelabo), Summary of Product Characteristics; August 2003.
11. Slozem Capsules (Merck), Summary of Product Characteristics; February 2001.
12. Allen L, Erickson M. Stability of baclofen, captopril, diltiazem hydrochloride, dipyridamole and flecanide acetate in extemporaneously compounded oral liquids. *Am J Health Syst Pharm.* 1996; 53: 2179–2184.
13. Dilzem SR (Elan), Summary of Product Characteristics; March 2001.
14. Dilzem XL (Elan), Summary of Product Characteristics; March 2001.

Dipyridamole

Formulations available[1]

Brand name (Manufacturer)	Formulation and strength	Product information/Administration information
Dipyridamole (Alpharma, Hillcross, IVAX)	Tablets 25 mg, 100 mg	Coated. Tablets can be crushed but the coating may not pulverise;[2] there is a risk of tube blockage. Tablets do not crush readily owing to the coating.[3]
Dipyridamole (Rosemont)	Oral suspension 50 mg/5 mL	Sugar-free suspension. Doses should be given 3–4 times daily. Does not contain sorbitol.[5] Rosemont advises to take before meals.
Persantin (Boehringer Ingelheim)	Tablets 25 mg, 100 mg	Sugar-coated tablets. Tablets may be crushed.[4]
Persantin (Boehringer Ingelheim)	Injection 5 mg/mL (2 mL)	Licensed for diagnostic use only. pH of solution is 2.5–3. The injection solution could be administered via the tube,[4] but this would require a large number of ampoules.
Persantin Retard (Boehringer Ingelheim)	Capsules 200 mg	Hard gelatin capsule containing modified-release granules. Capsule may be opened and granules flushed through the tube. Boehringer comments that the granules easily block the tube and the procedure should be attempted with caution.[4]
Asasantin Retard (Boehringer Ingelheim)	Capsules 200 mg dipyridamole + 25 mg aspirin	Hard gelatin capsule containing modified-release granules. Capsule may be opened and granules flushed through the tube. Boehringer comments that the granules easily block the tube and the procedure should be attempted with caution.[4]

Site of absorption (oral administration)

Dipyridamole is mainly absorbed in the small intestine.[4] Peak plasma concentration occurs 0.5–2 hours after oral dosing with immediate-release preparations.[5]

Alternative routes available

Parenteral route is not used for therapeutic purposes.

Interactions

There is no documented interaction with food.[5]

Health and safety

Standard precautions apply.

Suggestions/recommendations

- Use a liquid preparation. Dilute before use if administering into the jejunum.
- If converting from a modified-release preparation, divide total daily dose into four equal doses.
- A prolonged break in feeding is not required.

Intragastric administration

1. Stop the enteral feed.
2. Flush the enteral feeding tube with the recommended volume of water.
3. Shake the medication bottle thoroughly to ensure adequate mixing.
4. Draw the medication suspension into an appropriate size and type of syringe.
5. Flush the medication dose down the feeding tube.
6. Finally, flush with the recommended volume of water.
7. Re-start the feed, unless a prolonged break is required.

Alternatively, at step (4) measure the medicine in a suitable container and then add an equal volume of water and mix thoroughly. Draw this into an appropriate syringe. Ensure that the measure is rinsed and that this rinsing water is administered also to ensure that the total dose is given. **Do not** measure liquid medicines using a catheter-tipped syringe as this results in excessive dosing owing to the volume of the tip.

Intrajejunal administration

There are no specific reports relating to the jejunal administration of dipyridamole; however, as there is a modified-release preparation that releases dipyridamole into the small bowel, it is unlikely that jejunal administration will adversely affect pharmacokinetics.

Administer using the above method.

References

1. *BNF 50*, September 2005.
2. Personal communication, Alpharma; 21 January 2003.
3. BPNG data on file, 2004.
4. Personal communication, Boehringer Ingelheim; 6 March 2003.
5. Dipyridamole Suspension (Rosemont), Summary of Product Characteristics; September 2002.

Docusate sodium

Formulations available[1]

Brand name (Manufacturer)	Formulation and strength	Product information/Administration information
Dioctyl (Schwarz)	Capsules 100 mg	Soft gelatin capsules. The viscous liquid inside the capsule can be aspirated and suspended in water. Such a transfer is likely to result in inaccurate dosing and therefore is not recommended.[4]

Formulations available [1] (continued)

Brand name (Manufacturer)	Formulation and strength	Product information/Administration information
Docusol (Typharm)	Adult oral solution 50 mg/5 mL Paediatric oral solution 12.5 mg/5 mL	Adult solution: Slightly viscous clear solution; flushes through a fine-bore tube with slight resistance. Mixes well with an equal volume of water. [2]

Site of absorption (oral administration)

Docusate sodium functions as a faecal softener by acting as a wetting agent in the colon; only minimal quantities are absorbed. [3]

Alternative routes available

Not applicable.

Interactions

No significant interaction with food.

Health and safety

Standard precautions apply.

Suggestions/recommendations

- Use a liquid preparation; dilute.
- Administration into the jejunum will not affect pharmacological response.
- A prolonged break in feeding is not required.

Intragastric administration

1. Stop the enteral feed.
2. Flush the enteral feeding tube with the recommended volume of water.
3. Draw the medication solution into an appropriate size and type of syringe.
4. Flush the medication dose down the feeding tube.
5. Finally, flush with the recommended volume of water.
6. Re-start the feed, unless a prolonged break is required.

Alternatively, at step (3) measure the medicine in a suitable container and then add an equal volume of water and mix thoroughly. Draw this into an appropriate syringe. Ensure that the measure is rinsed and that this rinsing water is administered also to ensure that the total dose is given. **Do not** measure liquid medicines using a catheter-tipped syringe as this results in excessive dosing owing to the volume of the tip.

Intrajejunal administration

Administration directly into the jejunum will not affect the pharmacological response. Administer using the above method.

References

1. *BNF 50*, September 2005.
2. BPNG data on file, 2004.
3. Dioctyl (Schwarz), Summary of Product Characteristics; August 2005.
4. Personal communication, Schwarz Pharma; 17 February 2003.

Domperidone

Formulations available[1]

Brand name (Manufacturer)	Formulation and strength	Product information/Administration information
Domperidone (Arrow, Co-pharma, CP, Hillcross, Sterwin)	Tablets 10 mg	Domperidone maleate. Tablets will disperse in water, although the time taken is variable. Co-pharma and CP brands both produce dispersion that does not block an 8Fr NG tube.[3]
Motilium (Sanofi-Synthelabo)	Tablets 10 mg	Domperidone maleate. Film-coated. 10–20 mg every 4–8 hours. Tablets can be crushed.[2]
Motilium (Sanofi-Synthelabo)	Suspension 5 mg/5 mL	Suspension flushes via an 8Fr NG tube with little resistance. Mixes easily with an equal volume of water to reduce viscosity and osmolarity.[3] Contains sorbitol[5] 2.275 g/5 mL dose.[6]
Motilium (Sanofi-Synthelabo)	Suppositories 30 mg	30–60 mg every 4–8 hours. Rectal administration.

Site of absorption (oral administration)

Specific site of administration is not documented. Peak plasma concentration occurs within 30 minutes following oral administration, and 1–4 hours following rectal administration.[4]

Alternative routes available

Rectal route is available.

Interactions

Administration 90 minutes after a meal increases bioavailability.[4]

Health and safety

Standard precautions apply.

Suggestions/recommendations

- Use the suspension formulation, although the total daily dose of sorbitol should be considered. If administering into the jejunum, dilute the suspension with at least an equal volume of water immediately prior to administration. Alternatively, the suppositories can be used rectally.
- A prolonged break in feeding is not required.

Intragastric administration

1. Stop the enteral feed.
2. Flush the enteral feeding tube with the recommended volume of water.
3. Shake the medication bottle thoroughly to ensure adequate mixing.
4. Draw the medication suspension into an appropriate size and type of syringe.
5. Flush the medication dose down the feeding tube.
6. Finally, flush with the recommended volume of water.
7. Re-start the feed, unless a prolonged break is required.

Alternatively, at step (3) measure the medicine in a suitable container and then draw into an appropriate syringe. Ensure that the measure is rinsed and that this rinsing water is administered also to ensure that the total dose is given. **Do not** measure liquid medicines using a catheter-tipped syringe as this results in excessive dosing owing to the volume of the tip.

Intrajejunal administration

1. Stop the enteral feed.
2. Flush the enteral feeding tube with the recommended volume of water.
3. Shake the medication bottle thoroughly to ensure adequate mixing.
4. Draw the medication suspension into an appropriate size and type of syringe.
5. Draw an equal volume of water and a little air into the syringe and shake to mix thoroughly.
6. Flush the medication dose down the feeding tube.
7. Finally, flush with the recommended volume of water.
8. Re-start the feed, unless a prolonged break is required.

Alternatively, at step (4) measure the medicine in a suitable container and then add an equal volume of water and mix thoroughly. Draw this into an appropriate syringe. Ensure that the measure is rinsed and that this rinsing water is administered also to ensure that the total dose is given. **Do not** measure liquid medicines using a catheter-tipped syringe as this results in excessive dosing owing to the volume of the tip.

References

1. *BNF 50*, September 2005.
2. Personal communication, Sanofi-Synthelabo; 3 February 2003.
3. BPNG data on file, 2004.
4. Dollery C. *Therapeutic Drugs*, 2nd edn. London: Churchill Livingstone; 1998.
5. Motilium Suspension (Sanofi), Summary of Product Characteristics; August 2003.
6. Personal communication, Sanofi-Synthelabo; 18 February 2005.

Donepezil

Formulations available[1]

Brand name (Manufacturer)	Formulation and strength	Product information/Administration information
Aricept (Pfizer, Eisai)	Tablets 5 mg, 10 mg	Tablets can be crushed and suspended in water immediately prior to administration.[2,4] Tablets disintegrate within 5 minutes when placed in 10 mL of water to give a fine dispersion that which flushes via an 8Fr NG tube without blockage.[3]

Site of absorption (oral administration)

Aricept is absorbed in the small intestine.[2] Peak plasma concentration occurs 3–4 hours following oral dosing.[5]

Alternative routes available

None available.

Interactions

The absorption of donepezil is unaffected by food.[5]

Health and safety

Standard precautions apply.

Suggestions/recommendations

- Disperse the tablets in water immediately prior to administration.
- Consider changing to an alternative therapy available as a liquid preparation, such as galantamine, memantine or rivastigmine. Seek specialist advice before changing therapy.
- A prolonged break is feeding is not required.

Intragastric administration

1. Stop the enteral feed.
2. Flush the enteral feeding tube with the recommended volume of water.
3. Place the tablet in the barrel of an appropriate size and type of syringe.
4. Draw 10 mL of water into the syringe and allow the tablet to disperse, shaking if necessary.
5. Flush the medication dose down the feeding tube.
6. Draw another 10 mL of water into the oral syringe and also flush this via the feeding tube (this will rinse the syringe and ensure that the total dose is administered).
7. Finally, flush with the recommended volume of water.
8. Re-start the feed, unless a prolonged break is required.

Alternatively, at step (3) place the tablet into a medicine pot, add 10 mL of water and allow the tablet to disperse. Draw this into an appropriate syringe. Ensure that the measure is rinsed and that this rinsing water is administered also to ensure that the total dose is given.

Intrajejunal administration

There are no specific data relating to the jejunal administration of donepezil. Administer using the above method. Monitor for increased side-effects or loss of efficacy.

References

1. *BNF 50*, September 2005.
2. Personal communication, Eisai; 15 January 2003.
3. BPNG data on file, 2005.
4. Personal communication, Pfizer; 23 June 2003.
5. Aricept (Eisai), Summary of Product Characteristics; January 2002.

Dosulepin (Dothiepin) hydrochloride

Formulations available[1]

Brand name (Manufacturer)	Formulation and strength	Product information/Administration information
Dosulepin (Alpharma, APS, Ashbourne, Berk, Generics, Hillcross, IVAX, Kent, Sandoz, Sanofi-Synthelabo, Sovereign, Sterwin)	Capsules 25 mg	Capsules contains insoluble excipients. Can be dispersed in 30 mL of water.[2]
Dosulepin (Alpharma, APS, Ashbourne, Berk, Cox, Generics, Hillcross, IVAX, Kent, Sandoz, Sanofi-Synthelabo, Sovereign, Sterwin)	Tablets 75 mg	**Do not** crush tablets and mix with water as there is a risk of blocking tube with fragments of film coating.[2] Cox brand tablets disperse in 10 mL of water if shaken for 5 minutes, resulting in a pink milky dispersion that flushes via an 8Fr NG tube without blockage but leaves traces of red coating on the syringe and tube.[3] APS brand tablets do not disperse readily in water; they are difficult to crush owing to the sugar coating, but with persistence they can be crushed and mixed with water. Once the coating has dissolved the dispersion will flush via an 8Fr NG tube without blockage.[3]
Prothiaden (Abbott)	Capsules 25 mg	No specific data on enteral tube administration are available for this formulation.
Prothiaden (Abbott)	Tablets 75 mg	No specific data on enteral tube administration are available for this formulation.
Dosulepin (Rosemont)	Oral solution 25 mg/5 mL, 75 mg/5 mL	Available as manufactured 'special'. Contains sorbitol[4] 1.14 g/5 mL.

Site of absorption (oral administration)

Specific site of absorption and time to peak plasma concentration are not documented in SPC[5].

Alternative routes available

None available.

Interactions

No specific interaction with food are documented.[5]

Health and safety

Standard precautions apply.

Suggestions/recommendations

- Consider changing to an alternative tricyclic antidepressant available in liquid formulation such as amitriptyline (see monograph). Alternatively, use the manufactured 'special' liquid preparation.
- A prolonged break in feeding is not required.

Intragastric administration

1. Stop the enteral feed.
2. Flush the enteral feeding tube with the recommended volume of water.
3. Draw the medication liquid into an appropriate size and type of syringe.
4. Flush the medication dose down the feeding tube.
5. Finally, flush with the recommended volume of water.
6. Re-start the feed, unless a prolonged break is required.

Alternatively, at step (3) measure the medicine in a suitable container. Draw this into an appropriate syringe. Ensure that the measure is rinsed and that this rinsing water is administered also to ensure that the total dose is given. **Do not** measure liquid medicines using a catheter-tipped syringe as this results in excessive dosing owing to the volume of the tip.

Intrajejunal administration

There are no specific data relating to the jejunal administration of dosulepin. Administer using the above method, or alternatively disperse the capsule contents in water.

1. Stop the enteral feed.
2. Flush the enteral feeding tube with the recommended volume of water.
3. Open the capsule and pour the contents into a medicine pot.
4. Add 15 mL of water.
5. Stir to disperse the powder.
6. Draw into the syringe and administer via the feeding tube.
7. Add a further 15 mL of water to the medicine pot; stir to ensure that any powder remaining in the pot is mixed with water.
8. Draw up this dispersion and flush down the tube. This will ensure that the whole dose is given.
9. Flush the tube with recommended volume of water.
10. Re-start the feed, unless a prolonged break is required.

References

1. *BNF* 50, September 2005.
2. Personal communication, Alpharma; 21 January 2003.
3. BPNG data on file, 2004.
4. Personal communication, Rosemont Pharma; 20 January 2005.
5. Prothiaden (Abbott), Summary of Product Characteristics; February 2002.

Doxazosin

Formulations available[1]

Brand name (Manufacturer)	Formulation and strength	Product information/Administration information
Doxazosin (APS, Dexcel, Discovery, Generics, Sterwin)	Tablets 1 mg, 2 mg, 4 mg	Tablets disperse within 2 minutes in 10 mL of water to give a coarse dispersion; this flushes via an 8Fr NG tube without blockage.[2]
Cardura (Pfizer)	Tablets 1 mg, 2 mg	Tablets can be crushed and mixed with water immediately prior to administration.[3] The water must not contain excessive chloride ions as this may cause the drug to precipitate out.[3]
Cardura XL (Pfizer)	Tablets 4 mg, 8 mg	Modified-release tablets. Should not be crushed.[3] Unsuitable for administration via the feeding tube. Bioavailability compared to conventional tablets is 54% for 4 mg and 59% for 8 mg;[4] therefore, when converting to conventional tablets it is advisable to halve the dose and titrate upwards according to response.

Site of absorption (oral administration)

Specific site of absorption is unknown.[3]

Alternative routes available

No alternative route is available.

Interactions

No reported interaction with food.[3]

Health and safety

Standard precautions apply.

Suggestions/recommendations

- Disperse the tablets in water immediately prior to administration.
- A prolonged break in feeding is not required.

Intragastric administration

1. Stop the enteral feed.
2. Flush the enteral feeding tube with the recommended volume of water.
3. Place the tablet in the barrel of an appropriate size and type of syringe.
4. Draw 10 mL of water into the syringe and allow the tablet to disperse, shaking if necessary.
5. Flush the medication dose down the feeding tube.
6. Draw another 10 mL of water into the syringe and also flush this via the feeding tube (this will rinse the syringe and ensure that the total dose is administered).
7. Finally, flush with the recommended volume of water.
8. Re-start the feed, unless a prolonged break is required.

Alternatively, at step (3) place the tablet into a medicine pot, add 10 mL of water and allow the tablet to disperse. Draw this into an appropriate syringe. Ensure that the measure is rinsed and that this rinsing water is administered also to ensure that the total dose is given.

Intrajejunal administration

There are no documented reports of jejunal administration of doxazosin. Administer using the above method. Titrate dose to effect.

References

1. *BNF* 50, September 2005.
2. BPNG data on file, 2004.
3. Personal communication, Pfizer; 23 June 2003.
4. Cardura XL (Pfizer), Summary of Product Characteristics; January 2001.

Doxepin hydrochloride

Formulations available[1]

Brand name (Manufacturer)	Formulation and strength	Product information/Administration information
Sinequan (Pfizer)	Capsules 10 mg, 25 mg, 50 mg, 75 mg	Capsules may be opened and the contents mixed with water.[2]

Site of absorption (oral administration)

Not known.[2]

Alternative routes available

None available for doxepin.

Interactions

There is no reported interaction with food.[2]

Health and safety

Standard precautions apply.

Suggestions/recommendations

- Open the capsules and disperse the contents in water immediately prior to administration.
- Consider changing to an alternative tricyclic antidepressant available as a liquid preparation.
- A prolonged break in feeding is not required.

Intragastric administration

1. Stop the enteral feed.
2. Flush the enteral feeding tube with the recommended volume of water.
3. Open the capsule and pour the contents into a medicine pot.
4. Add 15 mL of water.
5. Stir to disperse the powder.
6. Draw into the syringe and administer via the feeding tube.
7. Add a further 15 mL of water to the medicine pot; stir to ensure that any powder remaining in the pot is mixed with water.
8. Draw up this dispersion and flush down the tube. This will ensure that the whole dose is given.
9. Flush the tube with recommended volume of water.
10. Re-start the feed, unless prolonged break required.

Intrajejunal administration

There are no specific data relating to the jejunal administration of doxepin. Administer using the above method. Monitor for loss of efficacy or increased side-effects.

References

1. *BNF 50*, September 2005.
2. Personal communication, Pfizer; 23 June 2003.

Doxycycline

Formulations available[1]

Brand name (Manufacturer)	Formulation and strength	Product information/Administration information
Doxycycline (Alpharma, APS, Hillcross, IVAX, Kent, PLIVA, Sandoz)	Capsules 50 mg, 100 mg	Do not open capsules as the contents are irritant.[2]
Vibramycin (Pfizer)	Capsules 50 mg, 100 mg	The capsules should not be opened as they contain the hyclate salt which is highly irritant to the oesophagus.[3]
Vibramycin-D (Pfizer)	Dispersible tablets 100 mg	Tablet disintegrates within 1 minute when placed in 10 mL of water; disintegrates further when drawn into the syringe. Produces some visible particles but does not block an 8Fr NG tube.[4]

Site of absorption (oral administration)

Doxycycline is rapidly absorbed following oral absorption; it is suggested that peak absorption occurs in the duodenum.[3]

Alternative routes available

None available for doxycycline.

Interactions

Unlike with other tetracyclines, doxycycline absorption is not influenced by simultaneous ingestion of food or milk;[3] however, absorption may be reduced by antacids containing high concentrations of aluminium, calcium or magnesium.[5]

Health and safety

Standard precautions apply.

Suggestions/recommendations

- Use dispersible tablets. Disperse in 10 mL of water immediately prior to administration.
- A prolonged break in feeding does not appear to be necessary; however, it is possible that there may be a reduction in absorption and therefore the dose should be administered during a break in feeding if practical. Alternatively, the higher end of the dose range should be used.

Intragastric administration

1. Stop the enteral feed.
2. Flush the enteral feeding tube with the recommended volume of water.
3. Administer during a break in the feeding regimen if possible.
4. Place the tablet in the barrel of an appropriate size and type of syringe.
5. Draw 10 mL of water into the syringe and allow the tablet to disperse, shaking if necessary.
6. Flush the medication dose down the feeding tube.
7. Draw an equal volume of water into the syringe and also flush this via the feeding tube (this will rinse the syringe and ensure that the total dose is administered).
8. Finally, flush with the recommended volume of water.
9. Re-start the feed, unless a prolonged break is required.

Alternatively, at step (4) place the tablet into a medicine pot, add 10 mL of water and allow the tablet to disperse. Draw this into an appropriate syringe. Ensure that the measure is rinsed and that this rinsing water is administered also to ensure that the total dose is given.

Intrajejunal administration

As peak absorption may occur in the duodenum, it is possible that bioavailability may be reduced by jejunal administration. Consider using alternative antibiotic or monitor for loss of efficacy. Administer as above.

References

1. *BNF* 50, September 2005.
2. Personal communication, Alpharma; 21 January 2003.
3. Personal communication, Pfizer; 23 June 2003.
4. BPNG data on file, 2004.
5. Vibramycin (Pfizer), Summary of Product Characteristics; July 2002.

Efavirenz

Formulations available

Brand name (Manufacturer)	Formulation and strength	Product information/Administration information
Sustiva Hard Capsules (Bristol-Myers Squibb)	Capsules.[1] 50 mg 100 mg 200 mg	The contents of three 200 mg capsules can be mixed with at least 5 mL of medium chain triglyceride oil or 15 mL of any aqueous vehicle. Polyethylene glycol should not be used as a vehicle because it affects the bioavailability of Sustiva.[3] *Effect of food:* The bioavailability of a single 600 mg dose of efavirenz in uninfected volunteers was increased 22% and 17%, respectively, when given with a meal of high fat or normal composition, relative to the bioavailability of a 600 mg dose given under fasted conditions.[1] *200 mg capsules:* Contents empty easily from capsule, mix with water and flush via an 8Fr NG tube without blockage.[6]
Sustiva Tablets (BMS)	Film-coated tablet[1] 600 mg	*Effect of food:* The AUC and C_{max} of a single 600 mg dose of efavirenz film-coated tablets in uninfected volunteers was increased by 28% and 79%, respectively, when given with a high-fat meal, relative to fasted conditions.[5]
Sustiva Oral Solution (BMS)	Solution 30 mg/mL[1]	Excipients include medium chain triglycerides and benzoic acid.[4] The C_{max} and AUC of a 240 mg dose of Sustiva oral solution were 78% and 97%, respectively, of the values measured when Sustiva was given as a 200 mg hard capsule.[4] *Effect of food:* The AUC and C_{max} of a single 240 mg dose of oral solution in uninfected adult volunteers were increased by 30% and 43%, respectively, when given with a high-fat meal compared to fasted conditions.[4] Clear liquid, flushes easily via NG tube. Nonaqueous; does not mix with water.[6]

Site of absorption (oral administration)

Specific site of absorption is not documented. Peak plasma concentration occurs 3–5 hours following oral dose.[1]

Alternative routes available

None.

Interactions

- Food: see notes above on individual formulations.
- Grapefruit juice: plasma concentration of efavirenz are possibly increased by grapefruit juice.[2]

Health and safety

Standard precautions apply.

Suggestions/recommendations

- Liquid formulation is preferable in terms of ease of manipulation and cost; however, a difference in bioavailability should be noted.
- Because of differences in bioavailability, formulations are not interchangeable.
- No break in feeding is necessary, as bioavailability is increased when given with food.

Intragastric administration

1. Stop the enteral feed.
2. Flush the enteral feeding tube with the recommended volume of water.
3. Draw the medication solution into an appropriate size and type of syringe.
4. Flush the medication dose down the feeding tube.
5. Finally, flush with the recommended volume of water.
6. Re-start the feed, unless a prolonged break is required.

Alternatively, at step (3) measure the medicine in a suitable container and then draw into an appropriate syringe. Ensure that the measure is rinsed and that this rinsing water is administered also to ensure that the total dose is given. **Do not** measure liquid medicines using a catheter-tipped syringe as this results in excessive dosing owing to the volume of the tip.

Intrajejunal administration

There is no specific information relating to jejunal administration of efavirenz. Administer using the above method. Monitor for adverse effects or loss of efficacy.

References

1. Sustiva Hard Capsules, Summary of Product Characteristics; 30 September 2002.
2. *BNF 50*, September 2005.
3. Personal communication, Medical Information Department, Bristol-Myers Squibb; 24 January 2003.
4. Sustiva Oral Solution, Summary of Product Characteristics; 30 September 2002.
5. Sustiva Tablets, Summary of Product Characteristics; 22 August 2002.
6. BPNG data on file, 2005.

Enalapril maleate

Formulations available[1]

Brand name (Manufacturer)	Formulation and strength	Product information/Administration information
Innovace (MSD)	Tablets 2.5 mg, 5 mg, 10 mg, 20 mg	Once-daily dosing in hypertension and heart failure.[1] Enalapril has high solubility in water.[2] No specific data on enteral tube administration are available for this formulation.
Enalapril (Alpharma)	Tablets 2.5 mg, 5 mg, 10 mg, 20 mg	Tablets can be crushed/suspended and administered via PEG/NG tube.[3]

Formulations available[1] (continued)

Brand name (Manufacturer)	Formulation and strength	Product information/Administration information
Enalapril (Dexcel)	Tablets 2.5 mg, 5 mg, 10 mg, 20 mg	Tablets dissolve in 10 mL of water within 5 minutes if agitated; lower strengths disperse more rapidly than higher strengths. The fine suspension flushes easily down an 8Fr NG tube.[4]
Enalapril (IVAX, Opus, PLIVA, Sterwin, Milpharm)	Tablets 2.5 mg, 5 mg, 10 mg, 20 mg	Milpharm 10 mg tablets disperse in water within 5 minutes to give fine dispersion that flushes easily via an 8Fr NG tube.[4]
Enalapril (extemporaneous suspension)	Suspension 1 mg/mL	*Extemporaneous enalapril suspension 1 mg/mL:* Enalapril 5 mg tablet 20 tablets Cherry syrup to 100 mL Store at room temperature or refrigerate. Expiry 60 days.[5]

Site of absorption (oral administration)

Specific site of absorption is not documented. Peak plasma concentration occurs within 1 hour of oral dosing.[6]

Alternative routes available

None available for any of the ACE inhibitors.

Interactions

Absorption of enalapril is not affected by food.[6]

Health and safety

Standard precautions apply.

Suggestions/recommendations

- Tablets can be dispersed in water immediately before administration.
- A prolonged break in feeding is not necessary.
- If a liquid preparation is preferred, therapy can be changed to lisinopril (see monograph).

Intragastric administration

1. Stop the enteral feed.
2. Flush the enteral feeding tube with the recommended volume of water.
3. Place the tablet in the barrel of an appropriate size and type of syringe.
4. Draw 10 mL of water into the syringe and allow the tablet to disperse, shaking if necessary.
5. Flush the medication dose down the feeding tube.
6. Draw another 10 mL of water into the syringe and also flush this via the feeding tube (this will rinse the syringe and ensure that the total dose is administered).
7. Finally, flush with the recommended volume of water.
8. Re-start the feed, unless a prolonged break is required.

Alternatively, at step (3) place the tablet into a medicine pot, add 10 mL of water and allow the tablet to disperse. Draw this into an appropriate syringe. Ensure that the measure is rinsed and that this rinsing water is administered also to ensure that the total dose is given.

Intrajejunal administration

There are no specific data relating to jejunal administration of enalapril. Administer using the above method. Monitor for increased side-effects or loss of efficacy and titrate dose accordingly.

References

1. *BNF* 50, September 2005.
2. Dollery C. *Therapeutic Drugs*, 2nd edn. London: Churchill Livingstone; 1998.
3. Personal communication, Medical Information, Alpharma Ltd; 21 January 2003.
4. BPNG data on file, 2004.
5. Nahata M, Morosco R, Hipple T. Stability of enalapril maleate in three extemporaneously prepared oral liquids. *Am J Health Syst Pharm*. 1998; 55: 1155–1157.
6. Innovace Tablets (MSD), Summary of Product Characteristics; May 2002.

Entacapone

Formulations available[1]

Brand name (Manufacturer)	Formulation and strength	Product information/Administration information
Comtess (Orion)	Tablets 200 mg	Film-coated tablets. Tablets disintegrate when shaken in 10 mL of water for 5 minutes, to give a bright orange, cloudy dispersion that flushes via an 8Fr NG tube without blockage.[2] The dispersion will stain and therefore crushing tablets to a dry powder should be avoided.

Site of absorption (oral administration)

Specific site of absorption is not documented. Peak plasma concentration occurs 1 hour following oral dosing.[3]

Alternative routes available

None available.

Interactions

Food does not significantly affect the bioavailability of entacapone. Can be taken with or without food, but should be administered at the same time as the levodopa/dopa-decarboxylase dose.[3]

Health and safety

Standard precautions apply.

Suggestions/recommendations

- Disperse the tablets in water immediately prior to dosing.
- Administer during or immediately after feed.

Intragastric administration

1. Stop the enteral feed.
2. Flush the enteral feeding tube with the recommended volume of water.
3. Place the tablet in the barrel of an appropriate tipped syringe.
4. Draw 10 mL of water into the syringe and allow the tablet to disperse, shaking as required.
5. Flush the medication dose down the feeding tube.
6. Draw another 10 mL of water into the syringe and also flush this via the feeding tube (this will rinse the syringe and ensure that the total dose is administered).
7. Finally, flush with the recommended volume of water.
8. Re-start the feed, unless a prolonged break is required.

Alternatively, at step (3) place the tablet into a medicine pot, add 10 mL of water and allow the tablet to disperse. Draw this into an appropriate syringe. Ensure that the measure is rinsed and that this rinsing water is administered also to ensure that the total dose is given.

Intrajejunal administration

There are no specific data on jejunal administration of entacapone. Administer using the above method. Monitor for increased side-effects or loss of efficacy.

References

1. *BNF* 50, September 2005.
2. BPNG data on file, 2005.
3. Comptess (Orion), Summary of Product Characteristics; September 2002.

Eprosartan mesilate

Formulations available[1]

Brand name (Manufacturer)	Formulation and strength	Product information/Administration information
Teveten (Solvay)	Tablets 300 mg, 400 mg, 600 mg	Solvay has no information on the effect on absorption and bioavailability of crushing Teteven tablets.[3] The tablets do not disperse readily in water, but will crush and mix with water and flush via a fine-bore tube without blockage.[5]

Site of absorption (oral administration)

Specific site of absorption is not documented. Peak plasma concentration occurs 1–2 hours post dose in the fasted state.[2]

Alternative routes available

No other routes of administration are available for any of the angiotensin II receptor antagonists.

Interactions

Absorption of eprosartan is reduced and delayed by food; although this is considered unlikely to have clinical consequences, it is recommended that the dose be taken before food.[4]

Health and safety

Standard precautions apply.

Suggestions/recommendations

- Owing to lack of data, consider changing to irbesartan (see monograph).
- A prolonged break in feeding is not required.

Intragastric administration

1. Stop the enteral feed.
2. Flush the enteral feeding tube with the recommended volume of water.
3. Place the tablet in a mortar and crush to a fine powder using the pestle.
4. Add a few millilitres of water and mix to form a paste.
5. Add up to 15 mL of water and mix thoroughly ensuring that there are no visible lumps of tablet.
6. Draw this into an appropriate size and type of syringe.
7. Flush the medication dose down the feeding tube.
8. Add another 15 mL of water to the mortar and stir to ensure that any remaining drug is rinsed from the container. Draw this water into the syringe and also flush this via the feeding tube (this will rinse the mortar and syringe and ensure that the total dose is administered).
9. Finally, flush the enteral feeding tube with the recommended volume of water.
10. Re-start the feed, unless prolonged break required.

Intrajejunal administration

There are no specific data on Intrajejunal administration of eprosartan. Administer using the above method. Monitor for increased side-effects or loss of efficacy.

References

1. *BNF 50*, September 2005.
2. Teteven (Solvay), Summary of Product Characteristics; January 2002.
3. Personal communication, Solvay Healthcare; 19 February 2003.
4. Tenero D. Pharmacokinetics of intravenously and orally administered eprosartan in healthy males: absolute bioavailability and effect of food. *Biopharm Drug Dispos.* 1998; 19: 351–356.
5. BPNG data on file, 2005.

Ergometrine maleate

Formulations available[1]

Brand name (Manufacturer)	Formulation and strength	Product information/Administration information
Ergometrine (IVAX, Celltech)	Tablets 500 microgram	Tablets are uncoated and can be crushed. The manufacturers have no bioavailability data from crushed tablets.[2]
Ergometrine (Antigen, Phoenix)	Injection 500 microgram/mL	No specific data on enteral tube administration are available for this formulation.

Site of absorption (oral administration)

Specific site of absorption is not documented. Peak plasma concentration occurs 60–90 minutes following oral dose.[3]

Alternative routes available

Parenteral route is available.

Interactions

No documented interactions with food.

Health and safety

Inhalation of powder from crushed tablets can cause headaches, vertigo, tinnitus, abdominal pain, nausea, vomiting, hypertension, chest pains, palpitations, dyspnoea, and heart irregularities.[2] A closed system should be used where possible.

Suggestions/recommendations

- Seek advice on alternative therapy.
- If indicated, crush tablets and disperse in water immediately prior to administration.

Intragastric administration

1. Stop the enteral feed.
2. Flush the enteral feeding tube with the recommended volume of water.
3. Place the tablet in a mortar and crush to a fine powder using the pestle.
4. Add a few millilitres of water and mix to form a paste.
5. Add up to 15 mL of water and mix thoroughly, ensuring that there are no large particles of tablet.
6. Draw this into an appropriate size and type of syringe.
7. Flush the medication dose down the feeding tube.
8. Add another 15 mL of water to the mortar and stir to ensure that any remaining drug is rinsed from the container. Draw this water into the syringe and also flush this via the feeding tube (this will rinse the mortar and syringe and ensure that the total dose is administered).
9. Finally, flush the enteral feeding tube with the recommended volume of water.
10. Re-start the feed, unless prolonged break necessary.

Intrajejunal administration

There are no specific data on jejunal administration of ergometrine. Administer using the above method. Monitor for loss of efficacy or increased side-effects.

References

1. *BNF* 50, September 2005.
2. Personal communication, Celltech; 31 March 2003.
3. Ergometrine Tablets (Celltech), Summary of Product Characteristics; October 2001.

Erythromycin

Formulations available[1]

Brand name (Manufacturer)	Formulation and strength	Product information/Administration information
Erythromycin (PLIVA, Tillomed)	Capsules 250 mg	Contains enteric coated granules. Capsules are not suitable for opening.
Erythromycin (Alpharma, APS, Ashbourne, Generics, IVAX, Kent)	Tablets 250 mg	Enteric coated tablets. Should not be crushed.
Erythromycin (Alpharma, APS, Generics, Hillcross, IVAX, Kent, Pinewood)	Suspension 125 mg/5 mL, 250 mg/5 mL, 500 mg/5 mL	Erythromycin ethyl succinate. Sugar-free versions are available.
Erythromycin (Abbott, Mayne)	Injection 1 g	Erythromycin lactobionate. No specific data on enteral tube administration are available for this formulation.
Erymax (Elan)	Capsules 250 mg	Capsules contain enteric coated granules; not suitable for tube administration.[2]
Erythrocin (Abbott)	Tablets 250 mg	Film-coated. No specific data on enteral tube administration are available for this formulation.
Erythroped (Abbott)	Suspension 125 mg/5 mL, 250 mg/5 mL, 500 mg/5 mL	Erythromycin ethyl succinate granules for suspension. Doses may be administered 2, 3 or 4 times a day. Contains sorbitol.[3] When reconstituted forms a creamy, viscous liquid, resistant to flushing. This mixes with an equal volume of water if shaken, which reduces resistance to flushing.[4]
Erythroped A (Abbott)	Tablets 500 mg	Film-coated. No specific data on enteral tube administration are available for this formulation.

Site of absorption (oral administration)

Erythromycin ethyl succinate is less susceptible to the adverse effect of gastric acid. It is absorbed from the small intestine.[4] Peak plasma concentration occurs within 1 hour of dosing using the erythromycin ethyl succinate suspension.[4]

Alternative routes available

Parenteral route is available.

Interactions

No specific interaction with food is documented.[4]

Health and safety

Standard precautions apply.

Suggestions/recommendations

- For serious infections, use the parenteral route. For administration via enteral feeding tubes, use the liquid preparation. Use a twice-daily dosing regimen.
- A prolonged break in feeding is not required.

Intragastric administration

1. Stop the enteral feed.
2. Flush the enteral feeding tube with the recommended volume of water.
3. Shake the medication bottle thoroughly to ensure adequate mixing.
4. Draw the medication suspension into an appropriate size and type of syringe.
5. Draw an equal volume of water and a little air into the syringe and shake to mix thoroughly.
6. Flush the medication dose down the feeding tube.
7. Finally, flush with the recommended volume of water.
8. Re-start the feed, unless a prolonged break is required.

Alternatively, at step (4) measure the medicine in a suitable container and then add an equal volume of water and mix thoroughly. Draw this into an appropriate syringe. Ensure that the measure is rinsed and that this rinsing water is administered also to ensure that the total dose is given. **Do not** measure liquid medicines using a catheter-tipped syringe as this results in excessive dosing owing to the volume of the tip.

Intrajejunal administration

There are no specific data, but, as an enteric-coated preparation is available, jejunal administration is unlikely to affect bioavailability. Administer using the above method.

References

1. *BNF* 50, September 2005.
2. Personal communication, Elan; 16 January 2003.
3. BPNG data on file, 2005.
4. Erythroped (Abbott), Summary of Product Characteristics; August 1998.

Escitalopram

Formulations available[1]

Brand name (Manufacturer)	Formulation and strength	Product information/Administration information
Cipralex (Lundbeck)	Tablets 5 mg, 10 mg, 20 mg	Escitalopram oxalate. Film coated tablets.[2] No specific data on enteral tube administration are available for this formulation.

Site of absorption (oral administration)

Specific site of absorption is not documented. Peak plasma concentration occurs 4 hours following oral dosing.[2]

Alternative routes available

Not applicable.

Interactions

Absorption is unaffected by food.[2]

Health and safety

Standard precautions apply.

Suggestions/recommendations

- Change to citalopram and use the oral drops (see monograph). Escitalopram 10 mg is approximately therapeutically equivalent to 20 mg of citalopram.

References

1. *BNF* 50, September 2005.
2. Cipralex (Lundbeck), Summary of Product Characteristics; June 2002.

Esomeprazole

Formulations available[1]

Brand name (Manufacturer)	Formulation and strength	Product information/Administration information
Nexium (AstraZeneca)	Tablet 20 mg, 40 mg	Gastro-resistant tablet.[2] The formulation is a film-coated tablet containing a compressed core of enteric coated microgranules. Nexium is licensed for administration via a gastric tube.[2]
Nexium (AstraZeneca)	Injection 40 mg	No specific data on enteral tube administration are available for this formulation.

Site of absorption (oral administration)

Delivery into the small bowel does not affect absorption as the formulation is enteric-coated.[2] Peak plasma concentration occurs 1–2 hours following oral dosing.

Alternative routes available

Parenteral route is available and is indicated when oral intake is not appropriate.[5]

Interactions

Food intake both delays and decreases the absorption of esomeprazole, although this has no significant influence on the effect of esomeprazole on intragastric acidity.[2]

Health and safety

Standard precautions apply.

Suggestions/recommendations

- Follow instructions in SPC.
- A prolonged break in feeding is not required.
- Alternative proton pump inhibitors include lansoprazole and omeprazole (see monographs).

Intragastric administration

Administration through gastric tube[2]

1. Put the tablet into an appropriate syringe and fill the syringe with approximately 25 ml of water and approximately 5 mL of air. For some tubes, dispersion in 50 mL of water is needed to prevent the pellets from clogging the tube.
2. Immediately shake the syringe for approximately 2 minutes to disperse the tablet.
3. Hold the syringe with the tip up and check that the tip has not clogged.
4. Attach the syringe to the tube while maintaining the above position.
5. Shake the syringe and position it with the tip pointing down. Immediately inject 5–10 mL into the tube. Invert the syringe after injection and shake (the syringe must be held with the tip pointing up to avoid clogging of the tip).
6. Turn the syringe with the tip down and immediately inject another 5–10 mL into the tube. Repeat this procedure until the syringe is empty.
7. Fill the syringe with 25 mL of water and 5 mL of air and repeat step (5) if necessary to wash down any sediment left in the syringe. For some tubes, 50 mL water is needed.
8. Finally, flush with recommended volume of water.
9. Re-start feed, unless a prolonged break is required.

Tubes tested by AstraZeneca were fine-bore 10Fr and 8Fr NG tubes.[3]
Non-adherence to this procedure will result in tube blockage.[4]

Intrajejunal administration

Although they are not licensed via this route, intrajejunal administration of the enteric coated microgranules is unlikely to affect the pharmacokinetic response to esomeprazole.

References

1. *BNF* 50, September 2005.
2. Nexium Tablets (AstraZeneca), Summary of Product Characteristics; January 2003.
3. Personal communication, AstraZeneca; 18 June 2003.
4. BPNG data on file, 2004.
5. Nexium Injection (AstraZeneca), Summary of Product Characteristics; January 2004.

Ethambutol

Formulations available[1]

Brand name (Manufacturer)	Formulation and strength	Product information/Administration information
Ethambutol (Genus)	Tablets 100 mg, 400 mg	Ethambutol hydrochloride. Film-coated tablets.[2] The tablets can be crushed and mixed with water, the coating takes a few minutes to dissolve.
Myambutol (imported by IDIS)	Injection 1000 mg	Unlicensed in UK. Imported by IDIS. No specific data on enteral tube administration are available for this formulation.
Ethambutol (extemporaneous preparation)	Suspension	A formulation for suspension is available; this formula uses ethambutol powder.[2]

Site of absorption (oral administration)

Specific site of absorption is not documented. Peak plasma concentration occurs within 4 hours of oral dosing.[3]

Alternative routes available

A parenteral formulation not licensed in the UK is available, see above.

Interactions

The absorption of ethambutol is not considered to be significantly affected by food.[3] However, it has been shown that peak plasma concentrations may be delayed and reduced by a high fat-meal or antacid therapy.[4]

Health and safety

Standard precautions apply.

Suggestions/recommendations

- Crush tablets and mix with water.
- A prolonged break in feeding is not required.
- If gastrointestinal function is compromised, consider parenteral therapy.

Intragastric administration

1. Stop the enteral feed.
2. Flush the enteral feeding tube with the recommended volume of water.
3. Place the tablet in a mortar and crush to a fine powder using the pestle.
4. Add a few millilitres of water and mix to form a paste.
5. Add up to 15 mL of water and mix thoroughly ensuring that there are no large particles of tablet or coating.
6. Draw this into an appropriate syringe.
7. Flush the medication dose down the feeding tube.
8. Add another 15 mL of water to the mortar and stir to ensure that any remaining drug is rinsed from the container. Draw this water into the syringe and also flush this via the feeding tube (this will rinse the mortar and syringe and ensure that the total dose is administered).
9. Finally, flush the enteral feeding tube with the recommended volume of water.
10. Re-start the feed, unless a prolonged break is required.

Intrajejunal administration

There are no specific data relating to jejunal administration of ethambutol. Administer using the above method. Monitor for loss of efficacy or increased side-effects.

References

1. *BNF 50*, September 2005.
2. Dollery C. *Therapeutic Drugs*, 2nd edn. London: Churchill Livingstone; 1998.
3. Sweetman SC, ed. *Martindale*, 34th edn. London: Pharmaceutical Press; 2005.
4. Peloquin CA, Bulpitt AE, Jaresko GS, *et al.* Pharmacokinetics of ethambutol under fasting conditions, with food, and with antacids. *Antimicrob Agents Chemother.* 1999; 43(3): 568–572.

Ethinylestradiol

Formulations available [1]

Brand name (Manufacturer)	Formulation and strength	Product information/Administration information
Ethinylestradiol (Celltech)	Tablets 10 microgram, 50 microgram, 1 mg	Tablets are uncoated and can be crushed; the manufacturer has no bioavailability data for this method of administration. Ethinylestradiol is insoluble in water. [2]

Site of absorption (oral administration)

Ethinylestradiol is absorbed in the gut but undergoes some first-pass metabolism in the gut wall. [3] Peak plasma concentration occurs 2–3 hours after oral dosing.

Alternative routes available

Topical patches are available for alternative estrogens for contraceptive and hormone replacement use.

Interactions

There is no documented interaction with food.

Health and safety

Use a closed system to crush or disperse tablet, e.g. a crushing syringe. Ensure that adequate precautions are taken to minimise operator exposure.

Suggestions/recommendations

- Use transdermal patches where clinically appropriate.
- A prolonged break in feeding is not required.

Intragastric administration

See notes above.

1. Stop the enteral feed.
2. Flush the enteral feeding tube with the recommended volume of water.
3. Place the tablet in the barrel of an appropriate size and type of syringe.
4. Draw 10 mL of water into the syringe and allow the tablet to disperse, shaking if necessary.
5. Flush the medication dose down the feeding tube.
6. Draw another 10 mL of water into the syringe and also flush this via the feeding tube (this will rinse the syringe and ensure that the total dose is administered).
7. Finally, flush with the recommended volume of water.
8. Re-start the feed, unless a prolonged break is required.

Alternatively, at step (3) place the tablet into a medicine pot, add 10 mL of water and allow the tablet to disperse. Draw this into an appropriate syringe. Ensure that the measure is rinsed and that this rinsing water is administered also to ensure that the total dose is given.

Intrajejunal administration

Ethinylestradiol pharmacokinetics are unlikely to be affected by jejunal administration. Administer using the above method.

References

1. *BNF* 50, September 2005.
2. Personal communication, Celltech; 31 March 2003.
3. Ethinylestradiol (Celltech), Summary of Product Characteristics; August 2004.

Ethosuximide

Formulations available [1]

Brand name (Manufacturer)	Formulation and strength	Product information/Administration information
Emeside (LAB)	Capsules 250 mg	No specific data on enteral tube administration are available for this formulation.
Emeside (LAB)	Syrup 250 mg/5 mL	Blackcurrant syrup base. [2]

Formulations available [1] (continued)

Brand name (Manufacturer)	Formulation and strength	Product information/Administration information
Zarontin (Parke-Davis)	Capsules 250 mg	No specific data on enteral tube administration are available for this formulation.
Zarontin (Parke-Davis)	Syrup 250 mg/5 mL	Raspberry flavoured syrup and saccharin base. [3] Slightly viscous liquid; mixes easily with water to reduce resistance to flushing. [4]

Site of absorption (oral administration)

No specific site of absorption documented. Peak plasma concentration occurs 1–4 hours after oral dosing. [2]

Alternative routes available

No alternative routes for ethosuximide.

Interactions

There are no documented interactions with food. [3]

Health and safety

Standard precautions apply.

Suggestions/recommendations

- Use a liquid preparation diluted with an equal quantity of water immediately prior to administration.
- A prolonged break in feeding is not necessary.

Intragastric administration

1. Stop the enteral feed.
2. Flush the enteral feeding tube with the recommended volume of water.
3. Draw the medication liquid into an appropriate size and type of syringe.
4. Draw an equal volume of water and a little air into the syringe and shake to mix thoroughly.
5. Flush the medication dose down the feeding tube.
6. Finally, flush with the recommended volume of water.
7. Re-start the feed, unless a prolonged break is required.

Alternatively, at step (4) measure the medicine in a suitable container and then add an equal volume of water and mix thoroughly. Draw this into an appropriate syringe. Ensure that the measure is rinsed and that this rinsing water is administered also to ensure that the total dose is given. **Do not** measure liquid medicines using a catheter-tipped syringe as this results in excessive dosing owing to the volume of the tip.

Intrajejunal administration

There are no specific data relating to the jejunal administration of ethosuximide. Administer using the above method. Monitor for increased side-effects or loss of efficacy.

References

1. *BNF* 50, September 2005.
2. Emeside Syrup (LAB), Summary of Product Characteristics; June 2001.
3. Zarontin Syrup (Parke-Davis), Summary of Product Characteristics; June 2003.
4. BPNG data on file, 2004.

Etidronate

Formulations available[1]

Brand name (Manufacturer)	Formulation and strength	Product information/Administration information
Didronel (Procter & Gamble)	Tablets 200 mg	Avoid giving food for at least 2 hours before and after oral treatment, particularly calcium-containing products such as milk; also avoid iron and mineral supplements and antacids.[1] The manufacturers have anecdotal data of patients crushing tablets and mixing them with water immediately prior to administration. The tablets should only be mixed with plain water owing to the risk of interaction.[2] The tablets do not disperse readily in water but crush easily and suspend in water; the suspension flushes via an 8Fr NG tube without blockage.[4]

Site of absorption (oral administration)

Specific site of absorption is not documented.[3]

Alternative routes available

None available for etidronate. Other bisphosphonates are available in parenteral formulations, although indications and doses differ: consult product literature for dosing guidelines.

Interactions

Etidronate absorption may be decreased by food in the stomach or upper portions of the small intestine, particularly materials with a high calcium content such as milk.[3]

Health and safety

Standard precautions apply.

Suggestions/recommendations

- Consider changing to an alternative therapy.
- If continued treatment with etidronate is necessary, stop the enteral feed 2 hours prior to administration. Crush the tablet and disperse in water immediately prior to administration. Flush the tube well. Do not restart the feed for 2 hours.

Intragastric administration

1. Stop the enteral feed.
2. Flush the enteral feeding tube with the recommended volume of water.
3. Allow a 2-hour break.
4. Place the tablet in a mortar and crush to a fine powder using the pestle.
5. Add a few millilitres of water and mix to form a paste.
6. Add up to 15 mL of water and mix thoroughly, ensuring that there are no large particles of tablet.
7. Draw this into an appropriate size and type of syringe.
8. Flush the medication dose down the feeding tube.
9. Add another 15 mL of water to the mortar and stir to ensure that any remaining drug is rinsed from the container. Draw this water into the syringe and also flush this via the feeding tube (this will rinse the mortar and syringe and ensure that the total dose is administered).
10. Finally, flush the enteral feeding tube with the recommended volume of water.
11. Wait for at least 2 hours before re-starting the feed.

Intrajejunal administration

There are no specific data relating to the jejunal administration of etidronate. Administer using the above method.

References

1. *BNF* 50, September 2005.
2. Personal communication, Procter & Gamble; 22 January 2003.
3. Didronel (P&G), Summary of Product Characteristics; October 2002.
4. BPNG data on file, 2005.

Etodolac

Formulations available [1]		
Brand name (Manufacturer)	**Formulation and strength**	**Product information/Administration information**
Lodine SR (Shire)	M/R tablets 600 mg	Modified-release tablets; do not crush. [2]
Etodolac (Viatris)	Capsules 300 mg	No specific data on enteral tube administration are available for this formulation.

Site of absorption (oral administration)

Specific site of absorption is not documented. Peak plasma concentration occurs 1 hour following oral dosing. [3]

Alternative routes available

None available for etodolac. Meloxicam (also COXII-selective) is available as a suppository.

Interactions

Food reduces the rate but not the extent of absorption.[3]

Health and safety

Standard precautions apply.

Suggestions/recommendations

- As there are no data available for etodolac administered via enteral feeding tubes, consider changing to meloxicam suppositories or tablets or etoricoxib tablets (see monographs).

References

1. *BNF* 50, September 2005.
2. Personal communication, Shire Pharmaceuticals; 17 February 2003.
3. Dollery C. *Therapeutic Drugs*, 2nd edn. London: Churchill Livingstone; 1998.

Etoposide

Formulations available[1]

Brand name (Manufacturer)	Formulation and strength	Product information/Administration information
Vepesid (BMS)	Capsules 50 mg, 100 mg	Oral dose is double the intravenous dose.[1] It is not appropriate to open capsules; the soft gelatin capsule contains liquid.[2]
Vepesid (BMS)	Injection 20 mg/mL (5 mL)	Generic version is also available from APS, Mayne and Medac. No specific data on enteral tube administration are available for this formulation.
Etopophos (BMS)	Injection 100 mg	Powder for reconstitution. No specific data on enteral tube administration are available for this formulation.
Extemporaneous preparation	Solution 10 mg/mL	*Extemporaneous etoposide solution 10 mg/mL:* Etoposide 20 mg/mL injection 60 mL Sodium Chloride 0.9% Injection to 120 mL Stability data support 22-day expiry at room temperature;[3] however, as this solution does not contain a preservative, a shelf-life of 7 days may be considered more appropriate. This solution should be prepared in a suitable containment facility. The solution should not be refrigerated as this may lead to precipitation. It should be stored in a glass bottle.

Site of absorption (oral administration)

Specific site of absorption is not documented. Peak plasma concentration occurs 2 hours after oral dosing. Absorption is incomplete (50%) and variable (25–80%).[4]

Alternative routes available

Parenteral route is available.

Interactions

No specific interaction with food is documented.[4]

Health and safety

Etoposide is cytotoxic. Protective clothing should be worn. Etoposide should not be handled by pregnant women. Administration equipment, e.g. syringes, should be disposed of as cytotoxic waste.

Suggestions/recommendations

- Use an extemporaneously prepared solution preparation. This should be prepared in appropriate facilities.
- A prolonged break in feeding is not required.

Intragastric administration

1. Stop the enteral feed.
2. Flush the enteral feeding tube with the recommended volume of water.
3. Draw the medication solution into an appropriate size and type of syringe.
4. Flush the medication dose down the feeding tube.
5. Finally, flush with the recommended volume of water.
6. Re-start the feed, unless a prolonged break is required.

Alternatively, at step (3) measure the medicine in a suitable container and then draw into an appropriate syringe. Ensure that the measure is rinsed and that this rinsing water is administered also to ensure that the total dose is given. **Do not** measure liquid medicines using a catheter-tipped syringe as this results in excessive dosing owing to the volume of the tip.

Intrajejunal administration

There are no specific data relating to the jejunal administration of etoposide. Administer using the above method. Monitor for increased side-effects or loss of efficacy.

References

1. *BNF* 50, September 2005.
2. Personal communication, Bristol-Myers Squibb; 24 January 2003.
3. McLeod HL, Relling MV. Stability of etoposide solution for oral use. *Am J Hosp Pharm.* 1992; 49: 2784–2785.
4. Dollery C. *Therapeutic Drugs*, 2nd edn. London: Churchill Livingstone; 1998.

Etoricoxib

Formulations available[1]

Brand name (Manufacturer)	Formulation and strength	Product information/Administration information
Arcoxia (MSD)	Tablets 60 mg, 90 mg, 120 mg	Film-coated tablets. When placed in 10 mL of water, tablets swell rapidly then disintegrate to give fine granules that settle quickly but disperse easily and flush down an 8Fr NG tube without blockage.[2]

Site of absorption (oral administration)

Specific site of absorption is not documented. Peak plasma concentration occurs 1 hour after oral dosing in fasted adults.[3]

Alternative routes available

Meloxicam (COXII-selective) is available as suppositories. Rectal, topical and parenteral routes are available for other NSAIDs.

Interactions

Administration with food delays but does not reduce absorption; this effect is not clinically important.[3]

Health and safety

Standard precautions apply.

Suggestions/recommendations

- Disperse the tablets in water immediately prior to administration.
- A prolonged break in feeding is not necessary.
- Alternatively change to meloxicam suppositories.

Intragastric administration

1. Stop the enteral feed.
2. Flush the enteral feeding tube with the recommended volume of water.
3. Place the tablet in the barrel of an appropriate size and type of syringe.
4. Draw 10 mL of water into the syringe and allow the tablet to disperse, shaking if necessary.
5. Flush the medication dose down the feeding tube.
6. Draw another 10 mL of water into the syringe and also flush this via the feeding tube (this will rinse the syringe and ensure that the total dose is administered).
7. Finally, flush with the recommended volume of water.
8. Re-start the feed, unless a prolonged break is required.

Alternatively, at step (3) place the tablet into a medicine pot, add 10 mL of water and allow the tablet to disperse. Draw this into the syringe. Ensure that the measure is rinsed and that this rinsing water is administered also to ensure that the total dose is given.

Intrajejunal administration

There are no specific data relating to the jejunal administration of etoricoxib. Administer as above and monitor for lack of efficacy or increased side-effects.

References

1. *BNF* 50, September 2005.
2. BPNG data on file, 2005.
3. Arcoxia (MSD), Summary of Product Characteristics; May 2005.

Ezetimibe

Formulations available [1]

Brand name (Manufacturer)	Formulation and strength	Product information/Administration information
Ezetrol (MSD)	Tablets 10 mg	Tablets disperse in 10 mL of water within 5 minutes if shaken. The fine white dispersion flushes via an 8Fr NG tube without blockage. [2]

Site of absorption (oral administration)

Ezetimibe is rapidly absorbed, with the peak plasma concentration of the active metabolite occurring 1–2 hours following oral dosing. [3]

Alternative routes available

Parenteral route is available.

Interactions

Food does not affect the bioavailability of ezetimibe. [3]

Health and safety

Standard precautions apply.

Suggestions/recommendations

• Disperse the tablets in water immediately prior to administration.
• A prolonged break in feeding is not necessary.

Intragastric administration

1. Stop the enteral feed.
2. Flush the enteral feeding tube with the recommended volume of water.
3. Place the tablet in the barrel of an appropriate size and type of syringe.
4. Draw 10 mL of water into the syringe and allow the tablet to disperse, shaking if necessary.
5. Flush the medication dose down the feeding tube.
6. Draw another 10 mL of water into the syringe and also flush this via the feeding tube (this will rinse the syringe and ensure that the total dose is administered).
7. Finally, flush with the recommended volume of water.
8. Re-start the feed, unless a prolonged break is required.

Alternatively, at step (3) place the tablet into a medicine pot, add 10 mL of water and allow the tablet to disperse. Draw this into an appropriate syringe. Ensure that the measure is rinsed and that this rinsing water is administered also to ensure that the total dose is given.

Intrajejunal administration

There are no specific reports relating to the jejunal administration of ezetimibe. Administer using the above method. Monitor for loss of efficacy or increased side-effects.

References

1. *BNF* 50, September 2005.
2. BPNG data on file, 2005.
3. Ezetrol (MSD), Summary of Product Characteristics; June 2005.

Famciclovir

Formulations available[1]

Brand name (Manufacturer)	Formulation and strength	Product information/Administration information
Famvir (Novartis)	Tablets 125 mg, 250 mg, 500 mg, 750 mg	Film-coated tablets. The tablets do not disperse readily in water even if agitated for 5 minutes. The tablets are very hard and difficult to crush owing to their unusual shape. They can be crushed with persistence and will suspend in water, although the granules settle quickly. The dispersion will flush through an 8Fr NG tube without blockage.[3]

Site of absorption (oral administration)

Specific site of absorption is not documented. Peak plasma concentration of the active metabolite of famciclovir occurs within 1 hour of oral dosing.[2]

Alternative routes available

None.

Interactions

Food does not have a significant effect on the bioavailability of famciclovir.[2]

Health and safety

Standard precautions apply.

Suggestions/recommendations

- Consider using aciclovir (see monograph). Alternatively crush tablets and disperse in water immediately prior to administration.
- A prolonged break in feeding is not required.

Intragastric administration

1. Stop the enteral feed.
2. Flush the enteral feeding tube with the recommended volume of water.
3. Place the tablet in a mortar and crush to a fine powder using the pestle.
4. Add a few millilitres of water and mix to form a paste.
5. Add up to 15 mL of water and mix thoroughly ensuring that there are no large particles of tablet.
6. Draw this into an appropriate size and type of syringe.
7. Flush the medication dose down the feeding tube.
8. Add another 15 mL of water to the mortar and stir to ensure that any remaining drug is rinsed from the container. Draw this water into the syringe and also flush this via the feeding tube (this will rinse the mortar and syringe and ensure that the total dose is administered).
9. Finally, flush the enteral feeding tube with the recommended volume of water.
10. Re-start the feed, unless prolonged break is required.

Intrajejunal administration

There are no specific data relating to the jejunal administration of famciclovir. Administer using the above method. Monitor for increased incidence of adverse effects or loss of efficacy.

References

1. *BNF* 50, September 2005.
2. Dollery C. *Therapeutic Drugs*, 2nd edn. London: Churchill Livingstone; 1998.
3. BPNG data on file, 2004.

Famotidine

Formulations available[1]

Brand name (Manufacturer)	Formulation and strength	Product information/Administration information
Pepcid (MSD)	Tablets 20 mg, 40 mg	Film-coated. No specific data on enteral tube administration are available for this formulation.
Famotidine (APS, Arrow, Generics, Niche, Sandoz)	Tablets 20 mg, 40 mg	No specific data. No specific data on enteral tube administration are available for this formulation.

Site of absorption (oral administration)

Specific site is not documented. Peak plasma concentration occurs 1–3 hours after dosing.[2]

Alternative routes available

None available for famotidine, ranitidine and cimetidine as injection.

Interactions

Bioavailability is unaffected by food.[2]

Health and safety

Standard precautions apply

Suggestions/recommendations

- As no liquid preparation is available for famotidine, change therapy to ranitidine. Famotidine 40 mg is equivalent to 300 mg ranitidine (see monograph).

References

1. *BNF* 50, September 2005.
2. Pepcid (MSD), Summary of Product Characteristics; July 2003.

Felodipine

Formulations available[1]

Brand name (Manufacturer)	Formulation and strength	Product information/Administration information
Plendil (AstraZeneca)	M/R tablets 2.5 mg, 5 mg, 10 mg	Extended-release tablets. Tablets must not be chewed or crushed.[2]
Felodipine (Generics, Genus)	M/R tablets 5 mg, 10 mg	Swallow whole, do not chew.[1]

Site of absorption (oral administration)

Specific site of absorption is not documented.

Alternative routes available

None for felodipine.

Interactions

No documented interaction with food.[2]

Health and safety

Standard precautions apply.

Suggestions/recommendations

- Felodipine tablets are modified release and therefore unsuitable. Change to amlodipine (see monograph) and titrate dose to response.

References

1. *BNF* 50, September 2005.
2. Plendil 2.5 mg (AstraZeneca), Summary of Product Characteristics; September 2003.

Fexofenadine hydrochloride

Formulations available[1]

Brand name (Manufacturer)	Formulation and strength	Product information/Administration information
Telfast (Aventis)	Tablets 30 mg, 120 mg, 180 mg	Aventis has no data to support crushing the tablets and has no data on enteral tube administration.[2]

Site of absorption (oral administration)

Specific site of absorption is not documented. Peak plasma concentration occurs 1–3 hours following oral absorption.[3]

Alternative routes available

None.

Interactions

No specific interaction with food is documented. SPC recommends that the dose be taken before a meal.[3]

Health and safety

Standard precautions apply.

Suggestions/recommendations

- Owing to lack of data, consider changing to an alternative nonsedating antihistamine available as a liquid, such as cetirazine, desloratidine or loratidine.

References

1. *BNF* 50, September 2005.
2. Personal communication, Aventis, 2 January 2003.
3. Telfast (Aventis), Summary of Product Characteristics; April 2003.

Finasteride

Formulations available[1]

Brand name (Manufacturer)	Formulation and strength	Product information/Administration information
Proscar (MSD)	Tablets 5 mg	Film-coated. Tablets disperse within 5 minutes when placed in 10 mL of water. The resulting pale blue, milky dispersion draws up and flushes easily via an 8Fr NG tube.[2]

Site of absorption (oral administration)

Specific site is unknown. Peak plasma concentration occurs 2 hours following oral dosing.[3]

Alternative routes available

None available.

Interactions

Bioavailability is unaffected by food.[3]

Health and safety

Women should not handle crushed or broken tablets if they are or may be pregnant owing to the potential risk to a male fetus.[3] For this reason a 'closed system' should be used to disperse tablet (see chapter 9).

Suggestions/recommendations

- Tablets can be dispersed in water immediately prior to administration; a closed system should be used to minimise operator exposure.
- A prolonged break in feeding is not required.

Intragastric administration

1. Stop the enteral feed.
2. Flush the enteral feeding tube with the recommended volume of water.
3. Place the tablet in the barrel of an appropriate size and type of syringe.
4. Draw 10 mL of water into the syringe and allow the tablet to disperse, shaking if necessary.
5. Flush the medication dose down the feeding tube.
6. Draw another 10 mL of water into the syringe and also flush this via the feeding tube (this will rinse the syringe and ensure that the total dose is administered).
7. Finally, flush with the recommended volume of water.
8. Re-start the feed, unless a prolonged break is required.

Intrajejunal administration

There are no specific data relating to the jejunal administration of finasteride. Administer as above. Monitor efficacy and side-effects.

References

1. *BNF 50*, September 2005.
2. BPNG data on file, 2004.
3. Proscar (MSD), Summary of Product Characteristics; April 2002.

Flavoxate hydrochloride

Formulations available[1]

Brand name (Manufacturer)	Formulation and strength	Product information/Administration information
Urispas 200 (Shire)	Tablets 200 mg	Sugar-coated tablets.[2] The tablets do not disperse readily in water. The tablets are very hard to crush, but with persistence can be ground to a fine powder, which mixes well with water to form a milky dispersion that flushes via an 8Fr NG tube without blockage.[3]

Site of absorption (oral administration)

Specific site of absorption is not documented. Peak plasma concentrations of the active metabolite of flavoxate appear in the plasma 30–60 minutes following oral dosing.[4]

Alternative routes available

None available.

Interactions

No specific interaction with food is documented.[4]

Health and safety

Standard precautions apply.

Suggestions/recommendations

- Although the tablets can be crushed and mixed with water, there are no stability data to support this. Consideration should be given to changing to an alternative such as oxybutynin or tolterodine (see monographs).
- A prolonged break in feeding is not required.

Intragastric administration

1. Stop the enteral feed.
2. Flush the enteral feeding tube with the recommended volume of water.
3. Place the tablet in mortar and crush to a fine powder using the pestle.
4. Add a few millilitres of water and mix to form a paste.
5. Add up to 15 mL of water and mix thoroughly, ensuring that there are no large particles of tablet.
6. Draw this into an appropriate size and type of syringe.
7. Flush the medication dose down the feeding tube.
8. Add another 15 mL of water to the mortar and stir to ensure that any remaining drug is rinsed from the container. Draw this water into the syringe and also flush this via the feeding tube (this will rinse the mortar and syringe and ensure that the total dose is administered).
9. Finally, flush the enteral feeding tube with the recommended volume of water.
10. Re-start the feed, unless a prolonged break is required.

Intrajejunal administration

There are no data relating to jejunal administration of flavoxate. Administer using the above method. Monitor for loss of efficacy or increased side-effects.

References

1. *BNF* 50, September 2005.
2. Personal communication, Shire Ltd; 17 February 2003.
3. BPNG data on file, 2005.
4. Urispas 200 (Shire), Summary of Product Characteristics; December 2002.

Flecanide

Formulations available[1]

Brand name (Manufacturer)	Formulation and strength	Product information/Administration information
Flecainide (Alpharma, APS, Generics, Sterwin)	Tablets 50 mg, 100 mg	Tablets can be crushed.[2] Generics brand tablets disintegrate within 2 minutes when placed in 10 mL of water to give very fine dispersion that draws up and flushes via an 8Fr NG tube without blockage.[3]
Tambacor (3M)	Tablets 50 mg, 100 mg	No specific data on enteral tube administration are available for this formulation.
Tambacor (3M)	Injection 10 mg/mL (15 mL)	No specific data on enteral tube administration are available for this formulation.

Site of absorption (oral administration)

Flecanide is rapidly and almost completely absorbed following oral absorption, although the specific site of absorption is not documented.[4]

Alternative routes available

Parenteral route is available.

Interactions

Food reduces the rate but not the extent of absorption.[4]

Health and safety

Standard precautions apply.

Suggestions/recommendations

- Disperse tablet in water immediately prior to administration.
- A prolonged break in feeding is not required.
- The parenteral route can be used in acute situations and when gastrointestinal absorption is compromised.

Intragastric administration

1. Stop the enteral feed.
2. Flush the enteral feeding tube with the recommended volume of water.
3. Place the tablet in the barrel of an appropriate size and type of syringe.
4. Draw 10 mL of water into the syringe and allow the tablet to disperse, shaking if necessary.
5. Flush the medication dose down the feeding tube.
6. Draw another 10 mL of water into the syringe and also flush this via the feeding tube (this will rinse the syringe and ensure that the total dose is administered).
7. Finally, flush with the recommended volume of water.
8. Re-start the feed, unless a prolonged break is required.

Alternatively, at step (3) place the tablet into a medicine pot, add 10 mL of water and allow the tablet to disperse. Draw this into an appropriate syringe. Ensure that the measure is rinsed and that this rinsing water is administered also to ensure that the total dose is given.

Intrajejunal administration

There are no specific data relating to jejunal administration. Administer as above. Monitor closely for loss of efficacy or increased side-effects. Plasma concentration can be measured.

References

1. *BNF* 50, September 2005.
2. Personal communication, Alpharma Ltd; 21 January 2003.
3. BPNG data on file, 2005.
4. Dollery C. *Therapeutic Drugs*, 2nd edn. London: Churchill Livingstone; 1998.

Flucloxacillin

Formulations available[1]

Brand name (Manufacturer)	Formulation and strength	Product information/Administration information
Flucloxacillin (various manufacturers)	Capsules 250 mg, 500 mg	Avoid opening capsules owing to the risk of operator sensitisation. As sodium salt.
Flucloxacillin (various manufacturers)	Oral solution 125 mg/5 mL, 250 mg/5 mL	As sodium salt. *Kent brand:* Pink nongranular liquid, slightly viscous. Flushes with little resistance. Mixes easily with water to reduce viscosity.[4]
Flucloxacillin (Berk, CP)	Injection 250 mg, 500 mg, 1 g	As sodium salt. Can be administered enterally.[3]
Floxapen (GSK)	Capsules 250 mg, 500 mg, 1 g	Avoid opening capsules owing to the risk of operator sensitisation. As sodium salt.

Formulations available[1] (continued)

Brand name (Manufacturer)	Formulation and strength	Product information/Administration information
Floxapen (GSK)	Syrup 125 mg/5 mL, 250 mg/5 mL	As magnesium salt. Contains sucrose.
Floxapen (GSK)	Injection 250 mg, 500 mg, 1 g	As sodium salt. Contains no other excipients.[2] No specific data on enteral tube administration are available for this formulation.

Site of absorption (oral administration)

Flucloxacillin is absorbed in the upper small bowel with the peak plasma concentration occurring after 1 hour.[2] Administration directly into the jejunum is not expected to reduce bioavailability.[3]

Alternative routes available

Injection available, can be given intramuscularly or intravenously.

Interactions

Oral doses should be administered half to one hour before food.[2]

Health and safety

Standard precautions apply. Avoid inhalation of the dry powder.

Suggestions/recommendations

- Flucloxacillin requires four daily doses and a break in feeding is required around the dose. This dosing regimen may be suitable for patients on bolus feeding, but may be impractical in patients on continuous feeds. Consider using an alternative antibiotic or increasing the dose used if prolonged breaks in feeding are not possible.
- Feed should be stopped 1 hour prior to dose and the tube flushed; use the liquid preparations for intragastric administration. Consider using the injection for intrajejunal administration as the osmolarity is lower,[3] or alternatively dilute the suspension with at least an equal volume of water to reduce osmolarity.
- Restart feed half to 1 hour after the dose.

Intragastric administration

1. Stop the enteral feed.
2. Flush the enteral feeding tube with the recommended volume of water.
3. Allow at least 1 hour before administering dose.
4. Draw the medication solution into an appropriate size and type of syringe.
5. Flush the medication dose down the feeding tube.
6. Finally, flush with the recommended volume of water.
7. Do not restart the feed for at least 30 minutes.

Alternatively, at step (4) measure the medicine in a suitable container and then draw into the syringe. Ensure that the measure is rinsed and that this rinsing water is administered also to ensure that the total dose is given. **Do not** measure liquid medicines using a catheter-tipped syringe as this results in excessive dosing owing to the volume of the tip.

Intrajejunal administration

1. Stop the enteral feed.
2. Flush the enteral feeding tube with the recommended volume of water.
3. Allow at least 1 hour before administering dose.
4. Shake the medication bottle thoroughly to ensure adequate mixing.
5. Draw the medication suspension into an appropriate size and type of syringe.
6. Draw an equal volume of water and a little air into the syringe and shake to mix thoroughly.
7. Flush the medication dose down the feeding tube.
8. Finally, flush with the recommended volume of water.
9. Do not restart the feed for at least 30 minutes.

Alternatively, at step (5) measure the medicine in a suitable container and then add an equal volume of water and mix thoroughly. Draw this into an appropriate syringe. Ensure that the measure is rinsed and that this rinsing water is administered also to ensure that the total dose is given. **Do not** measure liquid medicines using a catheter-tipped syringe as this results in excessive dosing owing to the volume of the tip.

References

1. *BNF* 50, September 2005.
2. Floxapen (GSK), Summary of Product Characteristics; April 2003.
3. Adams D. Administration of drugs through a jejunostomy tube. *Br J Intensive Care*. 1994; 4(1): 10–17.
4. BPNG data on file, 2004.

Fluconazole

Formulations available[1]

Brand name (Manufacturer)	Formulation and strength	Product information/Administration information
Diflucan (Pfizer)	Capsules 50 mg, 150 mg, 200 mg	If the suspension is not available, the capsules can be opened and washed down the tube with plenty of water.[2] Powder from 150 mg capsules does not mix well with water.[3]
Diflucan (Pfizer)	Suspension 50 mg/5 mL 200 mg/5 mL	Orange-flavoured suspension when reconstituted.[4]
Diflucan (Pfizer)	Intravenous infusion 2 mg/mL (100 mL)	Not suitable for enteral administration owing to large volume.
Fluconazole (Alpharma, APS, Generics, IVAX, PLIVA, Sandoz, Sterwin)	50 mg, 150 mg, 200 mg	Powder from 50 mg capsules can be mixed with water (PLIVA and Medimpex tested).[3]

Formulations available[1] (continued)

Brand name (Manufacturer)	Formulation and strength	Product information/Administration information
Fluconazole (PLIVA)	Intravenous infusion 2 mg/mL (100 mL)	Not suitable for enteral administration owing to large volume.

Site of absorption (oral administration)

Specific site is not documented. Peak plasma concentration occurs 1–2 hours after oral dosing indicating absorption high in the GI tract.[5]

Alternative routes available

Parenteral route is available.

Interactions

Food and gastric pH do not affect absoprtion.[5]

Health and safety

Standard precautions apply.

Suggestions/recommendations

- Fluconazole is absorbed when administered via both gastric and post-pyloric enteral feeding tubes and demonstrates similar pharmacokinetics to oral administration.[6] There is no interaction with enteral feed.[6]
- The suspension should be used and the tube flushed well with water after the dose.
- A prolonged break in feeding is not necessary.

Intragastric administration

1. Stop the enteral feed.
2. Flush the enteral feeding tube with the recommended volume of water.
3. Shake the medication bottle thoroughly to ensure adequate mixing.
4. Draw the medication suspension into an appropriate size and type of syringe.
5. Flush the medication dose down the feeding tube.
6. Finally, flush with the recommended volume of water.
7. Re-start the feed, unless a prolonged break is required.

Alternatively, at step (4) measure the medicine in a suitable container and then add an equal volume of water and mix thoroughly. Draw this into an appropriate syringe. Ensure that the measure is rinsed and that this rinsing water is administered also to ensure that the total dose is given. **Do not** measure liquid medicines using a catheter-tipped syringe as this results in excessive dosing owing to the volume of the tip.

Intrajejunal administration

Bioavailability is unaffected by jejunal administration; see notes above. Administer using the above method.

References

1. *BNF 50*, September 2005.
2. Personal communication, Pfizer; 23 June 2003.
3. BPNG data on file, 2004.
4. Diflucan (Pfizer), Summary of Product Characteristics; July 2000.
5. Dollery C. *Therapeutic Drugs*, 2nd edn. London: Churchill Livingstone; 1998.
6. Nicolau DP, Crowe H, Nightingale CH, Quintiliani R. Bioavailability of fluconazole administered via a feeding tube in intensive care unit patients. *J Antimicrob Chemother*. 1995; 36: 395–401.

Fludrocortisone acetate

Formulations available[1]

Brand name (Manufacturer)	Formulation and strength	Product information/Administration information
Florinef (Squibb)	Tablets 100 microgram	Fludrocortisone is practically insoluble in water (0.04 mg/mL).[2, 5] However, the usual dose of 100 micrograms will dissolve in 2.5 mL of water. Tablet disintegrates within 2 minutes when placed in 10 mL of water; the fine dispersion settles quickly but flushes via an 8Fr NG tube without blockage.[3]

Site of absorption (oral administration)

Specific site of absorption is not documented. Peak plasma concentration occurs 4–8 hours following oral dosing.[4]

Alternative routes available

None available for fludrocortisone. General steroid replacement can be achieved using parenteral hydrocortisone.

Interactions

No specific interaction with food is documented.

Health and safety

Mineralocorticoid steroid: avoid exposure to crushed tablets. Standard precautions should be sufficient.

Suggestions/recommendations

- Disperse tablet in water immediately prior to administration.
- A prolonged break in feeding is not required.

Intragastric administration

1. Stop the enteral feed.
2. Flush the enteral feeding tube with the recommended volume of water.
3. Place the tablet in the barrel of an appropriate size and type of syringe.
4. Draw 10 mL of water into the syringe and allow the tablet to disperse, shaking if necessary.
5. Flush the medication dose down the feeding tube.
6. Draw another 10 mL of water into the oral syringe and also flush this via the feeding tube (this will rinse the syringe and ensure that the total dose is administered).
7. Finally, flush with the recommended volume of water.
8. Re-start the feed, unless a prolonged break is required.

Alternatively, at step (3) place the tablet into a medicine pot, add 10 mL of water and allow the tablet to disperse. Draw this into an appropriate syringe. Ensure that the measure is rinsed and that this rinsing water is administered also to ensure that the total dose is given.

Intrajejunal administration

There are no specific data relating to jejunal administration of fludrocortisone. Administer using the above method. Monitor for increased side-effects or loss of efficacy.

References

1. *BNF* 50, September 2005.
2. Personal communication, Bristol-Myers Squibb; 24 January 2003.
3. BPNG data on file, 2004.
4. Florinef (Squibb), Summary of Product Characteristics; January 1999
5. Trissel LA, ed. *Stability of Compounded Formulations*, 2nd edn. Washington, DC: American Pharmaceutical Association; 2000.

Fluoxetine hydrochloride

Formulations available[1]

Brand name (Manufacturer)	Formulation and strength	Product information/Administration information
Fluoxetine (Alpharma, APS, Arrow, CP, Generics, Genus, IVAX, Sandoz, Sterwin)	Capsules 20 mg, 60 mg	Capsules can be opened and the contents mixed with 10 mL of water, although this requires a degree of manual dexterity owing to the small size of the capsules.[2] There are no stability data to support this method, so this should be done immediately prior to administration.
Fluoxetine (APS)	Liquid 20 mg/5 mL	No specific data on enteral tube administration are available for this formulation.
Prozac (Dista)	Capsules 20 mg, 60 mg	No specific data on enteral tube administration are available for this formulation.
Prozac (Dista)	Liquid 20 mg/5 mL	Clear, colourless liquid. Does not contain sorbitol.[3]

Site of absorption (oral administration)

Specific site of absorption is not documented. Peak plasma concentration occurs 6–8 hours following oral absorption.[3]

Alternative routes available

No alternative routes for fluoxetine.

Interactions

Absorption is delayed by 3–4 hours by the presence of food.[4] Can be taken with or without food.[3]

Health and safety

Standard precautions apply.

Suggestions/recommendations

- Use the liquid preparation.
- A prolonged break in feeding is not necessary.

Intragastric administration

1. Stop the enteral feed.
2. Flush the enteral feeding tube with the recommended volume of water.
3. Draw the medication liquid into an appropriate size and type of syringe.
4. Flush the medication dose down the feeding tube.
5. Finally, flush with the recommended volume of water.
6. Re-start the feed, unless a prolonged break is required.

Alternatively, at step (3) measure the medicine in a suitable container. Draw this into the syringe. Ensure that the measure is rinsed and that this rinsing water is administered also to ensure that the total dose is given. **Do not** measure liquid medicines using a catheter-tipped syringe as this results in excessive dosing owing to the volume of the tip.

Intrajejunal administration

There are no specific reports of jejunal administration of fluoxetine. Administer using the above method. Monitor for loss of efficacy or increased side-effects.

References

1. *BNF* 50, September 2005.
2. BPNG data on file, 2004.
3. Prozac (Dista), Summary of Product Characteristics; August 2003.
4. Oxactin Capsules (Discovery), Summary of Product Characteristics; April 2001.

Flupentixol (Flupenthixol)

Formulations available[1]

Brand name (Manufacturer)	Formulation and strength	Product information/Administration information
Fluanxol (Lundbeck)	Tablets 500 microgram, 1 mg	Flupenthixol dihydrochloride. Sugar-coated. No specific data on enteral tube administration are available for this formulation.
Depixol (Lundbeck)	Tablets 3 mg	Flupenthixol dihydrochloride. Sugar-coated. Tablets do not disperse readily owing to the sugar coating, but disintegrate if shaken in water for 5 minutes to give a pale pink, very fine dispersion that flushes via an 8Fr NG tube without blockage.[2]
Depixol (Lundbeck)	Injection 20 mg/mL	Flupenthixol decanoate. Depot injection. No specific data on enteral tube administration are available for this formulation.
Depixol Conc (Lundbeck)	Injection 100 mg/mL	Flupenthixol decanoate. Depot injection. No specific data on enteral tube administration are available for this formulation.
Depixol Low Volume (Lundbeck)	Injection 200 mg/mL	Flupenthixol decanoate. Depot injection. No specific data on enteral tube administration are available for this formulation.

Site of absorption (oral administration)

Specific site of absorption is not documented. Flupentixol is absorbed via the GI tract with the peak plasma concentration occurring 4 hours following oral dosing.[3]

Alternative routes available

Depot injection is available.

Interactions

No specific interaction with food is documented.[3, 4]

Health and safety

Standard precautions apply.

Suggestions/recommendations

- Flupentixol should not be stopped abruptly.[4]
- Disperse the tablets in water immediately prior to administration. A prolonged break in feeding is not required. Consider changing to an alternative therapy available in suitable formulation; alternatively, use depot injection every 2 weeks. Seek specialist advice.

Intragastric administration

1. Stop the enteral feed.
2. Flush the enteral feeding tube with the recommended volume of water.
3. Place the tablet in the barrel of an appropriate size and type of syringe.
4. Draw 10 mL of water into the syringe and allow the tablet to disperse, shaking if necessary.
5. Flush the medication dose down the feeding tube.
6. Draw another 10 mL of water into the syringe and also flush this via the feeding tube (this will rinse the syringe and ensure that the total dose is administered).
7. Finally, flush with the recommended volume of water.
8. Re-start the feed, unless a prolonged break is required.

Alternatively, at step (3) place the tablet into a medicine pot, add 10 mL of water and allow the tablet to disperse. Draw this into an appropriate syringe. Ensure that the measure is rinsed and that this rinsing water is administered also to ensure that the total dose is given.

Intrajejunal administration

There are no specific data relating to jejunal administration. Administer as above. Monitor for loss of efficacy or increased side-effects.

References

1. *BNF* 50, September 2005.
2. BPNG data on file, 2005.
3. Dollery C. *Therapeutic Drugs*, 2nd edn. London: Churchill Livingstone; 1998.
4. Depixol (Lundbeck), Summary of Product Characteristics; July 2002.

Fluphenazine

Formulations available[1]

Brand name (Manufacturer)	Formulation and strength	Product information/Administration information
Moditen (Sanofi-Synthelabo)	Tablets 1 mg, 2.5 mg, 5 mg	Fluphenazine hydrochloride. Sugar-coated. Tablets do not disperse readily in water even when shaken. They are quite difficult to crush owing to the coating, but once crushed will suspend in water and will flush via an 8Fr NG tube without blockage.[2]
Modecate (Sanofi-Synthelabo)	Injection 25 mg/mL	Fluphenazine decanoate. Depot injection. Also available from Antigen, Mayne and Hillcross. No specific data on enteral tube administration are available for this formulation.
Modecate Conc (Sanofi-Synthelabo)	Injection 100 mg/mL	Fluphenazine decanoate. Depot injection. Also available from Antigen, Mayne and Hillcross. No specific data on enteral tube administration are available for this formulation.

Site of absorption (oral administration)

Specific site of absorption is not documented. Peak plasma concentration occurs within 3 hours of oral dosing.[3]

Alternative routes available

Depot injection is available for parenteral administration.

Interactions

No specific interaction with food is documented[3, 4].

Health and safety

Standard precautions apply.

Suggestions/recommendations

- Fluphenazine should not be stopped abruptly.[4]
- Consider changing to alternative therapy available in suitable formulation; alternatively use depot injection every 2 weeks. Seek specialist advice.
- If alternative therapy is not appropriate, crush the tablets and suspend in water immediately prior to administration. A prolonged break in feeding is not required.

Intragastric administration

1. Stop the enteral feed.
2. Flush the enteral feeding tube with the recommended volume of water.
3. Place the tablet in a mortar and crush to a fine powder using the pestle.
4. Add a few millilitres of water and mix to form a paste.
5. Add up to 15 mL of water and mix thoroughly, ensuring that there are no large particles of tablet.
6. Draw this into an appropriate syringe.
7. Flush the medication dose down the feeding tube.
8. Add another 15 mL of water to the mortar and stir to ensure that any remaining drug is rinsed from the container. Draw this water into the syringe and also flush this via the feeding tube (this will rinse the mortar and syringe and ensure that the total dose is administered).
9. Finally, flush the enteral feeding tube with the recommended volume of water.
10. Re-start the feed, unless a prolonged break is required.

Intrajejunal administration

There is no specific information relating to jejunal administration. Administer as above. Monitor for loss of efficacy or increased side-effects.

References

1. *BNF 50*, September 2005.
2. BPNG data on file, 2004.
3. Dollery C. *Therapeutic Drugs*, 2nd edn. London: Churchill Livingstone; 1998.
4. Moditen (Sanofi), Summary of Product Characteristics; November 2001.

Flutamide

Formulations available[1]

Brand name (Manufacturer)	Formulation and strength	Product information/Administration information
Flutamide (Alpharma, Chiron, Generics, Hillcross, Tillomed)	Tablets 250 mg	*Generics brand:* Tablets are quite bulky and do not disintegrate readily, but will disperse if shaken in water for 5–10 minutes; this dispersion flushes via an 8Fr tube without blockage.[2]
Drogenil (Schering-Plough)	Tablets 250 mg	No specific data on enteral tube administration are available for this formulation.

Site of absorption (oral administration)

Specific site of absorption is not documented. Peak plasma concentration occurs 4–6 hours following oral dosing.[3]

Alternative routes available

None available.

Interactions

There is no documented interaction with food.[3]

Health and safety

Antiandrogen. Standard precautions apply.

Suggestions/recommendations

- Disperse the tablets in water immediately before administration.
- A prolonged break in feeding is not required.
- No liquid preparation and requires three times daily dosing; consider alternative treatment; seek specialist advice.

Intragastric administration

1. Stop the enteral feed.
2. Flush the enteral feeding tube with the recommended volume of water.
3. Place the tablet in the barrel of an appropriate size and type of syringe.
4. Draw 10 mL of water into the syringe and allow the tablet to disperse, shaking if necessary.
5. Flush the medication dose down the feeding tube.
6. Draw another 10 mL of water into the syringe and also flush this via the feeding tube (this will rinse the syringe and ensure that the total dose is administered).
7. Finally, flush with the recommended volume of water.
8. Re-start the feed, unless a prolonged break is required.

Alternatively, at step (3) place the tablet into a medicine pot, add 10 mL of water and allow the tablet to disperse. Draw this into an appropriate syringe. Ensure that the measure is rinsed and that this rinsing water is administered also to ensure that the total dose is given.

Intrajejunal administration

There are no specific data on jejunal administration of flutamide. Administer as above and monitor for loss off effect or increased side-effects.

References

1. *BNF* 50, September 2005.
2. BPNG data on file, 2005.
3. Dollery C. *Therapeutic Drugs*, 2nd edn. London: Churchill Livingstone; 1998.

Fluvastatin

Formulations available[1]

Brand name (Manufacturer)	Formulation and strength	Product information/Administration information
Lescol (Novartis)	Capsules 20 mg, 40 mg	Sodium salt. Hard gelatin capsules. 20 mg = size 3 capsules. 40 mg = size 1 capsules.[2] Both the 20 mg and 40 mg capsules can be opened. The powder pours easily from the capsule and mixes readily with 10 mL of water to form a pale yellow, milky dispersion that flushes easily down an 8Fr NG tube.[5] The 20 mg capsules are more difficult to open owing to their small size.
Lescol XL (Novartis)	MR tablets 80 mg	Sodium salt. Swallow whole. Absorption is 60% slower than with capsules.[3] Not suitable for administration via feeding tube.

Site of absorption (oral administration)

Specific site of absorption is not documented. Fluvastatin is absorbed rapidly and completely (98%) following oral administration in fasted patients.[2] Time to peak plasma concentration is 0.5 hours;[4] it is therefore likely that fluvastatin is absorbed in the upper small intestine.

Alternative routes available

No alternative routes of administration are available for the 'statins'.

Interactions

Both total bioavailability and peak plasma concentration are reduced and time to reach peak is delayed when fluvastatin is taken with food, although this has no significant effect on the lipid-lowering effect of fluvastatin.[2]

Health and safety

Standard precautions apply

Suggestions/recommendations

- Consider changing to a tablet that disperses in water – atorvastatin or pravastatin (see monographs).
- If it is considered appropriate to continue fluvastatin therapy, open the capsules and mix the contents with water.
- A prolonged break in feeding is not necessary.
- The dose should be given at night;[2] however, if feeding overnight the dose should be given in the morning.

Intragastric administration

1. Stop the enteral feed.
2. Flush the enteral feeding tube with the recommended volume of water.
3. Open the capsule and pour the contents into a medicine pot.
4. Add 15 mL of water
5. Stir to disperse the powder
6. Draw into an appropriate syringe and administer via the feeding tube.
7. Add a further 15 mL of water to the medicine pot; stir to ensure that any powder remaining in the pot is mixed with water.
8. Draw up this dispersion and flush down the tube. This will ensure that the whole dose is given.
9. Flush the tube with the recommended volume of water.
10. Re-start the feed, unless a prolonged break is required.

Intrajejunal administration

There are no specific data relating to jejunal administration of fluvastatin. Administer using the above method. Monitor for increased side-effects or loss of efficacy.

References

1. *BNF* 50, September 2005.
2. Lescol (Novartis), Summary of Product Characteristics; March 2003.
3. Lescol XL80 mg (Novartis), Summary of Product Characteristics; March 2003.
4. Dollery C. *Therapeutic Drugs*, 2nd edn. London: Churchill Livingstone; 1998.
5. BPNG data on file, 2004.

Fluvoxamine maleate

Formulations available[1]

Brand name (Manufacturer)	Formulation and strength	Product information/Administration information
Fluvoxamine (APS, Arrow, IVAX, Ratiopharm)	Tablets 50 mg, 100 mg	No specific data on enteral tube administration are available for this formulation.
Faverin (Solvay)	Tablets 50 mg, 100 mg	Faverin tablets can be crushed and mixed with water, although the manufacturers have no data to support administration via enteral feeding tubes.[2]

Site of absorption (oral administration)

Specific site of absorption is not documented. Pharmacokinetic studies were performed using enteric coated preparations, so absorption occurs in small bowel. Peak plasma concentration occurred after 4–8 hours.[3] Peak plasma concentration occurs 3–8 hours following administration of Faverin.[4]

Alternative routes available

No alternative routes for fluvoxamine.

Interactions

Bioavailability is unaffected by food.[3]

Health and safety

Standard precautions apply.

Suggestions/recommendations

- Owing to lack of data, consider changing to an alternative SSRI antidepressant available as a liquid preparation. Seek specialist advice for the transfer regimen.

References

1. *BNF* 50, September 2005.
2. Personal communication, Solvay; 19 February 2003.
3. Dollery C. *Therapeutic Drugs*, 2nd edn. London: Churchill Livingstone; 1998.
4. Faverin Tablets (Solvay), Summary of Product Characteristics; November 2004.

Folic acid

Formulations available[1]

Brand name (Manufacturer)	Formulation and strength	Product information/Administration information
Folic acid (various manufacturers)	Tablets 400 microgram, 5 mg	No specific data on enteral tube administration are available for this formulation.
Folic acid (Hillcross, Rosemont)	Syrup 2.5 mg/5 mL, 400 microgram/ 5 mL	Does not contain sorbitol.[2]
Folic acid (BCM specials)	Injection 15 mg	Unlicensed; available as special order only. No specific data on enteral tube administration are available for this formulation.
Lexpec with Iron-M (Rosemont)	Syrup Iron 80 mg + folic acid 500 microgram/ 5 mL	Iron as ferric ammonium citrate Contains sorbitol 0.91 g/5 mL.[3]

Formulations available [1] (continued)

Brand name (Manufacturer)	Formulation and strength	Product information/Administration information
Lexpec with Iron (Rosemont)	Syrup Iron 80 mg + folic acid 2.5 mg/5 mL	Iron as ferric ammonium citrate Contains 0.91 g/5 mL of sorbitol.[3]

Site of absorption (oral administration)

Dietary folate is hydrolysed and absorbed in the duodenum; folic acid bound to milk proteins is absorbed in the ileum.

Alternative routes available

Injection is available (unlicensed product).

Interactions

There is no documented interaction with food affecting the absorption of folic acid.[4] Several drugs owe their pharmacological activity to their inhibition of dihydrofolate reductase, thereby causing a functional folate deficiency. Corrective therapy is dependent on the drug and desired outcome; for example, low-dose folic acid to reduce gastrointestinal side-effects of once-weekly methotrexate therapy compared with high-dose folinic acid therapy for rescue after high-dose methotrexate chemotherapy.[5]

Health and safety

Standard precautions apply.

Suggestions/recommendations

- Use a liquid preparation. Dilute with an equal volume of water to reduce osmolarity immediately prior to administration if administering into the jejunum.

Intragastric administration

1. Stop the enteral feed.
2. Flush the enteral feeding tube with the recommended volume of water.
3. Draw the medication solution into an appropriate size and type of syringe.
4. Flush the medication dose down the feeding tube.
5. Finally, flush with the recommended volume of water.
6. Re-start the feed, unless a prolonged break is required.

Alternatively, at step (3) measure the medicine in a suitable container and then draw into an appropriate syringe. Ensure that the measure is rinsed and that this rinsing water is administered also to ensure that the total dose is given. **Do not** measure liquid medicines using a catheter-tipped syringe as this results in excessive dosing owing to the volume of the tip.

Intrajejunal administration

1. Stop the enteral feed.
2. Flush the enteral feeding tube with the recommended volume of water.
3. Shake the medication bottle thoroughly to ensure adequate mixing.
4. Draw the medication suspension into an appropriate size and type of syringe.
5. Draw an equal volume of water and a little air into the syringe and shake to mix thoroughly.
6. Flush the medication dose down the feeding tube.
7. Finally, flush with the recommended volume of water.
8. Re-start the feed, unless a prolonged break is required.

Alternatively, at step (4) measure the medicine in a suitable container and then add an equal volume of water and mix thoroughly. Draw this into an appropriate syringe. Ensure that the measure is rinsed and that this rinsing water is administered also to ensure that the total dose is given. **Do not** measure liquid medicines using a catheter-tipped syringe as this results in excessive dosing owing to the volume of the tip.

References

1. *BNF 50*, September 2005.
2. Lexpec (Rosemont), Summary of Product Characteristics; October 2002.
3. Personal communication, Rosemont; 20 January 2005.
4. Dollery C. *Therapeutic Drugs*, 2nd edn. London: Churchill Livingstone; 1998.
5. White R, Ashworth A. How drug therapy can affect, threaten and compromise nutritional status. *J Hum Nutr Diet.* 2000; 13: 119–129.

Fosinopril

Formulations available[1]

Brand name (Manufacturer)	Formulation and strength	Product information/Administration information
Staril (Squibb)	Tablets 10 mg, 20 mg	Fosinopril is freely soluble in water.[2] No specific data on enteral tube administration are available for this formulation.
Fosinopril (nonproprietary)	Tablets 10 mg, 20 mg	Fosinopril sodium. No specific data on enteral tube administration are available for this formulation.

Site of absorption (oral administration)

Specific site of absorption is not documented. Peak plasma concentrations occur within 3 hours of an oral dose.[3]

Alternative routes available

None available for fosinopril.

Interactions

Absorption of fosinopril is not affected by the presence of food.[3]

Health and safety

Standard precautions apply.

Suggestions/recommendations

- No data are currently available; consider changing to alternative ACE inhibitors available in a suitable formulation.

References

1. *BNF* 50, September 2005.
2. Personal communication, Bristol-Myers Squibb; 24 January 2003.
3. Staril (Squibb), Summary of Product Characteristics; November 1995.

Furosemide (Frusemide)

Formulations available[1]

Brand name (Manufacturer)	Formulation and strength	Product information/Administration information
Furosemide (various manufacturers)	Tablets 20 mg, 40 mg, 500 mg	No specific data on enteral tube administration are available for this formulation.
Frusol (Rosemont)	Oral solution 4 mg/mL, 8 mg/mL, 10 mg/mL	Oral solution flushes down a fine-bore tube with very little resistance. Mixes easily with an equal volume of water if necessary.[2] Does not contain sorbitol.[4]
Furosemide (Antigen, Celltech, Phoenix)	Injection 10 mg/mL	No specific data on enteral tube administration are available for this formulation.
Lasix (Celltech)	Tablets 20 mg, 40 mg, 500 mg	No specific data on enteral tube administration are available for this formulation.
Lasix (Celltech)	Injection 10 mg/mL	No specific data on enteral tube administration are available for this formulation.

Site of absorption (oral administration)

The jejunum has a greater absorptive capacity for furosemide than does the ileum, and has been shown to give similar bioavailability to oral administration when given intrajejunally.[3]

Alternative routes available

Injection is available for parenteral administration.

Interactions

Food reduces the bioavailability of furosemide by 30%;[5] however, there are no specific recommendations for the timing of administration in relation to food intake. The liquid preparations and injection are alkaline (pH adjusted with sodium hydroxide).[4] There is risk of precipitation if mixed with acidic fluids, so special care should be taken to flush the tube before and after administration, especially if giving other liquid medication that may be acidic.

Health and safety

Standard precautions apply.

Suggestions/recommendations

- Use a liquid preparation. Flush the tube with water prior to administration.
- A prolonged break in feeding is not required.

Intragastric administration

1. Stop the enteral feed.
2. Flush the enteral feeding tube with the recommended volume of water.
3. Draw the medication solution into an appropriate size and type of syringe.
4. Flush the medication dose down the feeding tube.
5. Finally, flush with the recommended volume of water.
6. Re-start the feed, unless a prolonged break is required.

Alternatively, at step (3) measure the medicine in a suitable container and then draw into an appropriate syringe. Ensure that the measure is rinsed and that this rinsing water is administered also to ensure that the total dose is given. **Do not** measure liquid medicines using a catheter-tipped syringe as this results in excessive dosing owing to the volume of the tip.

Intrajejunal administration

Furosemide is absorbed well following jejunal administration. Administer using the method above.

References

1. *BNF 50*, September 2005.
2. BPNG data on file, 2004.
3. Adams D. Administration of drugs through a jejunostomy tube. *Br J Intensive Care*. 1994; 4(1): 10–17.
4. Frusol (Rosemont), Summary of Product Characteristics; October 2002.
5. McCrindle JL, Li Kam Wa TC, Barron W, Prescott LF. Effect of food on the absorption of frusemide and bumetanide in man. *Br J Clin Pharmacol*. 1996; 42(6): 743–746.

Gabapentin

Formulations available[1]

Brand name (Manufacturer)	Formulation and strength	Product information/Administration information
Neurontin (Parke-Davis)	Capsules 100 mg, 300 mg, 400 mg	Capsules can be opened and the contents mixed with 10 mL of water; the 100 mg capsule is quite fiddly owing to its small size. The powder mixes easily with water and flushes down an 8Fr NG tube without blockage.[2]
Neurontin (Parke-Davis)	Tablets 600 mg, 800 mg	No specific data on enteral tube administration are available for this formulation.
Gabapentin (nonproprietary)	Capsules 100 mg, 300 mg, 400 mg Tablets 600 mg, 800 mg	No specific data on enteral tube administration are available for these formulations.

Site of absorption (oral administration)

Specific site of absorption is not documented. Peak plasma concentration occurs 3 hours after oral dosing.[3]

Alternative routes available

No alternative routes for gabapentin.

Interactions

Food does not influence the absorption of gabapentin.[3]

Health and safety

Standard precautions apply.

Suggestions/recommendations

- Disperse the capsule contents in water immediately prior to administration.
- A prolonged break in feeding is not required.

Intragastric administration

1. Stop the enteral feed.
2. Flush the enteral feeding tube with the recommended volume of water.
3. Open the capsule and pour the contents into a medicine pot.
4. Add 15 mL of water.
5. Stir to disperse the powder
6. Draw into an appropriate syringe and administer via the feeding tube.
7. Add a further 15 mL of water to the medicine pot; stir to ensure that any powder remaining in the pot is mixed with water.
8. Draw up this dispersion and flush down tube. This will ensure that the whole dose is given.
9. Flush the tube with recommended volume of water.
10. Re-start feed, unless a prolonged break is required.

Intrajejunal administration

There are no specific data relating to jejunal administration of gabapentin. Administer using the above method. Monitor for loss of efficacy or increased side-effects.

References

1. *BNF* 50, September 2005.
2. BPNG data on file, 2004.
3. Neurontin (Parke-Davis), Summary of Product Characteristics; March 2003.

Galantamine hydrobromide

Formulations available[1]

Brand name (Manufacturer)	Formulation and strength	Product information/Administration information
Reminyl (Shire)	Tablets 4 mg, 8 mg, 12 mg	Tablets will dissolve in water.[2] Solubility of galantamine is 31 mg/mL in water.[3] Tablets disperse within 5 minutes when placed in 10 mL of water to give a fine dispersion that settles quickly but flushes easily via an 8Fr NG tube without blockage.[4]
Reminyl (Shire)	Oral solution 4 mg/mL	Does not contain sorbitol.[3] Oral solution can be mixed with water.[5] Shire does not have any specific information on the administration of the oral solution via enteral feeding tube.[5]
Reminyl (Shire)	M/R capsules 8 mg, 16 mg, 24 mg	Modified-release preparation. Not suitable for administration via enteral feeding tubes.

Site of absorption (oral administration)

Specific site of absorption is not documented. Absorption is rapid with both tablets and oral solution, with peak plasma concentrations occurring within 1 hour.[3]

Alternative routes available

None available.

Interactions

Co-administration of galantamine with food is recommended as this slows the rate, but not the extent, of absorption and reduces cholinergic side-effects.[3]

Health and safety

Standard precautions apply.

Suggestions/recommendations

- Use a liquid preparation; dilute with water prior to administration.
- Administer during or immediately after feed.
- Alternatively, tablets can be dispersed in water immediately prior to administration.

Intragastric administration

1. Stop the enteral feed.
2. Flush the enteral feeding tube with the recommended volume of water.
3. Draw the medication solution into an appropriate size and type of syringe.
4. Flush the medication dose down the feeding tube.
5. Finally, flush with the recommended volume of water.
6. Re-start the feed, unless a prolonged break is required.

Alternatively, at step (3) measure the medicine in a suitable container and then draw into an appropriate syringe. Ensure that the measure is rinsed and that this rinsing water is administered also to ensure that the total dose is given. **Do not** measure liquid medicines using a catheter-tipped syringe as this results in excessive dosing owing to the volume of the tip.

Intrajejunal administration

There are no specific data relating to jejunal administration of galantamine. Administer using the above method and monitor for increased side-effects or loss of efficacy.

References

1. *BNF* 50, September 2005.
2. Personal communication, Shire; 17 February 2003.
3. Reminyl (Shire), Summary of Product Characteristics; March 2003.
4. BPNG data on file, 2005.
5. Personal communication, Shire; 21 February 2005.

Ganciclovir

Formulations available[1]

Brand name (Manufacturer)	Formulation and strength	Product information/Administration information
Cymevene (Roche)	Infusion 500 mg vial	Sodium salt. Powder for reconstitution. No specific data on enteral tube administration are available for this formulation.
Cymevene (Roche)	Capsules 250 mg, 500 mg	Discontinued early 2004 – see valganciclovir.

Formulations available[1] (continued)

Brand name (Manufacturer)	Formulation and strength	Product information/Administration information
Extemporaneous preparation[2] (The pharmacokinetic and clinical efficacy of this preparation has not been tested.)	Suspension 25 mg/5 mL	Suspension should be prepared in area with appropriate preparation and containment facilities. 1. Aseptically reconstitute 5 vials of ganciclovir using 3 mL per vial. Shake well until dissolved. 2. Transfer the contents of the vials (total volume 15 mL) into a suitable measure. 3. Add 50 mL of Ora-sweet (US suspending agent) 4. Add 1 mL of 3% hydrogen peroxide solution. 5. Mix well. 6. Make to volume (100 mL) using Ora-sweet. 7. Mix thoroughly. 8. Dispense in amber bottle. Label 'shake well before each use'. 9. Assign an expiration date of 28 days.

Site of absorption (oral administration)

Ganciclovir is absorbed in the small bowel and absorption is not pH dependent.[2]

Alternative routes available

Parenteral route is available.

Interactions

Food delays peak plasma concentrations and increases overall bioavailability. It is proposed that food delays transit time and allows for increased paracellular diffusion,[2] therefore enteral feed may not increase bioavailability to the same extent.

Health and safety

Caution in handling:[1] Ganciclovir is toxic and personnel should be adequately protected during handling and administration. If the solution comes into contact with skin or mucosa, wash off immediately with soap and water.

Suggestions/recommendations

- Oral bioavailability is poor; consider changing to valganciclovir.
- Seek advice regarding alternative treatment.
- Use a parenteral formulation where clinically appropriate. Use of the extemporaneous suspension above should be considered a last resort because of the lack of supporting data.

References

1. *BNF 50*, September 2005.
2. Personal communication, Roche; 6 February 2003.

Glibenclamide

Formulations available[1]

Brand name (Manufacturer)	Formulation and strength	Product information/Administration information
Daonil (Hoechst Marion Roussel)	Tablets 5 mg	Scored. No specific data on enteral tube administration are available for this formulation.
Semi-Daonil (Hoechst Marion Roussel)	Tablets 2.5 mg	Scored. No specific data on enteral tube administration are available for this formulation.
Euglucon (Aventis Pharma)	Tablets 2.5 mg, 5 mg	No specific data on enteral tube administration are available for this formulation.
Glibenclamide (Alpharma, APS, Arrow, Ashbourne, CP, Generics, Hillcross, IVAX, Kent)	Tablets 2.5 mg, 5 mg	Alpharma advises caution because of the unknown effect of crushing tablets on efficacy.[3] APS brand tablets disperse in water within 5 minutes to give a very fine dispersion that flushes down an 8Fr NG tube without blockage.[4]

Site of absorption (oral administration)

Glibenclamide is rapidly absorbed, although no specific site of absorption is documented.[2]

Alternative routes available

None available for glibenclamide. Long-acting insulins are available for parenteral administration; seek specialist advice.

Interactions

No specific interaction with food is documented, although it is recommended that glibenclamide be taken with breakfast or the first main meal of the day.[2]

Health and safety

Standard precautions apply.

Suggestions/recommendations

- Disperse tablet in water immediately prior to administration. The dose should be given shortly after starting enteral feed. No break in feeding regimen is necessary, but the tube must be flushed before and after dosing to prevent blockage.

Intragastric administration

1. Stop the enteral feed.
2. Flush the enteral feeding tube with the recommended volume of water.
3. Place the tablet in the barrel of an appropriate size and type of syringe.
4. Draw 10 mL of water into the syringe and allow the tablet to disperse, shaking if necessary.
5. Flush the medication dose down the feeding tube.
6. Draw another 10 mL of water into the oral syringe and also flush this via the feeding tube (this will rinse the syringe and ensure that the total dose is administered).
7. Finally, flush with the recommended volume of water.
8. Re-start the feed, unless a prolonged break is required.

Alternatively, at step (3) place the tablet into a medicine pot, add 10 mL of water and allow the tablet to disperse. Draw this into the syringe with an appropriate adapter for the tube connector. Ensure that the measure is rinsed and that this rinsing water is administered also to ensure that the total dose is given.

Intrajejunal administration

There are no specific data relating to the jejunal administration of glibenclamide. Administer using the above method. Monitor for loss of efficacy or increased side-effects.

References

1. *BNF* 50, September 2005.
2. Daonil Tablets (Hoechst), Summary of Product Characteristics; April 2002.
3. Personal communication, Alpharma; 21 January 2003.
4. BPNG data on file, 2004.

Gliclazide

Formulations available[1]

Brand name (Manufacturer)	Formulation and strength	Product information/Administration information
Diamicron (Servier)	Tablets 80 mg	Scored. Tablets can be crushed and dispersed in water immediately prior to administration.[2]
Diamicron MR (Servier)	M/R tablets 30 mg	Diamicron MR 30 mg may be considered to be approximately equivalent in therapeutic effect to standard formulation diamicron 80 mg. Diamicron MR is a hydrophilic matrix formulation and should not be crushed.[2]

Formulations available[1] (continued)

Brand name (Manufacturer)	Formulation and strength	Product information/Administration information
Gliclazide (Alpharma, APS, Arrow, CP, Generics, Genus, Hillcross, IVAX, PLIVA)	Tablets 80 mg	Alpharma does not recommend crushing the tablets owing to the unknown effect on the pharmacokinetics and glycaemic control.[3] Alpharma and Generics brand disperse in 10 mL of water within 5 minutes to give a coarse dispersion. This flushes without blockage but leaves a residue on the syringe and may leave residue inside tube;[4] however, this is unlikely to be active drug as gliclazide is soluble in water.[5] CP brand takes 2–3 minutes to disperse when shaken in 10 mL of water; this forms a finer dispersion than the Alpharma and Generics brands, but also leaves a slight residue on the syringe.[4]

Site of absorption (oral administration)

Specific site of absorption is not documented. Average time to peak plasma concentration is 4 hours.[5]

Alternative routes available

No alternative route available. Insulin can be administered parenterally if clinically appropriate.

Interactions

No specific interaction with food is documented.

Health and safety

Standard precautions apply.

Suggestions/recommendations

- Disperse the tablets in water immediately prior to administration. As it is possible that some residue may be left in the syringe, ensure that blood glucose levels are monitored closely and the dose is adjusted according to response, until a stable drug and feeding regimen is determined.

Intragastric administration

1. Stop the enteral feed.
2. Flush the enteral feeding tube with the recommended volume of water.
3. Place the tablet in the barrel of an appropriate size and type of syringe.
4. Draw 10 mL of water into the syringe and allow the tablet to disperse, shaking if necessary.
5. Flush the medication dose down the feeding tube.
6. Draw another 10 mL of water into the syringe and also flush this via the feeding tube (this will rinse the syringe and ensure that the total dose is administered).
7. Finally, flush with the recommended volume of water.
8. Re-start the feed, unless a prolonged break is required.

Alternatively, at step (3) place the tablet into a medicine pot, add 10 mL of water and allow the tablet to disperse. Draw this into an appropriate syringe. Ensure that the measure is rinsed and that this rinsing water is administered also to ensure that the total dose is given.

Intrajejunal administration

There are no specific data relating to jejunal administration. Administer using the above method. Monitor for increased side-effects or loss of efficacy.

References

1. *BNF 50*, September 2005.
2. Personal communication, Servier Laboratories Ltd; 3 March 2003.
3. Personal communication, Alpharma Ltd; 21 January 2003.
4. BPNG data on file, 2004.
5. Dollery C. *Therapeutic Drugs*, 2nd edn. London: Churchill Livingstone; 1998.

Glimepiride

Formulations available[1]

Brand name (Manufacturer)	Formulation and strength	Product information/Administration information
Amaryl (Hoechst Marion Roussel)	Tablets 1 mg, 2 mg, 3 mg, 4 mg	Scored. Tablets disperse within 5 minutes when placed in 10 mL of water, to form a very fine dispersion that flushes down an 8Fr NG tube without blockage (only 3 mg strength tested).[2]

Site of absorption (oral administration)

Specific site of absorption is not documented. Peak plasma concentration occurs approximately 2.5 hours after oral dosing.[3]

Alternative routes available

No alternative route for any sulfonylureas. Insulin can be administered parenterally if clinically appropriate.

Interactions

There is no specific interaction with food, but to optimise effect the dose should be taken shortly before main meal of the day.[3]

Health and safety

Standard precautions apply.

Suggestions/recommendations

- Disperse tablet in water immediately prior to administration. This should be given immediately prior to the first bolus feed of the day, or before the feed infusion is started.

Intragastric administration

1. Stop the enteral feed.
2. Flush the enteral feeding tube with the recommended volume of water.
3. Place the tablet in the barrel of an appropriate size and type of syringe.
4. Draw 10 mL of water into the syringe and allow the tablet to disperse, shaking if necessary.
5. Flush the medication dose down the feeding tube.
6. Draw another 10 mL of water into the syringe and also flush this via the feeding tube (this will rinse the syringe and ensure that the total dose is administered).
7. Finally, flush with the recommended volume of water.
8. Re-start the feed, unless a prolonged break is required.

Alternatively, at step (4) place the tablet into a medicine pot, add 10 mL of water and allow the tablet to disperse. Draw this into an appropriate syringe. Ensure that the measure is rinsed and that this rinsing water is administered also to ensure that the total dose is given.

Intrajejunal administration

There are no specific data relating to the jejunal administration of glimepiride. Administer using the above method. Monitor for increased side-effects or loss of efficacy.

References

1. *BNF* 50, September 2005.
2. BPNG data on file, 2004.
3. Amaryl (Hoechst), Summary of Product Characteristics; March 2002.

Glipizide

Formulations available [1]

Brand name (Manufacturer)	Formulation and strength	Product information/Administration information
Glipizide (Alpharma, Generics, Hillcross, IVAX)	Tablets 5 mg	No specific data on enteral tube administration are available for this formulation.
Glibenese (Pfizer)	Tablets 5 mg	Tablets can be crushed and mixed with water immediately prior to administration. [2]
Minodiab (Pharmacia)	Tablets 2.5 mg, 5 mg	The tablets can be crushed and dispersed in water, but as there are no stability data it is recommended that this be done immediately prior to administration. [3]

Site of absorption (oral administration)

Specific site is not documented. Peak plasma concentration occurs 1–3 hours after oral dosing. [4]

Alternative routes available

None available for any of the sulfonylureas.

Interactions

Total bioavailability is not affected by food, but peak plasma concentrations are delayed by 40 minutes. Therefore, to obtain the greatest reduction in postprandial hyperglycaemia it is recommended that glipizide be given 30 minutes before food.[2]

Health and safety

Standard precautions apply.

Suggestions/recommendations

- Crush the tablets and disperse in water immediately prior to administration. This should be flushed down tube 30 minutes before enteral feed is commenced; blood sugar control persists for up to 24 hours after a single dose of glipizide.[4]

Intragastric administration

1. Administer the dose 30 minutes prior to starting enteral feed.
2. Flush the enteral feeding tube with the recommended volume of water.
3. Place the tablet in a mortar and crush to a fine powder using the pestle.
4. Add a few millilitres of water and mix to form a paste.
5. Add up to 15 mL of water and mix thoroughly, ensuring that there are no large particles of tablet.
6. Draw this into an appropriate size and type of syringe.
7. Flush the medication dose down the feeding tube.
8. Add another 15 mL of water to the mortar and stir to ensure that any remaining drug is rinsed from the container. Draw this water into the syringe and also flush this via the feeding tube (this will rinse the mortar and syringe and ensure total dose is administered).
9. Finally, flush the enteral feeding tube with the recommended volume of water.
10. Wait at least 30 minutes before starting the re-feed.

Intrajejunal administration

There are no specific data relating to the jejunal administration of glipizide. Administer using the above method. Monitor for loss of efficacy or increased side-effects.

References

1. *BNF* 50, September 2005.
2. Personal communication, Pfizer; 23 June 2003.
3. Personal communication, Pharmacia Ltd; 11 March 2003.
4. Glipizide Tablets (Pharmacia), Summary of Product Characteristics; March 2003.

Glyceryl trinitrate

Formulations available[1]

Brand name (Manufacturer)	Formulation and strength	Product information/Administration information
Short-acting preparations Glyceryl trinitrate (various manufacturers)	Sublingual tablets 300 microgram, 500 microgram, 600 microgram	Intended for sublingual administration; not suitable for administration via feeding tube. Peak plasma concentration occurs 6 minutes following sublingual administration.[2]
Glyceryl trinitrate (Alpharma, Roche, Sanofi, Merck, Servier)	Sublingual spray 400 microgram	Intended for sublingual administration; not suitable for administration via feeding tube.
Long-acting preparations Suscard (Forest)	Buccal tablets 2 mg, 3 mg, 5 mg	Modified-release buccal tablets. Intended for buccal administration, not suitable for administration via feeding tube. Peak plasma concentration occurs 1.52 hours following administration.[2]
Sustac (Forest)	Tablets 2.6 mg, 6.4 mg, 10 mg	Modified-release oral tablets. Must not be crushed.
Glyceryl trinitrate (Schwarz, 3M, Schering-Plough, Novartis, Goldshield)	Transdermal patches 5 mg/24 h, 10 mg/24 h, 15 mg/24 h	Transdermal application only. Deponit, Minitran, Nitro-Dur, Transiderm-Nitro, Trintek.
Percutol (PLIVA)	Ointment 0.2%	Topical use only.
Parenteral preparations Glyceryl trinitrate (Faulding, DBL, Schwarz, Merck)	Injection 1 mg/mL, 5 mg/mL	Parenteral use only.

Site of absorption (oral administration)

Peak plasma concentrations of the active metabolites of glyceryl trinitrate are detected 1 hour following oral administration of Sustac tablets.[3]

Alternative routes available

Sublingual, buccal, topical and parenteral routes are available.

Interactions

Not applicable.

Health and safety

Standard precautions apply.

Suggestions/recommendations

- Use topical or transdermal preparation for prophylactic therapy. The use of sublingual and buccal tablets may not be appropriate for patients with impaired local absorption following maxillofacial surgery or in patients with an impaired swallow; the sublingual spray should be considered in these patients.

References

1. *BNF* 50, September 2005.
2. Suscard Buccal (Forest), Summary of Product Characteristics; November 1997.
3. Sustac (Forest), Summary of Product Characteristics; September 2002.

Glycopyrronium

Formulations available[1]

Brand name (Manufacturer)	Formulation and strength	Product information/Administration information
Robinul Forte (First Horizon)	Tablets 2 mg	Unlicensed in UK. Tablets disperse in 10 mL of water within 5 minutes to give a coarse dispersion that settles quickly. Flushes via an 8Fr NG tube without blockage, but there is a risk of leaving drug in the syringe.[2]
Robinul (Anpharm)	Injection 200 microgram/mL	Intramuscular injection results in predictable peak plasma concentration at 30 minutes.[3] No specific data on enteral tube administration are available for this formulation.
Robinul (Antigen)	Powder 3 g	No specific data on enteral tube administration are available for this formulation.

Site of absorption (oral administration)

Specific site of absorption is not documented. Oral absorption is poor. Peak plasma concentration occurs 5 hours following oral dosing.[3]

Alternative routes available

Parenteral route is available.

Interactions

No specific interaction with food is documented.[4]

Health and safety

Standard precautions apply.

Suggestions/recommendations

- Disperse the tablets in water immediately prior to administration.
- A prolonged break in feeding is not required.

Intragastric administration

1. Stop the enteral feed.
2. Flush the enteral feeding tube with the recommended volume of water.
3. Place the tablet in the barrel of an appropriate size and type of syringe.
4. Draw 10 mL of water into the syringe and allow the tablet to disperse, shaking if necessary.
5. Flush the medication dose down the feeding tube.
6. Draw another 10 mL of water into the syringe and also flush this via the feeding tube (this will rinse the syringe and ensure that the total dose is administered).
7. Finally, flush with the recommended volume of water.
8. Re-start the feed, unless a prolonged break is required.

Alternatively, at step (3) place the tablet into a medicine pot, add 10 mL of water and allow the tablet to disperse. Draw this into an appropriate syringe. Ensure that the measure is rinsed and that this rinsing water is administered also to ensure that the total dose is given.

Intrajejunal administration

There are no specific data on jejunal administration of glycopyrronium. Administer using the above method. Monitor for loss of efficacy or increased side-effects.

References

1. *BNF* 50, September 2005.
2. BPNG data on file, 2005.
3. Dollery C. *Therapeutic Drugs*, 2nd edn. London: Churchill Livingstone; 1998.
4. Sweetman SC, ed. *Martindale*, 34th edn. London: Pharmaceutical Press; 2005.

Granisetron hydrochloride

Formulations available[1]		
Brand name (Manufacturer)	**Formulation and strength**	**Product information/Administration information**
Kytril (Roche)	Tablets 1 mg, 2 mg	Tablets can be crushed.[2] Tablet does not disintegrate readily but disperses in 10 mL of water if shaken for 5 minutes; this fine dispersion flushes via an 8Fr NG tube without blockage.[3]
Kytril (Roche)	Paediatric liquid 1 mg/5 mL	Contains sorbitol[4] 1 g/5 mL dose.[6]

Formulations available[1] (continued)		
Brand name (Manufacturer)	Formulation and strength	Product information/Administration information
Kytril (Roche)	Injection 1 mg/mL (1 mL, 3 mL)	Contains granisetron in isotonic saline, pH 5–7. This could be administered via the feeding tube if necessary.[2]

Site of absorption (oral administration)

Granisetron is rapidly absorbed. The specific site of absorption and time to peak plasma concentration are not documented.[4, 5]

Alternative routes available

Parenteral formulation is available. Can be administered by i.v. injection or infusion.

Interactions

The absorption of granisetron is not affected by food.[2]

Health and safety

Standard precautions apply.

Suggestions/recommendations

- Use a liquid preparation.
- A prolonged break is feeding is not required.

Intragastric administration

1. Stop the enteral feed.
2. Flush the enteral feeding tube with the recommended volume of water.
3. Draw the medication solution into an appropriate size and type of syringe.
4. Flush the medication dose down the feeding tube.
5. Finally, flush with the recommended volume of water.
6. Re-start the feed, unless a prolonged break is required.

Alternatively, at step (3) measure the medicine in a suitable container and then draw into an appropriate syringe. Ensure that the measure is rinsed and that this rinsing water is administered also to ensure that the total dose is given. **Do not** measure liquid medicines using a catheter-tipped syringe as this results in excessive dosing owing to the volume of the tip.

Intrajejunal administration

There are no specific data relating to jejunal administration of granisetron. Administer using the above method. Monitor for increased side-effects or loss of efficacy.

References

1. *BNF 50*, September 2005.
2. Personal communication, Roche; 6 February 2003.
3. BPNG data on file, 2004.
4. Kytril (Roche), Summary of Product Characteristics; August 2001.
5. Dollery C. *Therapeutic Drugs*, 2nd edn. London: Churchill Livingstone; 1998.
6. Personal communication, Roche; July 2005.

Griseofulvin

Formulations available[1]

Brand name (Manufacturer)	Formulation and strength	Product information/Administration information
Grisovin (GSK)	Tablets 125 mg, 250 mg	Film-coated tablets. Grisovin tablets are insoluble in water and it is likely that if crushed the dispersion of tablets in water would sediment rapidly. This may lead to inaccurate dosing.[2] Oral liquid preparation was discontinued in June 2000.

Site of absorption (oral administration)

No specific site is documented.

Alternative routes available

None for griseofulvin.

Interactions

Food ingestion alters the absorption of griseofulvin; relative bioavailability can be increased by 120% in the presence of fats.[3] As enteral feeds are relatively low in fat compared to the high-fat diet referred to in the literature,[4,5] in relation to griseofulvin absorption the significance of the interaction is uncertain.

Health and safety

Standard precautions apply.

Suggestions/recommendations

- Owing to lack of data, suitable formulation and the unpredictable affect of food on absorption, consider an alternative drug such as terbinafine (see monograph).

References

1. *BNF 50*, September 2005.
2. Personal communication, GSK; 22 January 2003.
3. Dollery C. *Therapeutic Drugs*, 2nd edn. London: Churchill Livingstone; 1998.
4. Crounse RG. Human pharmacology of griseofulvin: the effect of fat intake on gastrointestinal absorption. *J Invest Dermatol*. 1961; 37: 529.
5. Ogunbona FA, Smith IF, Olawoye OS, *et al*. Fat contents of meals and bioavailability of griseofulvin in man. *J Pharm Pharmacol*. 1985; 37: 283–284.

Haloperidol

Formulations available[1]

Brand name (Manufacturer)	Formulation and strength	Product information/Administration information
Haloperidol (various manufacturers)	Tablets 500 microgram, 1.5 mg, 5 mg, 10 mg, 20 mg	No specific data on enteral tube administration are available for this formulation.
Dozic (Rosemont)	Oral liquid 1 mg/mL	Sugar-free.
Haldol (Janssen-Cilag)	Tablets 5 mg, 10 mg	No specific data on enteral tube administration are available for this formulation.
Haldol (Janssen-Cilag)	Oral liquid 2 mg/mL	pH-adjusted oral solution.[2]
Haldol (Janssen-Cilag)	Injection 5 mg/mL (1 mL)	No specific data on enteral tube administration are available for this formulation.
Haldol (Janssen-Cilag)	Depot injection	Haloperidol decanoate. No specific data on enteral tube administration are available for this formulation.
Serenace (IVAX)	Capsules 500 microgram	ML held by Norton. Powder empties easily from capsule and disperses readily in water; quite fiddly owing to small capsule size.[3]
Serenace (IVAX)	Tablets 1.5 mg, 5 mg, 10 mg	No specific data on enteral tube administration are available for this formulation.
Serenace (IVAX)	Oral liquid 2 mg/mL	Sugar-free (ML held by Rosemont) Clear water-like consistency; flushes easily; no further dilution necessary.[3]
Serenace (IVAX)	Injection 5 mg/mL (1 mL), 10 mg/mL (2 mL)	No data relating to enteral tube administration of injection.

Site of absorption (oral administration)

Absorption is rapid following oral dosing;[2] no specific site of absorption is documented.

Alternative routes available

Injection is available for intravenous or intramuscular use.
Following intramuscular administration of 2 mg, peak plasma concentrations were similar to oral administration but were reached after 20 minutes.[4]

Interactions

There is no documented interaction with food. [2]

Health and safety

Standard precautions apply.

Suggestions/recommendations

- Use the oral liquids; all brands are oral solutions and do not require further dilution prior to administration.
- A prolonged break in feeding is not required.

Intragastric administration

1. Stop the enteral feed.
2. Flush the enteral feeding tube with the recommended volume of water.
3. Draw the medication solution into an appropriate size and type of syringe.
4. Flush the medication dose down the feeding tube.
5. Finally, flush with the recommended volume of water.
6. Re-start the feed, unless a prolonged break is required.

Alternatively, at step (3) measure the medicine in a suitable container and then draw into an appropriate syringe. Ensure that the measure is rinsed and that this rinsing water is administered also to ensure that the total dose is given. **Do not** measure liquid medicines using a catheter-tipped syringe as this results in excessive dosing owing to the volume of the tip.

Intrajejunal administration

There are no specific data relating to jejunal administration of haloperidol. Administer using the above method. Monitor for increased side-effects of loss of efficacy.

References

1. *BNF 50*, September 2005.
2. Haldol Tablets (Janssen-Cilag), Summary of Product Characteristics; 28 July 2003.
3. BPNG data on file, 2004.
4. Haldol Injection (Janssen-Cilag), Summary of Product Characteristics; September 2005.

Hydralazine hydrochloride

Formulations available [1]

Brand name (Manufacturer)	Formulation and strength	Product information/Administration information
Hydralazine (various manufacturers)	Tablets 25 mg, 50 mg	No specific data on enteral tube administration are available for this formulation.
Apresoline (Sovereign)	Tablets 25 mg, 50 mg	Sugar-coated. [2] No specific data on enteral tube administration are available for this formulation.

Formulations available[1] (continued)

Brand name (Manufacturer)	Formulation and strength	Product information/Administration information
Apresoline (Sovereign)	Injection 20 mg	Powder for reconstitution. Reconstituted injection can be given orally.[3]
Hydralazine (Special Products Limited)	Dispersible tablets 10 mg	Manufactured 'special'. The tablet can be dispersed in 10 mL of water and flushed down a feeding tube. The tablet contains microcrystalline cellulose, which is insoluble. The instructions indicate that the tablets should be stirred in water for 2 minutes to dissolve the active drug. The suspension should be allowed to settle for 1 minute, then the clear solution can be administered via the feeding tube.[4]

Site of absorption (oral administration)

Specific site of absorption is not documented. Peak plasma concentration occurs 0.5–1.5 hours following oral dosing.[2, 5]

Alternative routes available

Parenteral route is available.

Interactions

No specific interaction with food is documented.

Health and safety

Standard precautions apply.

Suggestions/recommendations

- Consider changing therapy.
- Use 'special' dispersible tablets if clinically indicated.

Intragastric administration

1. Stop the enteral feed.
2. Flush the enteral feeding tube with the recommended volume of water.
3. Place the tablet in the barrel of an appropriate size and type of syringe.
4. Draw 10 mL of water into the syringe and allow the tablet to disperse, shaking if necessary.
5. Flush the medication dose down the feeding tube.
6. Draw an equal volume of water into the syringe and also flush this via the feeding tube (this will rinse the syringe and ensure that the total dose is administered).
7. Finally, flush with the recommended volume of water.
8. Re-start the feed, unless a prolonged break is required.

Alternatively, at step (3) place the tablet into a medicine pot, add 10 mL of water and allow the tablet to disperse. Draw this into an appropriate syringe. Ensure that the measure is rinsed and that this rinsing water is administered also to ensure that the total dose is given.

Intrajejunal administration

There are no specific data relating to jejunal delivery of hydralazine. Administer using the above method. Monitor for increased side-effects or loss of efficacy.

References

1. *BNF* 50, September 2005.
2. Apresoline (Sovereign), Summary of Product Characteristics; April 2003.
3. *Medicines for Children*, 2nd edn. London: RCPCH Publication; 2003.
4. Personal communication, Special Products Ltd; 20 January 2003.
5. Sweetman SC, ed. *Martindale*, 34th edn. London: Pharmaceutical Press; 2005.

Hydrocortisone

Formulations available[1]

Brand name (Manufacturer)	Formulation and strength	Product information/Administration information
Hydrocortone (MSD)	Tablets 10 mg, 20 mg	Scored tablets. Tablets disintegrate readily in 10 mL of water within 2 minutes to give a fine dispersion that flushes down an 8Fr NG tube without blockage.[2]
Solu-Cortef (Pharmacia)	Injection 100 mg	Hydrocortisone as sodium succinate. No specific data on enteral tube administration are available for this formulation.

Site of absorption (oral administration)

Specific site is not documented; however, hydrocortisone is readily absorbed. The peak plasma concentration occurs 90 minutes after oral administration.[3]

Alternative routes available

Parenteral route is available. Rectal route is used for topical treatment only.

Interactions

No specific interaction with food is documented.[3]

Health and safety

Standard precautions apply.

Suggestions/recommendations

- Disperse the tablets in water immediately prior to administration. A prolonged break in feeding is not required.
- Injection can be used parenterally if enteral absorption is compromised.

Intragastric administration

1. Stop the enteral feed.
2. Flush the enteral feeding tube with the recommended volume of water.
3. Place the tablet in the barrel of an appropriate size and type of syringe.
4. Draw 10 mL of water into the syringe and allow the tablet to disperse, shaking if necessary.
5. Flush the medication dose down the feeding tube.
6. Draw another 10 mL of water into the syringe and also flush this via the feeding tube (this will rinse the syringe and ensure that the total dose is administered).
7. Finally, flush with the recommended volume of water.
8. Re-start the feed, unless a prolonged break is required.

Alternatively, at step (3) place the tablet into a medicine pot, add 10 mL of water and allow the tablet to disperse. Draw this into an appropriate syringe. Ensure that the measure is rinsed and that this rinsing water is administered also to ensure that the total dose is given.

Intrajejunal administration

There are no specific data available relating to jejunal administration. Use the method detailed above.

References

1. *BNF 50*, September 2005.
2. BPNG data on file, 2004.
3. Dollery C. *Therapeutic Drugs*, 2nd edn. London: Churchill Livingstone; 1998.

Hydromorphone hydrochloride

Formulations available[1]

Brand name (Manufacturer)	Formulation and strength	Product information/Administration information
Palladone (Napp)	Capsules 1.3 mg, 2.6 mg	No specific data on enteral tube administration are available for this formulation.
Palladone SR (Napp)	M/R capsules 2 mg, 4 mg, 8 mg, 16 mg, 24 mg	In-house studies conducted by Napp have given mixed results when administering the spheroids from the capsules via enteral feeding tubes. A common problem was blockage and therefore this route of administration is not recommended.[2]

Site of absorption (oral administration)

Specific site of absorption is not documented.[3]

Alternative routes available

None for hydromorphone. Other opioid analgesics are available in parenteral and topical formulations.

Interactions

No specific interaction with food is documented.[3]

Health and safety

Standard precautions apply.

Suggestions/recommendations

- Do not attempt to administer contents of modified-release capsules via the feeding tube owing to the high risk of blockage. Change to an alternative opiate available as liquid, e.g. morphine or oxycodone.
- Hydromorphone hydrochloride 1.3 mg oral is approximately equivalent to 10 mg of oral morphine or 5 mg of oral oxycodone.[1]
- For background maintenance analgesia, consider modified-release preparations with smaller granules (see Morphine monograph) or topical preparations, e.g. fentanyl or buprenorphine.

References

1. *BNF 50*, September 2005.
2. Personal communication, Napp; 29 January 2003.
3. Palladone (Napp), Summary of Product Characteristics; January 2006.

Hydroxycarbamide (Hydroxyurea)

Formulations available[1]

Brand name (Manufacturer)	Formulation and strength	Product information/Administration information
Hydroxycarbamide (Medac)	Capsules 500 mg	No specific data on enteral tube administration are available for this formulation.
Hydrea (Squibb)	Capsules 500 mg	Soluble 1 : 10–1 : 30 in water.[2] Excipients are not soluble.

Site of absorption (oral administration)

Specific site is not documented. Peak plasma concentration occurs 2 hours after oral dosing.[3]

Alternative routes available

None available for hydroxycarbamide.

Interactions

No specific interaction with food is documented.[3]

Health and safety

Hydroxycarbamide is cytotoxic. Suitable protective clothing should be worn. Contaminated equipment should be disposed of as cytotoxic waste. Steps should be taken to minimise operator exposure to the powder.

Suggestions/recommendations

- Capsules can be opened and the contents mixed with water immediately prior to administration; see notes above.
- A prolonged break in feeding is not required.

Intragastric administration

1. Stop the enteral feed.
2. Flush the enteral feeding tube with the recommended volume of water.
3. Open the capsule and pour the contents into a medicine pot.
4. Add 15 mL of water.
5. Stir to disperse the powder.
6. Draw into an appropriate syringe and administer via the feeding tube.
7. Add a further 15 mL of water to the medicine pot; stir to ensure that any powder remaining in the pot is mixed with water.
8. Draw up this dispersion and flush down tube. This will ensure that the whole dose is given.
9. Flush the tube with the recommended volume of water.
10. Re-start the feed, unless prolonged break is required.

Intrajejunal administration

There is no specific information relating to the jejunal administration of hydroxycarbamide. Administer as above.

References

1. *BNF* 50, September 2005.
2. Personal communication, BMS; 24 January 2003.
3. Hydrea (Squibb), Summary of Product Characteristics; July 2001.

Hydroxyzine hydrochloride

Formulations available[1]

Brand name (Manufacturer)	Formulation and strength	Product information/Administration information
Atarax (Pfizer)	Tablets 10 mg, 25 mg	Sugar-coated tablets; crushing may be difficult.[2]
Ucerax (UCB Pharma)	Syrup 10 mg/5 mL	Contains sucrose and alcohol (100 mg/5 mL), does not contain sorbitol.[4]

Site of absorption (oral administration)

Specific site is not documented. Hydroxyzine is rapidly absorbed following oral absorption; a therapeutic effect is achieved within 15–30 minutes.[3]

Alternative routes available

No alternative route available for hydroxyzine. Parenteral formulation is available for chlorphenamine.

Interactions

No specific interaction with food or feed.[2]

Health and safety

Standard precautions apply.

Suggestions/recommendations

- Use liquid preparation.
- A prolonged break in feeding is not required.

Intragastric administration

1. Stop the enteral feed.
2. Flush the enteral feeding tube with the recommended volume of water.
3. Draw the medication liquid into an appropriate size and type of syringe.
4. Flush the medication dose down the feeding tube.
5. Finally, flush with the recommended volume of water.
6. Re-start the feed, unless a prolonged break is required.

Alternatively, at step (3) measure the medicine in a suitable container. Draw this into an appropriate syringe. Ensure that the measure is rinsed and that this rinsing water is administered also to ensure that the total dose is given. **Do not** measure liquid medicines using a catheter-tipped syringe as this results in excessive dosing owing to the volume of the tip.

Intrajejunal administration

There are no specific data on jejunal administration. Administer as above; consider diluting the liquid preparation immediately prior to administration to reduce osmolarity. Monitor for lack of efficacy and increased side-effects.

References

1. *BNF* 50, September 2005.
2. Personal communication, Pfizer; 23 June 2003.
3. Atarax (Pfizer), Summary of Product Characteristics; March 2003.
4. Ucerax Syrup (UCB Pharma), Summary of Product Characteristics; February 2002.

Hyoscine butylbromide

Formulations available[1]

Brand name (Manufacturer)	Formulation and strength	Product information/Administration information
Buscopan (Boehringer Ingelheim)	Tablets 10 mg	Sugar-coated.[2] Tablets may be crushed but are sugar-coated.[3] Soluble 1 : 1 in water.[4]
Buscopan (Boehringer Ingelheim)	Injection 20 mg/mL	Injection can be given orally; pH is 3.7–5.5.[3]

Site of absorption (oral administration)

Hyoscine butylbromide has a low systemic absorption; it exhibits a predominantly local effect in the gut.[3, 4]

Alternative routes available

Parenteral formulation can be given i.v. or i.m.

Interactions

No documented interaction with food.[4]

Health and safety

Standard precautions apply.

Suggestions/recommendations

- Owing to the risk of tube blockage from crushing sugar-coated tablets, the buscopan injection should be used via enteral feeding tubes. A prolonged break in feeding is not necessary. If the tube exits in the jejunum, consider using parenteral therapy.
- Consider changing to dicycloverine liquid (see monograph) as an alternative therapy.

Intragastric administration

1. Stop the enteral feed.
2. Flush the enteral feeding tube with the recommended volume of water.
3. Draw up appropriate dose of injection into an appropriate size and type of syringe.
4. Flush the medication dose down the feeding tube.
5. Finally, flush with the recommended volume of water.
6. Re-start the feed, unless a prolonged break is required.

Intrajejunal administration

No data are available relating to jejunal administration; however, jejunal administration is unlikely to affect therapeutic response.

Consider changing to parenteral therapy if enteral absorption is compromised.

References

1. *BNF* 50, September 2005.
2. Buscopan (Boehringer Ingelheim), Summary of Product Characteristics; October 2002.
3. Personal communication, Boehringer Ingelheim; 6 March 2003.
4. Dollery C. *Therapeutic Drugs*, 2nd edn. London: Churchill Livingstone; 1998.

Hyoscine hydrobromide

Formulations available[1]

Brand name (Manufacturer)	Formulation and strength	Product information/Administration information
Hyoscine hydrobromide (proprietary brands)	Tablets 300 microgram	No specific data on enteral tube administration are available for this formulation. Joy-rides, Kwells.

Formulations available[1] (continued)

Brand name (Manufacturer)	Formulation and strength	Product information/Administration information
Scopaderm TTS (Novartis Consumer Health)	Patch 1 mg	Apply behind the ear to a hairless patch of skin; replace every 72 hours.
Hyoscine (various manufacturers)	Injection 400 microgram/mL, 600 microgram/mL	No specific data on enteral tube administration are available for this formulation.

Site of absorption (oral administration)

Hyoscine hydrobromide is readily absorbed from the GI tract; it is also well absorbed following application to the skin.[2]

Alternative routes available

Topical patch and parenteral formulation.

Interactions

There is no documented interaction with food.

Health and safety

Standard precautions apply.

Suggestions/recommendations

• Use transdermal patch where clinically appropriate.

References

1. *BNF* 50, September 2005.
2. Sweetman SC, ed. *Martindale*, 34th edn. London: Pharmaceutical Press; 2005.

Ibuprofen

Formulations available[1]

Brand name (Manufacturer)	Formulation and strength	Product information/Administration information
Brufen (Abbott)	Tablets 200 mg, 400 mg, 600 mg	200 mg and 400 mg strength are sugar-coated. 600 mg strength are film-coated.
Brufen (Abbott)	Syrup 100 mg/5 mL	Contains sorbitol 500 mg/5 mL dose.[2] Brufen syrup is extremely viscous and should be mixed with an equal volume of water prior to administration via a feeding tube to reduce the viscosity and reduce resistance to flushing down the feeding tube.[3]

Formulations available[1] (continued)

Brand name (Manufacturer)	Formulation and strength	Product information/Administration information
Brufen (Abbott)	Granules 600 mg/sachet	Contains 9 mmol sodium per sachet. No specific data on enteral tube administration are available for this formulation.
Ibuprofen (various manufacturers)	Tablets 200 mg, 400 mg, 600 mg	Alpharma recommends that tablets should not be crushed.[4]
Ibuprofen (various manufacturers)	Oral suspension 100 mg/5 mL	No specific data on enteral tube administration are available for this formulation.

Site of absorption (oral administration)

Specific site of absorption is not documented. Peak plasma concentration occurs 1–2 hours after oral dosing.[5]

Alternative routes available

None for ibuprofen. Alternative routes are available for diclofenac, but the difference in efficacy and side-effect profile should be considered.

Interactions

Peak plasma concentrations are reduced and delayed when administered with food.[4]

Health and safety

Standard precautions apply.

Suggestions/recommendations

- Use a liquid preparation; dilute with an equal volume of water immediately prior to administration where possible. Alternatively, use the granules dispersed in 20 mL of water.
- A prolonged break in feeding is not required.

Intragastric administration

1. Stop the enteral feed.
2. Flush the enteral feeding tube with the recommended volume of water.
3. Shake the medication bottle thoroughly to ensure adequate mixing.
4. Draw the medication suspension into an appropriate size and type of syringe.
5. Draw an equal volume of water and a little air into the syringe and shake to mix thoroughly.
6. Flush the medication dose down the feeding tube.
7. Finally, flush with the recommended volume of water.
8. Re-start the feed, unless a prolonged break is required.

Alternatively, at step (4) measure the medicine in a suitable container and then add an equal volume of water and mix thoroughly. Draw this into an appropriate syringe. Ensure that the measure is rinsed and that this rinsing water is administered also to ensure that the total dose is given. **Do not** measure liquid medicines using a catheter-tipped syringe as this results in excessive dosing owing to the volume of the tip.

Intrajejunal administration

There are no specific data relating to jejunal administration of ibuprofen.

1. Stop the enteral feed.
2. Flush the enteral feeding tube with the recommended volume of water.
3. Shake the medication bottle thoroughly to ensure adequate mixing.
4. Draw the medication suspension into an appropriate size and type of syringe.
5. Draw 3–4 times the dose volume of water and a little air into the syringe and shake to mix thoroughly.
6. Flush the medication dose down the feeding tube.
7. Finally, flush with the recommended volume of water.
8. Re-start the feed, unless a prolonged break is required.

Alternatively, at step (4) measure the medicine in a suitable container and then add three to four times the dose volume of water and mix thoroughly. Draw this into an appropriate syringe. Ensure that the measure is rinsed and that this rinsing water is administered also to ensure that the total dose is given. **Do not** measure liquid medicines using a catheter-tipped syringe as this results in excessive dosing owing to the volume of the tip.

References

1. *BNF* 50, September 2005.
2. Personal communication, Abbott Laboratories; August 2005.
3. BPNG data on file, 2004.
4. Personal communication, Alpharma; 21 January 2003.
5. Dollery C. *Therapeutic Drugs*, 2nd edn. London: Churchill Livingstone; 1998.

Imipramine hydrochloride

Formulations available[1]

Brand name (Manufacturer)	Formulation and strength	Product information/Administration information
Imipramine (Alpharma, various manufacturers)	Tablets 10 mg, 25 mg	Alpharma brand tablets are difficult to crush owing to their small size and coating, but once crushed they disperse well in water and flush via an 8Fr NG tube without blockage, although inadequate crushing may lead to large particles that might block fine-bore tubes.[2]
Tofranil (Novartis)	Tablets 25 mg	Sugar-coated. No specific data on enteral tube administration are available for this formulation.

Site of absorption (oral administration)

Site of absorption is not specified.[3] Absorption is reduced when gastric pH is in the range 3.6–6.0.[4]

Alternative routes available

None available for imipramine.

Interactions

Food does not affect the bioavailability of imipramine;[3] however, the pH buffering effect of enteral feed may affect absorption (see note above).

Health and safety

Standard precautions apply.

Suggestions/recommendations

- Owing to lack of data and suitable formulation, consider changing to an alternative tricyclic antidepressant available as a liquid. Seek specialist advice for transference of therapy.

References

1. *BNF 50*, September 2005.
2. BPNG data on file, 2004.
3. Tofranil (Novartis), Summary of Product Characteristics; May 2001.
4. Dollery C. *Therapeutic Drugs*, 2nd edn. London: Churchill Livingstone; 1998.

Indapamide

Formulations available[1]

Brand name (Manufacturer)	Formulation and strength	Product information/Administration information
Indapamide (Alpharma, APS, Ashbourne, Hillcross, IVAX, Niche, Sterwin)	Tablet 2.5 mg	Sterwin and Generics brand tablets disperse in 10 mL of water within 2 minutes to give a fine dispersion that flushes via an 8Fr NG tube without blockage.[2]
Natrilix (Servier)	Tablet 2.5 mg	Film-coated tablet. Tablets can be crushed and mixed with water immediately prior to administration.[3]
Natrilix SR (Servier)	M/R tablet 1.5 mg	Sustained-release tablet, not suitable for administration via the feeding tube. Change to conventional-release tablet.

Site of absorption (oral administration)

Specific site of absorption is not documented. Rapidly and completely absorbed following oral administration. Peak plasma concentration occurs 1–2 hours following oral dose.[4]

Alternative routes available

None available for indapamide.

Interactions

No specific interaction with food is documented.[4]

Health and safety

Standard precautions apply.

Suggestions/recommendations

- Disperse conventional-release tablets in water immediately prior to administration.
- A prolonged break in feeding is not required.

Intragastric administration

1. Stop the enteral feed.
2. Flush the enteral feeding tube with the recommended volume of water.
3. Place the tablet in the barrel of an appropriate size and type of syringe.
4. Draw 10 mL of water into the syringe and allow the tablet to disperse, shaking if necessary.
5. Flush the medication dose down the feeding tube.
6. Draw another 10 mL of water into the syringe and also flush this via the feeding tube (this will rinse the syringe and ensure that the total dose is administered).
7. Finally, flush with the recommended volume of water.
8. Re-start the feed, unless a prolonged break is required.

Alternatively, at step (3) place the tablet into a medicine pot, add 10 mL of water and allow the tablet to disperse. Draw this into an appropriate syringe. Ensure that the measure is rinsed and that this rinsing water is administered also to ensure that the total dose is given.

Intrajejunal administration

There are no specific data relating to the jejunal administration of indapamide. Administer using the above method. Monitor for increased side-effects or loss of efficacy.

References

1. *BNF* 50, September 2005.
2. BPNG data on file, 2005.
3. Personal communication, Servier; 3 March 2003.
4. Natrilix (Servier), Summary of Product Characteristics; June 2003.

Indometacin (Indomethacin)

Formulations available [1]

Brand name (Manufacturer)	Formulation and strength	Product information/Administration information
Indometacin (Alpharma, Ranbaxy)	Capsules 25 mg, 50 mg	Alpharma advise against opening the capsules. [2]
Indometacin (Alpharma, Ivax)	Suppositories 100 mg	Rectal administration only.

Formulations available[1] (continued)

Brand name (Manufacturer)	Formulation and strength	Product information/Administration information
Indometacin M/R Preparations (various manufacturers)	Modified-release 25 mg, 50 mg, 75 mg	Not suitable for administration via enteral feeding tubes.
Indo-Paed (1A Pharma)	Suspension 25 mg/5 mL	Unlicensed in the UK. Import via IDIS. Slightly viscous suspension.

Site of absorption (oral administration)

Specific site of absorption is not documented. Peak plasma concentration occurs 30–120 minutes following oral dosing. Rectal administration produces earlier but lower peak concentrations.[3]

Alternative routes available

Suppositories are available for rectal administration.

Interactions

Absorption is delayed but not reduced by food.[3]

Health and safety

Standard precautions apply.

Suggestions/recommendations

- Change to suppositories administered once daily at night if clinically indicated. If the rectal route is not appropriate, consider changing to an alternative NSAID, e.g. diclofenac (see monograph).

References

1. *BNF* 50, September 2005.
2. Personal communication, Alpharma; 21 January 2003.
3. Dollery C. *Therapeutic Drugs*, 2nd edn. London: Churchill Livingstone; 1998.

Indoramin

Formulations available[1]

Brand name (Manufacturer)	Formulation and strength	Product information/Administration information
Baratol (Shire)	Tablet 25 mg	Indoramin hydrochloride. Readily soluble in water.[2] No specific data on enteral tube administration are available for this formulation.
Doralese (GSK)	Tablet 20 mg	Tablets disperse rapidly when placed in 10 mL of water; the dispersion settles quickly but flushes down an 8Fr NG tube without blockage.[3]

Site of absorption (oral administration)

Specific site is not documented. Peak plasma concentration occurs 1–2 hour following oral dosing.[4]

Alternative routes available

None available for indoramin.

Interactions

Alcohol increases the rate and extent of indoramin absorption. No interaction with food is documented.[5]

Health and safety

Standard precautions apply.

Suggestions/recommendations

- Disperse the tablets in water immediately prior to administration.
- A prolonged break in feeding is not necessary.

Intragastric administration

1. Stop the enteral feed.
2. Flush the enteral feeding tube with the recommended volume of water.
3. Place the tablet in the barrel of an appropriate size and type of syringe.
4. Draw 10 mL of water into the syringe and allow the tablet to disperse, shaking if necessary.
5. Flush the medication dose down the feeding tube.
6. Draw another 10 mL of water into the syringe and also flush this via the feeding tube (this will rinse the syringe and ensure that the total dose is administered).
7. Finally, flush with the recommended volume of water.
8. Re-start the feed, unless a prolonged break is required.

Alternatively, at step (3) place the tablet into a medicine pot, add 10 mL of water and allow the tablet to disperse. Draw this into an appropriate syringe. Ensure that the measure is rinsed and that this rinsing water is administered also to ensure that the total dose is given.

Intrajejunal administration

There is no specific information relating to jejunal administration of indoramin. Administer using the above method. Monitor for loss of efficacy and increased side-effects.

References

1. *BNF* 50, September 2005.
2. Personal communication, Shire; 17 February 2003.
3. BPNG data on file, 2004.
4. Doralese (GSK), Summary of Product Characteristics; October 2002.
5. Baratol (Shire), Summary of Product Characteristics, July 2003.

Inositol nicotinate

Formulations available[1]

Brand name (Manufacturer)	Formulation and strength	Product information/Administration information
Hexopa (Genus)	Tablets 500 mg	Tablets can be crushed; this is not expected to significantly affect the pharmacokinetics.[2]
Hexopal Forte (Genus)	Tablets 750 mg	As above.

Site of absorption (oral administration)

Specific site of absorption is not documented.[3]

Alternative routes available

None available for inositol.

Interactions

No specific interaction with food is documented.[3]

Health and safety

Standard precautions apply.

Suggestions/recommendations

- Crush the tablets and disperse in water immediately prior to administration.
- However, owing to the lack of data, consideration should be given to reviewing the therapy and advice sought regarding alternative treatment.

Intragastric administration

1. Stop the enteral feed.
2. Flush the enteral feeding tube with the recommended volume of water.
3. Place the tablet in a mortar and crush to a fine powder using the pestle.
4. Add a few millilitres of water and mix to form a paste.
5. Add up to 15 mL of water and mix thoroughly ensuring that there are no visible lumps of tablet.
6. Draw this into an appropriate size and type of syringe.
7. Flush the medication dose down the feeding tube.
8. Add another 15 mL of water to the mortar and stir to ensure that any remaining drug is rinsed from the container. Draw this water into the syringe and also flush this via the feeding tube (this will rinse the mortar and syringe and ensure total dose is administered).
9. Finally, flush the enteral feeding tube with the recommended volume of water.
10. Re-start the feed, unless a prolonged break is required.

Intrajejunal administration

There is no specific information relating to jejunal administration of inositol. If necessary, administer using the above method. Monitor for lack of efficacy or increased side-effects.

References

1. *BNF 50*, September 2005.
2. Personal communication, Sanofi-Synthelabo; 3 February 2003.
3. Hexopal (Sanofi), Summary of Product Characteristics; July 2003.

Irbesartan

Formulations available[1]

Brand name (Manufacturer)	Formulation and strength	Product information/Administration information
Aprovel (Bristol-Myers Squibb, Sanofi-Synthelabo)	Tablets 75 mg, 150 mg, 300 mg	Irbesartan is practically insoluble in water.[2] Tablets disperse in 10 mL water within 2–5 minutes to give fine milky dispersion with some larger particles; these break up when drawn into the syringe and flush down an 8Fr NG tube without blockage.[3]
CoAprovel (Bristol-Myers Squibb, Sanofi-Synthelabo)	Tablets Irbesartan 150 mg + hydrochlorthiazide 12.5 mg Irbesartan 300 mg + hydrochlorthiazide 12.5 mg	Film-coated. No specific data on enteral tube administration are available for this formulation.

Site of absorption (oral administration)

Specific site of absorption is not documented. Peak plasma concentration occurs 1–1.5 hours after oral dosing.[4]

Alternative routes available

No other routes of administration are available for any of the angiotensin II antagonists.

Interactions

There is no significant interaction with food.[4]

Health and safety

Standard precautions apply.

Suggestions/recommendations

- Disperse the tablets in water immediately prior to administration.
- A prolonged break in feeding is not necessary.

Intragastric administration

1. Stop the enteral feed.
2. Flush the enteral feeding tube with the recommended volume of water.
3. Place the tablet in the barrel of an appropriate size and type of syringe.
4. Draw 10 mL of water into the syringe and allow the tablet to disperse, shaking if necessary.
5. Flush the medication dose down the feeding tube.
6. Draw another 10 mL of water into the syringe and also flush this via the feeding tube (this will rinse the syringe and ensure that the total dose is administered).
7. Finally, flush with the recommended volume of water.
8. Re-start the feed, unless a prolonged break is required.

Alternatively, at step (3) place the tablet into a medicine pot, add 10 mL of water and allow the tablet to disperse. Draw this into an appropriate syringe. Ensure that the measure is rinsed and that this rinsing water is administered also to ensure that the total dose is given.

Intrajejunal administration

There are no specific data relating to the jejunal administration of irbesartan. Administer using the above method. Monitor for increased side-effects or loss of efficacy.

References

1. *BNF 50*, September 2005.
2. Personal communication, Bristol-Myers Squibb; 24 January 2003.
3. BPNG data on file, 2004.
4. Aprovel (Sanofi pharma Bristol-Myers Squibb SNC), Summary of Product Characteristics; 28 July 2003.

Iron preparations

Formulations available[1]

Brand name (Manufacturer)	Formulation and strength	Product information/Administration information
Ferrous sulphate (various manufacturers)	Tablets 200 mg	Sugar-coated tablets. 65 mg iron/tablet
Ironorm Drops (Wallace Mfg)	Oral drops 625 mg/5 mL	625 mg ferrous sulfate (125 mg iron)/5 mL. Usual adult dose 0.6 mL/day.
Ferrous gluconate (various manufacturers)	Tablets 300 mg	No liquid preparation. 35 mg iron/tablet.
Fersamal (Goldshield)	Suspension 140 mg/5 mL	Ferrous fumarate. 45 mg iron/5 mL. Orange/brown liquid, quite difficult to flush; mixes easily with an equal volume of water; this reduces viscosity and reduces resistance to flushing.[2]

Formulations available[1] (continued)

Brand name (Manufacturer)	Formulation and strength	Product information/Administration information
Galfer (Thornton & Ross)	Syrup 140 mg/5 mL	Ferrous fumarate. 45 mg iron/5 mL.
Plesmet (Link)	Syrup 25 mg iron/5 mL	Ferrous glycine sulfate. 25 mg iron/5 mL.
Niferex (Tillomed)	Elixir 100 mg/5 mL	Polysaccharide–iron complex. Dose 5 mL once or twice daily.
Sytron (Link)	Elixir 190 mg/5 mL	Sodium feredetate. 27.5 mg iron/5 mL. The complex is split in the upper GI tract to release elemental iron.[4] Contains sorbitol 40% w/v.[3]
Iron with folic acid Lexpec with Iron-M (Rosemont)	Syrup	80 mg iron/5 mL + 500 microgram folic acid/5 mL. Contains sorbitol 0.91 g/5 mL.
Lexpec with Iron (Rosemont)	Syrup	80 mg iron/5 mL + 2.5 mg folic acid/5 mL. Contains sorbitol 0.91 g/5 mL

Site of absorption (oral administration)

Iron is predominantly absorbed in the duodenum and proximal jejunum;[3] it is therefore possible that jejunal administration will reduce bioavailability.

Alternative routes available

Parenteral route is available, as CosmoFer and Venofer (see SPC for dosing information).

Interactions

Iron is best absorbed when taken between meals; however, owing to the high incidence of gastrointestinal side-effects, it is recommended that iron preparations be taken with food.

Health and safety

Standard precautions apply.

Suggestions/recommendations

- Ferrous sulfate 200 mg t.d.s. ~ ferrous fumarate liquid 10 mL b.d. ~ sodium feredetate 10 mL t.d.s. ~ Lexpec syrups 5 mL b.d. (also contains folic acid).
- Use a liquid preparation. The viscosity may necessitate dilution of the dose with water immediately prior to administration. It is not necessary to administer after feed, but this may reduce GI side-effects.

Intragastric administration

1. Stop the enteral feed.
2. Flush the enteral feeding tube with the recommended volume of water.
3. Shake the medication bottle thoroughly to ensure adequate mixing.
4. Draw the medication suspension into an appropriate size and type of syringe.
5. Flush the medication dose down the feeding tube.
6. Finally, flush with the recommended volume of water.
7. Re-start the feed, unless a prolonged break is required.

Alternatively, at step (4) measure the medicine in a suitable container and then add an equal volume of water and mix thoroughly. Draw this into an appropriate syringe. Ensure that the measure is rinsed and that this rinsing water is administered also to ensure that the total dose is given. **Do not** measure liquid medicines using a catheter-tipped syringe as this results in excessive dosing owing to the volume of the tip.

Intrajejunal administration

Jejunal administration is likely to result in reduced absorption; the dose should be titrated to response or the parenteral route should be considered. Administer as above.

References

1. *BNF 50*, September 2005.
2. BPNG data on file, 2004.
3. Personal communication, Link Pharmaceuticals; 4 February 2003.
4. Sytron (Link), Summary of Product Characteristics; June 2005.

Isoniazid

Formulations available[1]

Brand name (Manufacturer)	Formulation and strength	Product information/Administration information
Isoniazid (Celltech)	Tablets 50 mg, 100 mg	Tablets can be crushed.[2] Tablets disperse when shaken in 10 mL of water to form a fine white dispersion that flushes via an 8Fr NG tube without blockage.[3]
Isoniazid (Martindale, Rosemont, and local specials units)	Elixir (BPC) 50 mg/5 mL	Available as manufactured 'special'. *Isoniazid Elixir (BPC):*[4] Isoniazid 10.0 g Citric acid monohydrate 2.5 g Sodium citrate 12.0 g Concentrated anise water 10 mL Compound tartrazine solution 10 mL Glycerol 200 mL Chloroform water, double-strength 400 mL Water for preparations to 1000 mL This preparation is a non-viscous liquid that flushes easily via NG tube without further dilution.[3]

Formulations available[1] (continued)

Brand name (Manufacturer)	Formulation and strength	Product information/Administration information
Isoniazid (Cambridge)	Injection 25 mg/mL (2 mL)	No specific data on enteral tube administration are available for this formulation.

Site of absorption (oral administration)

Specific site of absorption is not documented. Peak plasma concentrations are achieved 1–2 hours after oral dosing.[5]

Alternative routes available

Parenteral route is available.

Interactions

The bioavailability of isoniazid is reduced by high-carbohydrate diet and by antacid therapy.[5] A high-carbohydrate diet also significantly prolongs the elimination half life in slow acetylators.[5]

Health and safety

Standard precautions apply.

Suggestions/recommendations

- Use liquid preparation.
- Give dose before food/feed if practical.

Intragastric administration

1. Stop the enteral feed.
2. Flush the enteral feeding tube with the recommended volume of water.
3. Allow 1 hour break if practical.
4. Draw the medication solution into an appropriate size and type of syringe.
5. Flush the medication dose down the feeding tube.
6. Finally, flush with the recommended volume of water.
7. Re-start the feed, unless a prolonged break is required.

Alternatively, at step (4) measure the medicine in a suitable container and then draw into an appropriate syringe. Ensure that the measure is rinsed and that this rinsing water is administered also to ensure that the total dose is given. **Do not** measure liquid medicines using a catheter-tipped syringe as this results in excessive dosing owing to the volume of the tip.

Intrajejunal administration

There are no specific data relating to jejunal administration of isoniazid. Administer using the above method. Monitor for increased side-effects or loss of efficacy.

References

1. *BNF 50*, September 2005.
2. Personal communication, Celltech; 31 March 2003.
3. BPNG data on file, 2005.
4. *The Pharmaceutical Codex*, 12th edn. London: Pharmaceutical Press; 1994.
5. Dollery C. *Therapeutic Drugs*, 2nd edn. London: Churchill Livingstone; 1998.

Isosorbide dinitrate

Formulations available[1]

Brand name (Manufacturer)	Formulation and strength	Product information/Administration information
Isosorbide dinitrate (Alpharma)	Tablets 10 mg, 20 mg	Crushing the tablets is not recommended; use an alternative route.[2]
Isosorbide dinitrate (Hillcross)	Tablets 10 mg, 20 mg	No specific data on enteral administration are available for this formulation.
Isosorbide dinitrate (IVAX)	Tablets 10 mg, 20 mg	No specific data on enteral administration are available for this formulation.
Cedocard Retard (Pharmacia)	Tablets M/R 20 mg, 40 mg	Modified-release matrix, not suitable for crushing.[3]
Isoket Retard (Schwarz)	Tablets M/R 20 mg, 40 mg	Modified-release tablets. Although these tablets can be halved, they unsuitable for administration via enteral feeding tube.[4]

Site of absorption (oral administration)

Specific site is not documented. Peak plasma concentration occurs 30–60 minutes following oral dosing.[5]

Alternative routes available

Isosorbide dinitrate aerosol spray (Angitak) is available for short-acting use; a parenteral formulation is also available, Isoket injection. Glyceryl trinitrate can be used as an alternative and is available as topical patches and injection (see BNF for available products).

Interactions

No specific interaction with food is documented.[5]

Health and safety

Standard precautions apply.

Suggestions/recommendations

- If intestinal absorption is uncertain and the drug is being used in a critical care situation, use glyceryl trinitrate or isosorbide dinitrate infusion. For all other situations, consider using glyceryl trinitrate patches (see BNF for dosing recommendations).

References

1. *BNF* 50, September 2005.
2. Personal communication, Alpharma; 21 January 2003.
3. Personal communication, Pharmacia; 11 March 2003.
4. Personal communication, Schwarz Pharma; 17 February 2003.
5. Dollery C. *Therapeutic Drugs*, 2nd edn. London: Churchill Livingstone; 1998.

Isosorbide mononitrate

Formulations available[1]

Brand name (Manufacturer)	Formulation and strength	Product information/Administration information
Immediate-release preparations Isosorbide mononitrate (Alpharma, APS, Berk, Dexcel, Hillcross, IVAX, Opus, PLIVA)	Tablets 10 mg, 20 mg, 40 mg	Alpharma does not recommend crushing the tablets.[2] Dexcel brand do not readily disperse in water. APS brand disperse in 10 mL of water within 5 minutes if agitated. The resulting dispersion flushes via an 8Fr NG tube without blockage.[3] Solubility in water 1 : 10–1 : 30.[6]
Elantan (Schwarz)	Tablets 10 mg, 20 mg, 40 mg	Crushing the tablets should be technically possible if clinically indicated.[4]
Ismo (Roche)	Tablets 10 mg, 20 mg, 40 mg	No specific data on enteral tube administration are available for this formulation.
Modified-release preparations Chemydur 60XL (Sovereign)	M/R tablets 60 mg	Modified-release tablets unsuitable for crushing.
Elantan LA (Schwarz)	Capsules 25 mg, 50 mg	Capsules containing slow-release microgranules. Schwarz has anecdotal data relating to the administration of the microgranules suspended in water immediately prior to administration via an enteral feeding tube.[4] There is no information on the bore size of the tubes or the incidence of blockage.
Imdur (AstraZeneca) Isib 60XL (Ashbourne)	Tablets 60 mg	Modified-release tablets; although they are suitable for halving, they must not be crushed.
Ismo Retard (Roche) Monit SR (Sanofi-Synthelabo)	Tablets 40 mg	Modified-release tablets unsuitable for crushing.
Isodur (Galen)	Capsules 25 mg, 50 mg	Modified-release capsules; no information available.
Isotard (Straken)	Tablets 25 mg, 40 mg, 50 mg, 60 mg	Modified-release tablets unsuitable for crushing.

Formulations available[1] *(continued)*

Brand name (Manufacturer)	Formulation and strength	Product information/Administration information
MCR-50 (Pharmacia)	Capsules 50 mg	Modified-release capsules; no information available.
Modisal XL (Sandoz) Monit XL (Sterwin) Monomax XL (Trinity) Monosorb XL 60 (Dexcel)	Tablets 60 mg	Modified-release tablets unsuitable for crushing.
Monomax SR (Trinity)	Capsules 40 mg, 60 mg	Modified-release capsules, no information available.

Site of absorption (oral administration)

Specific site is not documented. Peak plasma concentration occurs within 1 hour of oral dosing.[5]

Alternative routes available

Glyceryl trinitrate can be used as an alternative and is available as topical patches and injection (see BNF for available products).

Interactions

The rate of absorption is slowed by food but overall bioavailability is unchanged.[6]

Health and safety

Standard precautions apply.

Suggestions/recommendations

- If intestinal absorption is uncertain and the drug is being used in a critical care situation, use glyceryl trinitrate injection. For all other situations, consider using glyceryl trinitrate patches (see BNF for dosing recommendations).

References

1. *BNF* 50, September 2005.
2. Personal communication, Alpharma; 21 January 2003.
3. BPNG data on file, 2004.
4. Personal communication, Schwarz Pharma; 17 February 2003.
5. Elantan 10 (Schwarz), Summary of Product Characteristics; October 2002.
6. Dollery C. *Therapeutic Drugs*, 2nd edn. London: Churchill Livingstone; 1998.

Ispaghula husk

Formulations available[1]

Brand name (Manufacturer)	Formulation and strength	Product information/Administration information
Fybogel (R&C)	Granules 3.5 g/sachet	No specific data on enteral tube administration are available for this formulation.
Isogel (Pfizer)	Granules 90%	No specific data on enteral tube administration are available for this formulation.
Ispagel (Richmond)	Granules 3.5 g/sachet	No specific data on enteral tube administration are available for this formulation.
Fibrerelief (Manx)	Granules 3.5 g/sachet	No specific data on enteral tube administration are available for this formulation.
Regulan (Procter & Gamble)	Granules 3.4 g/sachet	No specific data on enteral tube administration are available for this formulation.

Site of absorption (oral administration)

Ispaghula husk is not absorbed from the GI tract; its pharmacological action is through its action as a bulking agent.[2]

Alternative routes available

Not applicable.

Interactions

No significant interaction with food.

Health and safety

Standard precautions apply.

Suggestions/recommendations

- Not recommended for use via the feeding tube owing the risk of blockage as the suspending agent begins to thicken.
- If chronic constipation is a problem, seek dietetic advice on the suitability of a fibre-enriched feed.

References

1. *BNF* 50, September 2005.
2. Fybogel (Britannia), Summary of Product Characteristics; June 2001.

Isradipine

Formulations available[1]

Brand name (Manufacturer)	Formulation and strength	Product information/Administration information
Prescal (Novartis)	Tablets 2.5 mg	Twice-daily dosing.[1] Uncoated tablets.[2] Solubility in water is very low.[3] No specific data on enteral tube administration are available for this formulation.

Site of absorption (oral administration)

Specific site of absorption is not documented. Detectable in plasma after 20 minutes, peak plasma concentration occurs 2 hours post dose.[2]

Alternative routes available

No alternative route is available for isradipine.

Interactions

Peak plasma concentrations are delayed by 1 hour, although total bioavailability is not affected by food.[2]

Health and safety

Standard precautions apply.

Suggestions/recommendations

- No data are currently available; consider changing to amlodipine (see monograph).

References

1. *BNF 50*, September 2005.
2. Plendil 2.5 mg (AstraZeneca), Summary of Product Characteristics; September 2003.
3. Dollery C. *Therapeutic Drugs*, 2nd edn. London: Churchill Livingstone; 1998.

Itraconazole

Formulations available[1]

Brand name (Manufacturer)	Formulation and strength	Product information/Administration information
Sporanox (Janssen-Cilag)	Capsules 100 mg	In past experience, patients who received the contents of capsules via NG tubes indicated reduced absorption. A published report of itraconazole administration via an NG tube shows that itraconazole capsules were dissolved in cranberry juice and administered. However, this is not recommended by Janssen-Cilag[2]
Sporanox (Janssen-Cilag)	Oral liquid 10 mg/mL	Pale yellow, slightly viscous liquid with pH of approximately 2. Will flush down the tube with some resistance.[3] Contains sorbitol.[4]
Sporanox (Janssen-Cilag)	Concentrate for infusion 10 mg/mL (25 mL)	No specific data on enteral tube administration are available for this formulation.

Site of absorption (oral administration)

Specific site of absorption is not documented. Peak plasma concentration occurs 2 hours after oral dose of the liquid preparation in fasted patients.[4]

Alternative routes available

Parenteral formulation is available and should be used if enteral absorption is compromised.

Interactions

Maximal absorption of itraconazole capsules occurs immediately after a meal. Ingestion of food increased the systemic bioavailability of itraconazole. However, impaired gastric acid secretion may reduce absorption, although this is not thought to be clinically important.[5]
The liquid formulation should be taken before food; when the oral solution is taken with food the absorption is reduced by 25%[4]

Health and safety

Standard precautions apply.

Suggestions/recommendations

- Stop feed at least 2 hours pre-dose and flush the tube well. Use a liquid preparation undiluted. Flush tube well after dose. Do not restart feed for at least 1 hour post dose.
- It is possible that absorption will be reduced with administration directly into the duodenum or jejunum owing to the higher pH; there are no data to support administration via this route.
- Use the parenteral route if reduced enteral absorption is suspected or if a break in enteral feeding is not possible.

Intragastric administration

1. Stop the enteral feed.
2. Flush the enteral feeding tube with the recommended volume of water.
3. Wait for 2 hours before administering dose.
4. Draw the medication solution into an appropriate size and type of syringe.
5. Flush the medication dose down the feeding tube.
6. Finally, flush with the recommended volume of water.
7. Do not restart the feed for at least 1 hour.

Alternatively, at step (4) measure the medicine in a suitable container and then draw into an appropriate syringe. Ensure that the measure is rinsed and that this rinsing water is administered also to ensure that the total dose is given. **Do not** measure liquid medicines using a catheter-tipped syringe as this results in excessive dosing owing to the volume of the tip.

Intrajejunal administration

There are no data on jejunal administration. See notes above. Consider using parenteral formulation.

References

1. *BNF 50*, September 2005.
2. Personal communication, Janssen-Cilag; 22 January 2003.
3. BPNG data on file, 2004.
4. Sporanox liquid (Janssen-Cilag), Summary of Product Characteristics; October 2001.
5. Dollery C. *Therapeutic Drugs*, 2nd edn. London: Churchill Livingstone; 1998.

Ketoconazole

Formulations available[1]

Brand name (Manufacturer)	Formulation and strength	Product information/Administration information
Nizoral (Janssen-Cilag)	Tablets 200 mg	Tablets disperse in 10 mL of water within 2 minutes to give a very fine dispersion that flushes easily via an 8Fr NG tube without blockage.[2]

Site of absorption (oral administration)

Specific site of absorption is not documented. Peak plasma concentration occurs approximately 2 hours after oral dosing.[3]

Ketoconazole requires an acidic pH for optimal absorption. Therefore, jejunal administration or administration in post-gastrectomy patients is likely to result in decreased bioavailability.[4]

Alternative routes available

None available for ketoconazole. Other antifungals are available in parenteral formulations.[1]

Interactions

The specific interaction with food is poorly defined, with conflicting data in the literature.[5]
The data sheet recommends taking ketoconazole with food to increase absorption;[3] however, as continuous feeding may cause a pH buffering effect in the stomach, it may be prudent to withhold feed for 2 hours following the dose as recommended for acid-neutralising medicines.[3]

Health and safety

Standard precautions apply.

Suggestions/recommendations

- Disperse the tablets in water immediately prior to administration.

Intragastric administration

1. Stop the enteral feed.
2. Flush the enteral feeding tube with the recommended volume of water.
3. Wait 30 minutes before administering dose.
4. Place the tablet in the barrel of an appropriate size and type of syringe.
5. Draw 10 mL of water into the syringe and allow the tablet to disperse, shaking if necessary.
6. Flush the medication dose down the feeding tube.
7. Draw another 10 mL of water into the syringe and also flush this via the feeding tube (this will rinse the syringe and ensure that the total dose is administered).
8. Finally, flush with the recommended volume of water.
9. Do not re-start feed for at least 2 hours.

Alternatively, at step (4) place the tablet into a medicine pot, add 10 mL of water and allow the tablet to disperse. Draw this into an appropriate syringe. Ensure that the measure is rinsed and that this rinsing water is administered also to ensure that the total dose is given.

Intrajejunal administration

Not suitable for jejunal administration. See notes above.

References

1. *BNF* 50, September 2005.
2. BPNG data on file, 2004.
3. Nizoral (Janssen-Cilag), Summary of Product Characteristics; May 2001.
4. Adams D. Administration of drugs through a jejunostomy tube. *Br J Intensive Care*. 1994; 4(1): 10–17.
5. Dollery C. *Therapeutic Drugs*, 2nd edn. London: Churchill Livingstone; 1998.

Ketoprofen

Formulations available[1]

Brand name (Manufacturer)	Formulation and strength	Product information/Administration information
Orudis (Hawgreen)	Capsules 50 mg, 100 mg	Take after food.[2] No specific data on enteral tube administration are available for this formulation.
Orudis (Hawgreen)	Suppositories 100 mg	Bioavailability of the suppositories is comparable to the capsule formulation.[3] However, the dosage recommendation is 100 mg at night.
Oruvail (Hawgreen)	Injection 50 mg/mL (2 mL)	Recommended for 3 days treatment only.[4] No specific data on enteral tube administration are available for this formulation.
Oruvail (Hawgreen)	Gel 2.5%	Only suitable for topical relief of mild musculoskeletal pain.[1]
Oruvail (Hawgreen)	M/R capsules 100 mg, 150 mg, 200 mg	Modified-release capsules; contents must not be crushed. Not suitable for administration via an enteral tube.
Ketoprofen (Sandoz)	Capsules 50 mg, 100 mg	No specific data on enteral tube administration are available for this formulation.
Ketoprofen (APS, Ashbourne, Goldshield, Sandoz, Tillomed, Trinity)	M/R capsules 100 mg, 200 mg	Modified-release capsules, contents must not be crushed. Not suitable for administration via an enteral tube.

Site of absorption (oral administration)

Specific site of absorption is not documented. Peak plasma concentration occurs 0.5–1 hour after oral dosing.[2]

Alternative routes available

Parenteral route is available; maximum course length of 3 days. Suppositories and topical gel are available; see SPC for dosing guidance.

Interactions

Food may reduce the bioavailability of ketoprofen, but this is unlikely to be clinically significant.[5] It is recommended that oral doses be taken after food to reduce the incidence of gastrointestinal side-effects.[2]

Health and safety

Standard precautions apply.

Suggestions/recommendations

- The rectal route can be used in the short term without dosage adjustment. However, the practicalities of the rectal route may make long-term treatment via this route inappropriate and an alternative equivalent nonsteroidal should be considered. Ibuprofen has similar anti-inflammatory properties.[1]

References

1. *BNF* 50, September 2005.
2. Orudis (Hawgreen), Summary of Product Characteristics; January 2002.
3. Orudis Suppositories (Hawgreen), Summary of Product Characteristics; January 2002.
4. Oruvail i.m. injection (Hawgreen), Summary of Product Characteristics; September 1998.
5. Dollery C. *Therapeutic Drugs*, 2nd edn. London: Churchill Livingstone; 1998.

Ketorolac trometamol

Formulations available[1]

Brand name (Manufacturer)	Formulation and strength	Product information/Administration information
Toradol (Roche)	Tablets 10 mg	Film-coated tablets. Tablets disperse if shaken in 10 mL of water for 5 minutes to give a fine dispersion that settles quickly but flushes down an 8Fr NG tube without blockage.[2]
Toradol (Roche)	Injection 10 mg/mL (1 mL), 30 mg/mL (1 mL)	No specific data on enteral tube administration are available for this formulation.

Site of absorption (oral administration)

Specific site of absorption is not documented. Peak plasma concentration occurs 30–60 minutes after oral dosing.[3]

Alternative routes available

Parenteral route can be used.

Interactions

A high-fat diet decreased the rate but not the extent of absorption.[4]

Health and safety

Standard precautions apply.

Suggestions/recommendations

- Ketorolac is only recommended for short-term use. The tablets can be dispersed in water immediately prior to administration and administered via an enteral feeding tube.
- A prolonged break in feeding is not required.

Intragastric administration

1. Stop the enteral feed.
2. Flush the enteral feeding tube with the recommended volume of water.
3. Place the tablet in the barrel of an appropriate size and type of syringe.
4. Draw 10 mL of water into the syringe and allow the tablet to disperse, shaking if necessary.
5. Flush the medication dose down the feeding tube.
6. Draw another 10 mL of water into the syringe and also flush this via the feeding tube (this will rinse the syringe and ensure that the total dose is administered).
7. Finally, flush with the recommended volume of water.
8. Re-start the feed, unless a prolonged break is required.

Alternatively, at step (3) place the tablet into a medicine pot, add 10 mL of water and allow the tablet to disperse. Draw this into an appropriate syringe. Ensure that the measure is rinsed and that this rinsing water is administered also to ensure that the total dose is given.

Intrajejunal administration

There are no specific data relating to jejunal administration of ketorolac. Administer as above and monitor for loss effect or side-effects.

References

1. *BNF* 50, September 2005.
2. BPNG data on file, 2004.
3. Dollery C. *Therapeutic Drugs*, 2nd edn. London: Churchill Livingstone; 1998.
4. Toradol Tablets (Roche), Summary of Product Characteristics; October 2002.

Labetalol hydrochloride

Formulations available[1]

Brand name (Manufacturer)	Formulation and strength	Product information/Administration information
Trandate (Celltech)	Tablets 50 mg, 100 mg, 200 mg, 400 mg	Celltech does not recommend crushing tablets for administration via a feeding tube as the tablets are film-coated and may block the feeding tube.[2] Tablets do not disperse readily in water. They are difficult to crush owing to the coating, but ground tablets do disperse in water. Adequate time must be allowed for the coating to dissolve. The resulting suspension can be administered via an 8Fr NG tube without blockage.[4]
Trandate (Celltech)	Injection 5 mg/mL (20 mL)	pH is 4. Can be given orally but has a bitter taste, which can be masked using fruit juice.[2]
Labetalol (Alpharma, Hillcross, IVAX)	Tablets 100 mg, 200 mg, 400 mg	Film-coated. No specific data on enteral tube administration are available for this formulation.

Formulations available [1] (*continued*)

Brand name (Manufacturer)	Formulation and strength	Product information/Administration information
Extemporaneous preparation	Suspension 10 mg/mL	*Extemporaneous labetalol suspension 10 mg/mL:* Labetalol tablets 400 mg 3 tablets Simple syrup to 120 mL Store in refrigerator. Expiration 28 days. [3]

Site of absorption (oral administration)

Site of absorption not documented.

Alternative routes available

Parenteral route is available; see SPC for dosing guidelines.

Interactions

There is no documented interaction with food.

Health and safety

Standard precautions apply.

Suggestions/recommendations

- Owing to the lack of data relating to administration via enteral feeding tubes, consider changing to an alternative beta-blocker such as atenolol or propranolol (see monographs) if clinically appropriate.
- If it is not appropriate to change therapy, crush the tablets and disperse in water immediately prior to administration. Alternatively, an extemporaneous suspension can be made.

Intragastric administration

See notes above.

1. Stop the enteral feed.
2. Flush the enteral feeding tube with the recommended volume of water.
3. Place the tablet in a mortar and crush to a fine powder using the pestle.
4. Add a few millilitres of water and mix to form a paste.
5. Add up to 15 mL of water and mix thoroughly, ensuring that there are no large particles of tablet.
6. Draw this into an appropriate size and type of syringe.
7. Flush the medication dose down the feeding tube.
8. Add another 15 mL of water to the mortar and stir to ensure that any remaining drug is rinsed from the container. Draw this water into the syringe and also flush this via the feeding tube (this will rinse the mortar and syringe and ensure that the total dose is administered).
9. Finally, flush the enteral feeding tube with the recommended volume of water.
10. Re-start the feed, unless a prolonged break is required.

Intrajejunal administration

There are no specific data relating to the jejunal administration of labetalol. Administer using the above method. Monitor for loss of efficacy or increased side-effects.

References

1. *BNF* 50, September 2005.
2. Personal communication, Celltech Pharmaceuticals; 31 March 2003.
3. Nahata MC. Stability of labetalol hydrochloride in distilled water, simple syrup, and three fruit juices. *DICP*. 1991; 25 :465–469.
4. BPNG data on file, 2005.

Lacidipine

Formulations available[1]

Brand name (Manufacturer)	Formulation and strength	Product information/Administration information
Motens (Boehringer Ingelheim)	Tablets 2 mg, 4 mg	Film-coated tablets.[2] Highly lipophilic drug, therefore very poorly soluble in water.[2] Light-sensitive.[2] No specific data on enteral tube administration are available for this formulation.

Site of absorption (oral administration)

Specific site of absorption is not documented. Peak plasma concentration occurs 30–150 minutes post oral dose.[2]

Alternative routes available

None.

Interactions

There is no documented interaction with food.[2]

Health and safety

Standard precautions apply.

Suggestions/recommendations

- Owing to poor solubility and light sensitivity, it is not appropriate to crush the tablets; consider changing to amlodipine (see monograph).

References

1. *BNF* 50, September 2005.
2. Motens (Boehringer Ingelheim), Summary of Product Characteristics; April 2001.

Lactulose

Formulations available[1]

Brand name (Manufacturer)	Formulation and strength	Product information/Administration information
Lactulose (Alpharma, APS, Arrow, CP, Hillcross, Intrapharm, IVAX, Novartis, Sandoz, Solvay)	Solution 3.1–3.7 g/5 mL	Lactulose liquid is sticky and may need to be diluted with water.[2] Undiluted lactulose liquid is very difficult to flush down a fine-bore feeding tube; the resistance is such that it is difficult to tell whether the tube is blocked. Dilution with 2–3 times the volume of water produces a solution that can be flushed down the tube with less resistance.[3]

Site of absorption (oral administration)

Lactulose is not broken down or absorbed in the stomach or small intestine. Its site of action is locally in the colon.[4]

Alternative routes available

Not applicable.

Interactions

No significant interaction with food is documented.

Health and safety

Standard precautions apply.

Suggestions/recommendations

- Dilution with 2–3 times the volume of water immediately prior to administration will reduce the viscosity and allow the solution to pass more easily down the feeding tube.
- A prolonged break in feeding is not required.

Intragastric administration

1. Stop the enteral feed.
2. Flush the enteral feeding tube with the recommended volume of water.
3. Draw the medication suspension into an appropriate size and type of syringe.
4. Draw twice the volume of water and a little air into the syringe and shake to mix thoroughly.
5. Flush the medication dose down the feeding tube.
6. Draw an equal volume of water into the syringe and also flush this via the feeding tube (this will rinse the syringe and ensure that the total dose is administered).
7. Finally, flush with the recommended volume of water.
8. Re-start the feed, unless a prolonged break is required.

Alternatively, at step (3) measure the medicine in a suitable container and then add twice the volume of water and mix thoroughly. Draw this into an appropriate syringe. Ensure that the measure is rinsed and that this rinsing water is administered also to ensure that the total dose is given. **Do not** measure liquid medicines using a catheter-tipped syringe as this results in excessive dosing owing to the volume of the tip.

Intrajejunal administration

As the site of action is the colon, lactulose will have a therapeutic effect if it is delivered directly into the stomach or jejunum. Administer using the above method.

References

1. *BNF* 50, September 2005.
2. Personal communication, Solvay; 19 February 2003.
3. BPNG data on file, 2004.
4. Lactulose (Novartis), Summary of Product Characteristics; November 2002.

Lamivudine

Formulations available[1]

Brand name (Manufacturer)	Formulation and strength	Product information/Administration information
Epivir (GSK)	Tablets 150 mg, 300 mg	Although there is no theoretical reason why the tablets cannot be crushed, GSK recommends using the liquid preparation in order to avoid exposure of the operator to active constituents of the crushed tablet.[2]
Epivir (GSK)	Oral solution 50 mg/5 mL	GSK is aware of anecdotal reports of Epivir being administered successfully via enteral feeding tubes.[2] Contains sucrose 1 g/5 mL.[2]
Zeffix (GSK)	Tablets 100 mg	Tablet disperses in 10 mL of water within 2 minutes to give a pale orange dispersion that settles quickly but re-disperses easily and flushes via an 8Fr NG tube without blockage.[3]
Zeffix (GSK)	Oral solution 25 mg/5 mL	GSK recommends using the oral solution instead of crushing the tablets[2] (this is outside the produce license).

With zidovudine – see Zidovudine
With abacavir and zidovudine – see Abacavir

Site of absorption (oral administration)

The specific site of absorption is not documented. Lamivudine is well absorbed orally, with peak plasma concentrations occurring within 1 hour.[4]

Alternative routes available

None available for lamivudine.

Interactions

Food delays the absorption and reduces the peak concentrations of lamivudine but does not affect bioavailability.[4]

Health and safety

Standard precautions apply.

Suggestions/recommendations

- Use oral solution for administration via the feeding tube. Alternatively, Zeffix tablets can be dispersed in water.
- A prolonged break in feeding is not required.

Intragastric administration

1. Stop the enteral feed.
2. Flush the enteral feeding tube with the recommended volume of water.
3. Draw the medication solution into an appropriate size and type of syringe.
4. Flush the medication dose down the feeding tube.
5. Finally, flush with the recommended volume of water.
6. Re-start the feed, unless a prolonged break is required.

Alternatively, at step (3) measure the medicine in a suitable container and then draw into an appropriate syringe. Ensure that the measure is rinsed and that this rinsing water is administered also to ensure that the total dose is given. **Do not** measure liquid medicines using a catheter-tipped syringe as this results in excessive dosing owing to the volume of the tip.

Intrajejunal administration

There are no specific data on jejunal administration of lamivudine. Administer using the above method. Alternatively, the tablets can be used, following the method below. Monitor for increased side-effects or loss of efficacy.

1. Stop the enteral feed.
2. Flush the enteral feeding tube with the recommended volume of water.
3. Place the tablet in the barrel of an appropriate size and type of syringe.
4. Draw 10 mL of water into the syringe and allow the tablet to disperse, shaking if necessary.
5. Flush the medication dose down the feeding tube.
6. Draw another 10 mL of water into the syringe and also flush this via the feeding tube (this will rinse the syringe and ensure that the total dose is administered).
7. Finally, flush with the recommended volume of water.
8. Re-start the feed, unless a prolonged break is required.

Alternatively, at step (3) place the tablet into a medicine pot, add 10 mL of water and allow the tablet to disperse. Draw this into an appropriate syringe. Ensure that the measure is rinsed and that this rinsing water is administered also to ensure that the total dose is given.

References

1. *BNF* 50, September 2005.
2. Personal communication, GlaxoSmithKline; 22 January 2003.
3. BPNG data on file, 2004.
4. Epivir Oral Solution (GSK), Summary of Product Characteristics; July 2003.

Lamotrigine

Formulations available[1]

Brand name (Manufacturer)	Formulation and strength	Product information/Administration information
Lamictal (GSK)	Tablets 25 mg, 50 mg, 100 mg, 200 mg	No specific data on enteral tube administration are available for this formulation.
Lamictal (GSK)	Dispersible tablets 2 mg, 5 mg, 25 mg, 100 mg	The tablets should be dispersed in a minimal amount of water and taken immediately.[2] Tablets disintegrate rapidly when placed in 10 mL of water; the resulting dispersion flushes down an 8Fr NG tube without blockage.[4]
Lamotrigine (nonproprietary)	Tablets 25 mg, 50 mg, 100 mg, 200 mg Dispersible tablets 5 mg, 25 mg, 100 mg	No specific data on enteral tube administration are available for these formulations. Dispersible formulation should be suitable for administration via the feeding tube.

Site of absorption (oral administration)

No specific site of absorption is documented. Peak plasma concentration occurs 2.5 hours after dosing.[3]

Alternative routes available

No alternative routes for lamotrigine.

Interactions

Lamictal dispersible tablets do not interact with enteral feeds.[2]

Health and safety

Standard precautions apply.

Suggestions/recommendations

- Disperse dispersible/chewable tablets in water immediately prior to administration.
- A prolonged break in feeding is not required.

Intragastric administration

1. Stop the enteral feed.
2. Flush the enteral feeding tube with the recommended volume of water.
3. Place the tablet in the barrel of an appropriate size and type of syringe.
4. Draw 10 mL of water into the syringe and allow the tablet to disperse, shaking if necessary.
5. Flush the medication dose down the feeding tube.
6. Draw an equal volume of water into the syringe and also flush this via the feeding tube (this will rinse the syringe and ensure that the total dose is administered).
7. Finally, flush with the recommended volume of water.
8. Re-start the feed, unless a prolonged break is required.

Alternatively, at step (3) place the tablet into a medicine pot, add 10 mL of water and allow the tablet to disperse. Draw this into an appropriate syringe. Ensure that the measure is rinsed and that this rinsing water is administered also to ensure that the total dose is given.

Intrajejunal administration

There are no specific data relating to jejunal administration of lamotrigine. Administer using the above method. Monitor for increased side-effects or loss of efficacy.

References

1. *BNF 50*, September 2005.
2. Personal communication, GSK; 22 January 2003.
3. Lamictal combined Tablets (GSK), Summary of Product Characteristics; June 2003.
4. BPNG data on file, 2004.

Lansoprazole

Formulations available[1]

Brand name (Manufacturer)	Formulation and strength	Product information/Administration information
Zoton (Wyeth)	Capsules 15 mg, 30 mg	Hard gelatin capsule containing gastro-resistant granules.[2] Granules can be emptied from capsules and mixed with 10 mL of 8.4% sodium bicarbonate;[6] this has been shown to be effective when administered nasogastrically[7] and has a shelf-life of 14 days when stored in the fridge.[8]
Zoton Suspension (Wyeth)	Suspension 30 mg/sachet	Gastroresistant granules for oral suspension.[3] Large granules are likely to block fine-bore enteral feeding tubes.
Zoton FasTab (Wyeth)	Orodispersible tablet 15 mg, 30 mg	This product is **not** absorbed sublingually. Orally dispersing gastro-resistant tablets speckled with orange to dark brown gastro-resistant microgranules.[4] FasTabs can be dispersed in 10 mL of water; the granules settle quickly but can be drawn into a syringe and administered via an 8Fr NG tube without blockage.[5]

Site of absorption (oral administration)

Enteric resistant granules ensure the drug is delivered to the small intestine. Peak plasma concentration occurs 1.5–2 hours following oral dosing.[2]

Alternative routes available

No alternative route is available for lansoprazole. Parenteral route is available for esomeprazole, omeprazole and pantoprazole.

Interactions

No specific interaction with food is documented.[2]

Health and safety

Standard precautions apply.

Suggestions/recommendations

- Do not use the suspension formulation as the granules are large and the suspending agent is viscous and this will block the feeding tube.
- For enteral feeding tubes larger than 8Fr, the FasTab formulation can be dispersed in 10 mL of water and flushed down the feeding tube using a push–pull technique to keep the granules suspended.
- For fine-bore tubes smaller than 8Fr, dissolve the contents of the capsule in 8.4% sodium bicarbonate before administration.
- If the tube becomes blocked, lock the tube using 8.4% sodium bicarbonate to dissolve any enteric coated granules lodged in the tube.

Intragastric administration

1. Stop the enteral feed.
2. Flush the enteral feeding tube with the recommended volume of water.
3. Place the FasTab tablet in the barrel of an appropriate size and type of syringe.
4. Draw 10 mL of water into the syringe and allow the tablet to disperse, shaking if necessary.
5. Flush the medication dose down the feeding tube using a push-pull technique to keep granules suspended.
6. Draw another 10 mL of water into the syringe and also flush this via the feeding tube (this will rinse the syringe and ensure that the total dose is administered).
7. Finally, flush with the recommended volume of water.
8. Re-start the feed, unless a prolonged break is required.

Alternatively, at step (3) place the tablet into a medicine pot, add 10 mL of water and allow the tablet to disperse. Draw this into an appropriate syringe, taking care to draw up all the enteric coated granules. Ensure that the measure is rinsed and that this rinsing water is administered also to ensure that the total dose is given.

Using capsules

1. Stop the enteral feed.
2. Flush the enteral feeding tube with the recommended volume of water.
3. Open the capsule and pour the contents into a medicine pot.
4. Add 15 mL of sodium bicarbonate 8.4%.
5. Stir to dissolve the granules.
6. Draw into the syringe and administer via the feeding tube.
7. Add a further 15 mL of water to the medicine pot; stir to ensure that any drug remaining in the pot is mixed with water.
8. Draw up this dispersion and flush down tube. This will ensure that the whole dose is given.
9. Flush the tube with the recommended volume of water.
10. Re-start the feed, unless a prolonged break is required.

Intrajejunal administration

Lansoprazole is absorbed in the small bowel; therefore, jejunal administration is not expected to reduce bioavailability. Administer using either of the methods above.

References

1. *BNF 50*, September 2005.
2. Zoton Capsules (Wyeth), Summary of Product Characteristics; 31 July 2005.
3. Zoton Suspension (Wyeth), Summary of Product Characteristics; 31 July 2005.
4. Zoton FasTab (Wyeth), Summary of Product Characteristics; 31 July 2005.
5. BPNG data on file, 2004.
6. Sharma VK, Vasudeva R, Howden CW. Simplified lansoprazole suspension – a liquid formulation of lansoprazole – effectively suppresses intragastric acidity when administered through a gastrostomy. *Am J Gastroenterol*. 1999; 94(7): 1813–1817.
7. Taubel JJ, Sharma VK, Chiu YL, Lukasik NL, Pilmer BL, Pan WJ. A comparison of simplified lansoprazole suspension administered nasogastrically and pantoprazole administered intravenously: effects on 24-h intragastric pH. *Aliment Pharmacol Ther*. 2001; 15(11): 1807–1817.
8. DiGiacinto JL, Olsen KM, Bergman KL, Hoie EB. Stability of suspension formulations of lansoprazole and omeprazole stored in amber-coloured plastic oral syringes. *Ann Pharmacother*. 2000; 34: 600–605.

Leflunomide

Formulations available[1]

Brand name (Manufacturer)	Formulation and strength	Product information/Administration information
Arava (Aventis Pharma)	Tablets 10 mg, 20 mg, 100 mg	Film-coated tablets. There is no theoretical reason why the tablets cannot be crushed. The manufacturer has no data to support this method of administration. Patients should be monitored for exaggerated or diminished response.[2] Tablets disperse if shaken in 10 mL of water for 5 minutes to form a cloudy dispersion that flushes via an 8Fr NG tube without blockage.[3]

Site of absorption (oral administration)

Specific site of absorption is not documented. Absorption is variable, with peak plasma concentrations of the active metabolites occurring between 1 and 24 hours following oral dosing.[4]

Alternative routes available

No alternative routes available.

Interactions

The effect of leflunomide is unaffected by food.[4]

Health and safety

Standard precautions apply.

Suggestions/recommendations

- Disperse in water immediately prior to administration.
- A prolonged break in feeding is not required.

Intragastric administration

1. Stop the enteral feed.
2. Flush the enteral feeding tube with the recommended volume of water.
3. Place the tablet in the barrel of an appropriate size and type of syringe.
4. Draw 10 mL of water into the syringe and allow the tablet to disperse, shaking if necessary.
5. Flush the medication dose down the feeding tube.
6. Draw another 10 mL of water into the syringe and also flush this via the feeding tube (this will rinse the syringe and ensure that the total dose is administered).
7. Finally, flush with the recommended volume of water.
8. Re-start the feed, unless a prolonged break is required.

Alternatively, at step (3) place the tablet into a medicine pot, add 10 mL of water and allow the tablet to disperse. Draw this into an appropriate syringe. Ensure that the measure is rinsed and that this rinsing water is administered also to ensure that the total dose is given.

Intrajejunal administration

There are no specific data on jejunal administration of leflunomide. Administer using the above method. Monitor for increased side-effects and loss of efficacy.

References

1. *BNF 50*, September 2005.
2. Personal communication, Aventis Pharma; 2 January 2003.
3. BPNG data on file, 2005.
4. Arava (Aventis), Summary of Product Characteristics; February 2003.

Lercanidipine hydrochloride

Formulations available[1]

Brand name (Manufacturer)	Formulation and strength	Product information/Administration information
Zanidip (Napp)	Tablets 10 mg	Film-coated tablets.[2] No specific data on enteral tube administration are available for this formulation.

Site of absorption (oral administration)

Specific site of absorption is not documented. Peak plasma concentrations occur 1.5–3 hours post oral dose.[2]

Alternative routes available

No alternative route available for lercanidipine.

Interactions

Oral availability of lercanidipine increased 4-fold when ingested 2 hours after a high-fat meal; for this reason lercanidipine should be taken before meals.[2]

Health and safety

Standard precautions apply.

Suggestions/recommendations

- Owing to lack of data and risk of variable absorption, consider changing to amlodipine (see monograph).

References

1. *BNF 50*, September 2005.
2. Zanidip (Napp), Summary of Product Characteristics; April 2002.

Levetiracetam

Formulations available[1]

Brand name (Manufacturer)	Formulation and strength	Product information/Administration information
Keppra (UCB Pharma)	Tablets 250 mg, 500 mg, 1 g	Film-coated tablets.[1] Keppra tablets are immediate-release and therefore may be crushed and sprinkled on food or given via enteral feeding tube. Keppra is water-soluble: 1.04 g/mL at room temperature. There are no stability data on the suspension of tablets in water and therefore this should be administered immediately.[2] 500 mg tablets (only strength tested) disperse in 10 mL of water if shaken for 5 minutes. This forms a milky, even dispersion that flushes down an 8Fr NG tube without blockage.[4]
Keppra (UCB Pharma)	Oral solution 100 mg/mL (300 mL)	Sugar-free, clear liquid. Contains maltitol.[5]

Site of absorption (oral administration)

Specific site of absorption is not documented. Oral bioavailability is close to 100% and peak plasma concentration occurs at 1.3 hours post dose.[3]

Alternative routes available

No alternative routes for levetiracetam.

Interactions

The extent of absorption is unaffected by food; the rate is slightly decreased.[3]

Health and safety

Standard precautions apply.

Suggestions/recommendations

- Use liquid preparation.
- A prolonged break in feeding is not required.

Intragastric administration

1. Stop the enteral feed.
2. Flush the enteral feeding tube with the recommended volume of water.
3. Shake the medication bottle thoroughly to ensure adequate mixing.
4. Draw the medication suspension into an appropriate size and type of syringe.
5. Draw twice the volume of water and a little air into the syringe and shake to mix thoroughly.
6. Flush the medication dose down the feeding tube.
7. Draw an equal volume of water into the syringe and also flush this via the feeding tube (this will rinse the syringe and ensure that the total dose is administered).
8. Finally, flush with the recommended volume of water.
9. Re-start the feed, unless a prolonged break is required.

Alternatively, at step (4) measure the medicine in a suitable container and then add twice the volume of water and mix thoroughly. Draw this into an appropriate syringe. Ensure that the measure is rinsed and that this rinsing water is administered also to ensure that the total dose is given. **Do not** measure liquid medicines using a catheter-tipped syringe as this results in excessive dosing owing to the volume of the tip.

Intrajejunal administration

There are no specific data relating to the jejunal administration of levetiracetam. Administer using the above method. Monitor for loss of efficacy or increased side-effects.

References

1. *BNF* 50, September 2005.
2. Personal communication, UCB Pharma; 16 January 2003.
3. Keppra (UCB), Summary of Product Characteristics; June 2001.
4. BPNG data on file, 2004.
5. Keppra Liquid (UCB), Summary of Product Characteristics; September 2005.

Levodopa

Formulations available[1]

Brand name (Manufacturer)	Formulation and strength	Product information/Administration information
Co-beneldopa (benserazide/ levodopa)		
Madopar (Roche)	Capsules '62.5' '125' '250'	12.5 mg benserazide + 50 mg levodopa. 25 mg benserazide + 100 mg levodopa. 50 mg benserazide + 200 mg levodopa. There are no stability data available for opening the capsules and dispersing in water; the dispersible tablets should be used.[2]
Madopar (Roche)	Dispersible tablets '62.5' '125'	12.5 mg benserazide + 50 mg levodopa. 25 mg benserazide + 100 mg levodopa. Tablets disperse in 10 mL of water within 2 minutes to give a cloudy white dispersion that flushes via an 8Fr NG tube without blockage.[2]
Madopar CR (Roche)	Capsules '125'	Modified-release capsules. Contain 25 mg benserazide + 100 mg levodopa. Not suitable for administration via enteral feeding tube.
Co-careldopa (carbidopa/ levodopa)		
Sinemet-62.5 (BMS)	Tablets 12.5 mg/50 mg	Tablets disperse readily when placed in 10 mL of water to form a pale yellow dispersion that settles quickly but flushes via an 8Fr NG tube without blockage. Care must be taken to administer whole dose owing to the tendency for settlement to the bottom of the container/syringe.[2]
Sinemet-110 (BMS)	Tablets 10 mg/100 mg	Tablets disperse readily when placed in 10 mL of water to form a bright blue dispersion that settles quickly but flushes via an 8Fr NG tube without blockage. Care must be taken to administer whole dose owing to the tendency for settlement to the bottom of the container/syringe.[2]
Sinemet-Plus (BMS)	Tablets 25 mg/100 mg	Tablets disperse readily when placed in 10 mL of water to form a bright yellow dispersion that settles quickly but flushes via an 8Fr NG tube without blockage. Care must be taken to administer whole dose owing to the tendency for settlement to the bottom of the container/syringe.[2]

Formulations available[1] (continued)

Brand name (Manufacturer)	Formulation and strength	Product information/Administration information
Sinemet-275 (BMS)	Tablets 25 mg/250 mg	Tablets disperse readily when placed in 10 mL of water to form a pale blue dispersion that settles quickly but flushes via an 8Fr NG tube without blockage. Care must be taken to administer whole dose owing to the tendency for settlement to the bottom of the container/syringe.[5]
Half Sinemet CR (BMS)	Tablets 25 mg/100 mg	Modified-release tablets. Do not crush; not suitable for administration via enteral feeding tube.
Sinemet CR (BMS)	Tablets 50 mg/200 mg	Modified-release tablets. Do not crush; not suitable for administration via enteral feeding tube.

Site of absorption (oral administration)

Levodopa is absorbed by the active transport system normally responsible for the absorption of large neutral amino acids in the upper small bowel.[6] Time to reach peak plasma concentrations of levodopa varies widely between individuals but peak concentrations generally occur within 2 hours of oral dosing.[4]

Alternative routes available

None available for levodopa. Apomorphine is available as a parenteral formulation.

Interactions

Protein in the diet and in the circulating system competes with levodopa for absorption and transport into the brain. Diets that do not exceed 0.8 g/kg of protein are reported to eliminate this problem.

Timing of feed and dosing of levodopa should be as consistent as possible to reduce fluctuations in daily response.[3] Administration after food delays the time to peak plasma concentration and reduces total bioavailability.[7]

Health and safety

Standard precautions apply.

Suggestions/recommendations

- Ensure that enteral diet is optimised and that, if appropriate, protein content does not exceed 0.8 g/kg.
- Use Madopar dispersible tablets or disperse Sinemet tablets in water immediately prior to administration.
- For patients on modified-release preparations, convert to dispersible tablets and increase dosing frequency.

Intragastric administration

1. Stop the enteral feed.
2. Flush the enteral feeding tube with the recommended volume of water.
3. Place the tablet in the barrel of an appropriate size and type of syringe.
4. Draw 10 mL of water into the syringe and allow the tablet to dissolve, shaking if necessary.
5. Flush the medication dose down the feeding tube.
6. Draw another 10 mL of water into the syringe and also flush this via the feeding tube (this will rinse the syringe and ensure that the total dose is administered).
7. Finally, flush with the recommended volume of water.
8. Re-start the feed, unless a prolonged break is required.

Alternatively, at step (3) place the tablet into a medicine pot, add 10 mL of water and allow the tablet to dissolve. Draw this into an appropriate syringe. Ensure that the measure is rinsed and that this rinsing water is administered also to ensure that the total dose is given.

Intrajejunal administration

Bioavailability should be unaffected by jejunal delivery of levodopa; time to peak may be shorter. Administer using the above method.

References

1. *BNF 50*, September 2005.
2. BPNG data on file, 2005.
3. Personal communication, Roche; 6 February 2003.
4. Levodopa Tablets (Cambridge), Summary of Product Characteristics; April 2000 (product discontinued).
5. BPNG data on file, 2004.
6. Lennernas H, Nilsson D, Aquilonius SM, Ahrenstedt O, Knutson L, Paalzow LK. The effects of L-leucine on the absorption of levodopa, studied by regional jejunal perfusion in man. *Br J Clin Pharmacol*. 1993; 35(3): 243–250.
7. Baruzzi A, Contin M, Riva R, *et al.* Influence of meal ingestion time on pharmacokinetics of orally administered levodopa in parkinsonian patients. *Clin Neuropharmacol*. 1987; 10(6): 527–537.

Levofloxacin

Formulations available[1]

Brand name (Manufacturer)	Formulation and strength	Product information/Administration information
Tavanic (Hoechst Marion Roussel)	Tablets 250 mg, 500 mg	Film-coated tablets.[2] Tablets do not disperse readily in water. The tablet can be crushed, but the flaky coating makes crushing difficult. It takes a few minutes for the coating to dissolve when mixed with water. The tablet then forms a milky dispersion that flushes via an 8Fr NG tube without blockage.[3]

Formulations available[1] (continued)

Brand name (Manufacturer)	Formulation and strength	Product information/Administration information
Tavanic (Hoechst Marion Roussel)	Infusion 5 mg/mL (100 mL)	No specific data on enteral tube administration are available for this formulation.

Site of absorption (oral administration)

Specific site of absorption is not documented. Peak plasma concentration occurs within 1 hour of oral dosing.[2]

Alternative routes available

Parenteral route is available.

Interactions

There is a documented in-vitro interaction between levofloxacin and Ensure, resulting in decreased plasma concentration,[4] although there are no in-vivo data.[5]

Health and safety

Standard precautions apply.

Suggestions/recommendations

- For serious infections use the parenteral formulation.
- As the tablets do not disperse readily in water, consider changing to an alternative antibiotic available in a liquid or dispersible tablet formulation.
- When continued therapy with oral levofloxacin is indicated, consider using the higher end of the dose range.
- Stop feed 1 hour pre-dose and restart feed 2 hours post dose.

Intragastric administration

See notes above.

1. Stop the enteral feed.
2. Flush the enteral feeding tube with the recommended volume of water.
3. Wait for at least 1 hour.
4. Place the tablet in a mortar and crush to a fine powder using the pestle.
5. Add a few millilitres of water and mix to form a paste.
6. Add up to 15 mL of water and mix thoroughly, ensuring that there are no visible lumps of tablet.
7. Draw this into an appropriate size and type of syringe.
8. Flush the medication dose down the feeding tube.
9. Add another 15 mL of water to the mortar and stir to ensure that any remaining drug is rinsed from the container. Draw this water into the syringe and also flush this via the feeding tube (this will rinse the mortar and syringe and ensure that the total dose is administered).
10. Finally, flush the enteral feeding tube with the recommended volume of water.
11. Wait for 2 hours before re-starting the feed.

Intrajejunal administration

There are no specific data on jejunal administration of levofloxacin. Consider an alternative antibiotic. Administer using the above method; use the higher end of dose range. Monitor for increased side-effects or loss of efficacy.

References

1. *BNF 50*, September 2005.
2. Tavanic (Hoechst), Summary of Product Characteristics; July 2003.
3. BPNG data on file, 2005.
4. Wright DH, Pietz SL, Konstantinides FN, Rotschafer JC. (2000) Decreased in vitro fluoroquinolone concentrations after admixture with an enteral feeding formulation. *JPEN J Parenter Enteral Nutr*. 2000; 24(1): 42–48.
5. Stockley IH. *Drug Interactions*, 4th edn. London: Pharmaceutical Press; 1996.

Levomepromazine (Methotrimeprazine)

Formulations available[1]

Brand name (Manufacturer)	Formulation and strength	Product information/Administration information
Nozinan (Link)	Tablets 25 mg	Levomepromazine maleate. Tablets disperse within 2 minutes when placed in 10 mL of water to give a coarse dispersion; some of the larger particles break up when drawn into the syringe. The dispersion flushes via an 8Fr NG tube without blockage, although it is likely to block finer tubes.[2]
Nozinan (Link)	Injection 25 mg/mL (1 mL)	Levomepromazine hydrochloride. pH 4.0–5.0 Can be administered orally if necessary.[3]

Site of absorption (oral administration)

There is no specific information on the site of absorption of levomepromazine.[3] Peak plasma concentration occurs 1–3 hours following oral dosing.[4]

Alternative routes available

Parenteral route is available; can be administered by i.v., i.m. or s.c. injection.

Interactions

There is no documented interaction with food or enteral feed.[3]

Health and safety

Standard precautions apply.

Suggestions/recommendations

- Disperse the tablets in water immediately prior to dosing.
- A prolonged break in feeding is not required.
- Alternatively, use the parenteral route.

Intragastric administration

1. Stop the enteral feed.
2. Flush the enteral feeding tube with the recommended volume of water.
3. Place the tablet in the barrel of an appropriate size and type of syringe.
4. Draw 10 mL of water into the syringe and allow the tablet to dissolve, shaking if necessary.
5. Flush the medication dose down the feeding tube.
6. Draw another 10 mL of water into the syringe and also flush this via the feeding tube (this will rinse the syringe and ensure that the total dose is administered).
7. Finally, flush with the recommended volume of water.
8. Re-start the feed, unless a prolonged break is required.

Alternatively, at step (3) place the tablet into a medicine pot, add 10 mL of water and allow the tablet to dissolve. Draw this into an appropriate syringe. Ensure that the measure is rinsed and that this rinsing water is administered also to ensure that the total dose is given.

Intrajejunal administration

There is no specific information relating to jejunal administration of levomepromazine. Administer using the above method. Monitor for loss of efficacy or increased side-effects.

References

1. *BNF* 50, September 2005.
2. BPNG data on file, 2005.
3. Personal communication, Link Pharmaceuticals; 4 February 2003.
4. Dollery C. *Therapeutic Drugs*, 2nd edn. London: Churchill Livingstone; 1998.

Levothyroxine sodium

Formulations available[1]

Brand name (Manufacturer)	Formulation and strength	Product information/Administration information
Levothyroxine (Alpharma, APS, CP, Goldshield, Hillcross, IVAX)	Tablets 25 microgram, 50 microgram, 100 microgram	Tablets can be crushed.[2] Care should be taken to avoid third-party contact.[3] Tablets disperse in 10 mL of water if shaken for 3–5 minutes to give a fine dispersion that flushes via an 8Fr NG tube without blockage.[4]
Extemporaneous preparation[5]		*Extemporaneous levothyroxine suspension 25 microgram/mL:* Levothyroxine tablets 100 microgram — 30 tablets; Glycerol — 48 mL; Sterile water for irrigation — to 120 mL. 'Shake well before use.' Store in refrigerator; 8-day expiry.

Site of absorption (oral administration)

Specific site of absorption is not documented. Some enterohepatic recirculation occurs.[6]

Alternative routes available

Anecdotal evidence exists for rectal administration of levothyroxine. Liothyronine injection is available for parenteral use when the oral route is not appropriate.

Interactions

There is no documented interaction with food.

Health and safety

Inhalation of crushed tablets should be avoided. Standard precautions apply.

Suggestions/recommendations

- Disperse the tablets in water immediately prior to administration.
- A prolonged break in feeding is not required.

Intragastric administration

1. Stop the enteral feed.
2. Flush the enteral feeding tube with the recommended volume of water.
3. Place the tablet in the barrel of an appropriate size and type of syringe.
4. Draw 10 mL of water into the syringe and allow the tablet to disperse, shaking if necessary.
5. Flush the medication dose down the feeding tube.
6. Draw another 10 mL of water into the syringe and also flush this via the feeding tube (this will rinse the syringe and ensure that the total dose is administered).
7. Finally, flush with the recommended volume of water.
8. Re-start the feed, unless a prolonged break is required.

Alternatively, at step (4) place the tablet into a medicine pot, add 10 mL of water and allow the tablet to dissolve. Draw this into an appropriate syringe. Ensure that the measure is rinsed and that this rinsing water is administered also to ensure that the total dose is given.

Intrajejunal administration

No specific data. Administer using the above method.

References

1. *BNF 50*, September 2005.
2. Personal communication, Alpharma; 21 January 2003.
3. Personal communication, Celltech; 31 March 2003.
4. BPNG data on file, 2004/2005.
5. Boulton DW, Fawcett P, Woods DJ. Stability of an extemporaneously compounded levothyroxine sodium oral liquid. *Am J Health Syst Pharm*. 1996; 52: 1157–1161.
6. Levothyroxine (Celltech), Summary of Product Characteristics; October 2001.

Linezolid

Formulations available [1]

Brand name (Manufacturer)	Formulation and strength	Product information/Administration information
Zyvox (Pharmacia)	Tablets 600 mg	Film-coated. No specific data on enteral tube administration are available for this formulation.
Zyvox (Pharmacia)	Suspension 100 mg/5 mL	Powder for reconstitution, 150 mL. Contains sucrose as base; contains sorbitol as additional sweetener only. [2]
Zyvox (Pharmacia)	Intravenous infusion 2 mg/mL (300 mL)	Not suitable for enteral administration.

Site of absorption (oral administration)

Absorption begins in the stomach although the majority of absorption takes place in the small intestine, so full absorption may not occur if linezolid is delivered directly into the jejunum. [3]

Alternative routes available

Parenteral route is available.

Interactions

Bioavailability is not affected by food. [3]

Health and safety

Standard precautions apply.

Suggestions/recommendations

- Use the liquid formulation.
- A prolonged break in feeding is not required.
- It is possible that absorption may be reduced following intrajejunal administration.
- Owing to the lack of data relating to the interaction with enteral feeding, plasma concentration should be monitored and the parenteral route used if treating a serious infection.

Intragastric administration

1. Stop the enteral feed.
2. Flush the enteral feeding tube with the recommended volume of water.
3. Shake the medication bottle thoroughly to ensure adequate mixing.
4. Draw the medication suspension into an appropriate size and type of syringe.
5. Flush the medication dose down the feeding tube.
6. Draw an equal volume of water into the syringe and also flush this via the feeding tube (this will rinse the syringe and ensure that the total dose is administered).
7. Finally, flush with the recommended volume of water.
8. Re-start the feed, unless a prolonged break is required.

Alternatively, at step (4) measure the medicine in a suitable container and then add an equal volume of water and mix thoroughly. Draw this into an appropriate syringe. Ensure that the measure is rinsed and that this rinsing water is administered also to ensure that the total dose is given. **Do not** measure liquid medicines using a catheter-tipped syringe as this results in excessive dosing owing to the volume of the tip.

Intrajejunal administration

See notes above. Consider monitoring plasma concentration or using parenteral therapy.

References

1. *BNF* 50, September 2005.
2. Zyvox Granules for Oral suspension (Pharmacia), Summary of Product Characteristics; February 2002.
3. Personal communication, Pharmacia; March 11 2003.

Lisinopril

Formulations available[1]

Brand name (Manufacturer)	Formulation and strength	Product information/Administration information
Carace (Bristol-Myers Squibb)	Tablets 2.5 mg, 5 mg, 10 mg, 20 mg	Lisinopril is soluble 1 : 10–1 : 30 of water.[2] No specific data on enteral tube administration are available for this formulation.
Zestril (AstraZeneca)	Tablets 2.5 mg, 5 mg, 10 mg, 20 mg	Lisinopril dihydrate. No specific data on enteral tube administration are available for this formulation.
Lisinopril (Rosemont)	Oral solution 5 mg/5 mL	Unlicensed special.
Lisinopril (APS, Generics, Sandoz)	Tablets 2.5 mg, 5 mg, 10 mg, 20 mg	Lisinopril dihydrate. No specific data on enteral tube administration are available for this formulation.

Formulations available[1] (continued)

Brand name (Manufacturer)	Formulation and strength	Product information/Administration information
Lisinopril (Ranbaxy)	Tablets 2.5 mg, 5 mg, 10 mg, 20 mg	All tablets disperse in 10 mL of water within 2 minutes to give a very fine dispersion that flushes easily via an 8Fr NG tube.[5]
Lisinopril (extemporaneous preparation)	Suspension 2 mg/mL	*Extemporaneous lisinopril syrup 2 mg/mL:* Lisinopril 5 mg tablet ... 48 tablets Sterile water for irrigation ... 5 mL Simple syrup ... to 120 mL Grind the tablets and add water to form a paste, then gradually add syrup to form a suspension. Store at room temperature or refrigerate. 30-day shelf-life.[6]
Carace Plus (Bristol-Myers Squibb)	Tablets	Carace 10 Plus = lisinopril 10 mg + hydrochlorothiazide 12.5 mg. Carace 20 Plus = lisinopril 20 mg + hydrochlorothiazide 12.5 mg. No specific data on enteral tube administration are available for this formulation.
Zestoretic (AstraZeneca)	Tablets	Zestoretic 10 tablets = lisinopril 10 mg + hydrochlorothiazide 12.5 mg. Zestoretic 20 tablets = lisinopril 20 mg + hydrochlorothiazide 12.5 mg. No specific data on enteral tube administration are available for this formulation.

Site of absorption (oral administration)

Specific site of absorption is not documented. Peak plasma concentration of lisinopril occurs within 6–8 hours of oral dosing.[3, 4]

Alternative routes available

None available.

Interactions

Absorption is unaffected by food.[3, 4]

Health and safety

Standard precautions apply.

Suggestions/recommendations

- Use 'special' liquid preparation or disperse tablets in water immediately prior to administration.
- A prolonged break in feeding is not necessary.

Intragastric administration

Instructions for administration of liquid formulations. For tablet formulations see method below.

1. Stop the enteral feed.
2. Flush the enteral feeding tube with the recommended volume of water.
3. Shake the medication bottle thoroughly to ensure adequate mixing.
4. Draw the medication suspension into an appropriate size and type of syringe.
5. Flush the medication dose down the feeding tube.
6. Finally, flush with the recommended volume of water.
7. Re-start the feed, unless a prolonged break is required.

Alternatively, at step (4) measure the medicine in a suitable container and then add an equal volume of water and mix thoroughly. Draw this into an appropriate syringe. Ensure that the measure is rinsed and that this rinsing water is administered also to ensure that the total dose is given. **Do not** measure liquid medicines using a catheter-tipped syringe as this results in excessive dosing owing to the volume of the tip.

Intrajejunal administration

There are no specific data relating to the jejunal administration of lisinopril. Owing to the higher osmolarity of liquid preparations, it is recommended that the tablets be used for jejunal administration.

1. Stop the enteral feed.
2. Flush the enteral feeding tube with the recommended volume of water.
3. Place the tablet in the barrel of an appropriate size and type of syringe.
4. Draw 10 mL of water into the syringe and allow the tablet to dissolve, shaking if necessary.
5. Flush the medication dose down the feeding tube.
6. Draw another 10 mL of water into the syringe and also flush this via the feeding tube (this will rinse the syringe and ensure that the total dose is administered).
7. Finally, flush with the recommended volume of water.
8. Re-start the feed, unless a prolonged break is required.

Alternatively, at step (3) place the tablet into a medicine pot, add 10 mL of water and allow the tablet to dissolve. Draw this into an appropriate syringe. Ensure that the measure is rinsed and that this rinsing water is administered also to ensure that the total dose is given.

References

1. *BNF 50*, September 2005.
2. Personal communication, Bristol-Myers Squibb; 24 January 2004.
3. Carace (Bristol-Myers Squibb), Summary of Product Characteristics; February 2003.
4. Zestril (AstraZeneca), Summary of Product Characteristics; June 2002.
5. BPNG data on file, 2004.
6. Webster A, English B, Rose D. The stability of lisinopril as an extemporaneous syrup. *Int J Pharm Compound*. 1997; 1: 352–353.

Lofepramine hydrochloride

Formulations available[1]

Brand name (Manufacturer)	Formulation and strength	Product information/Administration information
Lofepramine (Alpharma, APS, Ashbourne, Hillcross, Sandoz, Sterwin)	Tablets 70 mg	No specific data on enteral tube administration are available for this formulation.
Lomont (Rosemont)	Oral suspension 70 mg/5 mL	Sugar-free suspension, contains 1.36 g of sorbitol per 5 mL.[2] Pale yellow, cloudy suspension. Quite viscous and difficult to flush. Mixes well with an equal volume of water, which reduces flushing resistance.[3]
Gamanil (Merck)	Tablets 70 mg	Film-coated tablets. Gamanil tablets are coated but can be crushed.[4]

Site of absorption (oral administration)

Specific site of absorption is not documented. Peak plasma concentration occurs 1 hour following oral dosing.[5]

Alternative routes available

No alternative routes for lofepramine.

Interactions

No specific interaction with food is documented.[5]

Health and safety

Standard precautions apply.

Suggestions/recommendations

- Use the suspension formulation, shake well before use.
- Dilute with an equal volume of water immediately prior to administration.
- A prolonged break in feeding is not required.

Intragastric administration

1. Stop the enteral feed.
2. Flush the enteral feeding tube with the recommended volume of water.
3. Shake the medication bottle thoroughly to ensure adequate mixing.
4. Draw the medication suspension into an appropriate size and type of syringe.
5. Draw an equal volume of water and a little air into the syringe and shake to mix thoroughly.
6. Flush the medication dose down the feeding tube.
7. Finally, flush with the recommended volume of water.
8. Re-start the feed.

Alternatively, at step (4) measure the medicine in a suitable container and then add an equal volume of water and mix thoroughly. Draw this into an appropriate syringe. Ensure that the measure is rinsed and that this rinsing water is administered also to ensure that the total dose is given. **Do not** measure liquid medicines using a catheter-tipped syringe as this results in excessive dosing owing to the volume of the tip.

Intrajejunal administration

There are no specific data relating to the jejunal administration of lofepramine. Administer as above and monitor for loss of efficacy or increased side-effects.

References

1. *BNF* 50, September 2005.
2. Personal communication, Rosemont; 20 January 2005.
3. BPNG data on file, 2004.
4. Personal communication, Merck; 23 January 2003.
5. Lomont (Rosemont), Summary of Product Characteristics; January 2004.

Loperamide

Formulations available [1]

Brand name (Manufacturer)	Formulation and strength	Product information/Administration information
Imodium (Janssen Cilag)	Capsules 2 mg	No specific data on enteral tube administration are available for this formulation.
Imodium (Janssen Cilag)	Syrup 1 mg/5 mL	Loperamide syrup can be given undiluted into the small bowel. [2] Imodium liquid is not viscous and draws into a syringe and flushes down an NG tube without resistance; the liquid mixes well with water and flushes easily. [3]
Loperamide (Alpharma, APS, Berk, Generics, Hillcross, IVAX)	Capsules 2 mg	No specific data on enteral tube administration are available for this formulation.

Site of absorption (oral administration)

Imodium is absorbed in the gut and acts by binding the to the mu receptors all along the gut.[2] Owing to its high affinity for the gut wall and its high first-pass metabolism, very little loperamide reaches the systemic circulation.[4]

Alternative routes available

No alternative routes available for loperamide.

Interactions

There is no documented interaction with food.[4]

Health and safety

Standard precautions apply.

Suggestions/recommendations

- Use the liquid preparation undiluted. Flush well after dosing. Alternatively, the tablets can be used without risk of blockage, although efficacy is unknown.
- A prolonged break in feeding is not required.

Intragastric administration

1. Stop the enteral feed.
2. Flush the enteral feeding tube with the recommended volume of water.
3. Draw the medication solution into an appropriate size and type of syringe.
4. Flush the medication dose down the feeding tube.
5. Finally, flush with the recommended volume of water.
6. Re-start the feed, unless a prolonged break is required.

Alternatively, at step (3) measure the medicine in a suitable container and then draw into the syringe with appropriate adapter for tube connector. Ensure that the measure is rinsed and that this rinsing water is administered also to ensure that the total dose is given. **Do not** measure liquid medicines using a catheter-tipped syringe as this results in excessive dosing owing to the volume of the tip.

Intrajejunal administration

Jejunal administration will not affect the therapeutic response to loperamide. However, owing to the potential osmotic effect of the liquid preparation, it may be appropriate to further dilute the dose with water immediately prior to administration.

References

1. *BNF 50*, September 2005.
2. Personal communication, Janssen-Cilag; 22 January 2003.
3. BPNG data on file, 2004.
4. Imodium (Janssen-Cilag), Summary of Product Characteristics; September 2002.

Loratadine

Formulations available[1]

Brand name (Manufacturer)	Formulation and strength	Product information/Administration information
Loratadine (various manufacturers)	Tablets 10 mg	Alpharma tablets can be crushed.[2]
Loratadine (various manufacturers)	Syrup 5 mg/5 mL	No specific data on enteral tube administration are available for this formulation. However, no problem is envisaged with enteral administration of this formulation.
Clarityn (Schering Plough)	Tablets 10 mg	No specific data on enteral tube administration are available for this formulation.
Clarityn (Schering Plough)	Syrup 5 mg/5 mL	Contains sucrose; does not contain sorbitol.[3]

Site of absorption (oral administration)

Specific site of absorption is not documented. Peak plasma concentration occurs 1 hour following oral administration.[3]

Alternative routes available

No alternative route of administration is available for loratadine. A parenteral formulation is available for chlorpheniramine.

Interactions

No specific interaction with food is documented.[3]

Health and safety

Standard precautions apply.

Suggestions/recommendations

- Use the liquid preparation. Dilute with an equal volume of water prior to jejunal administration.
- A prolonged break in feeding is not required.

Intragastric administration

1. Stop the enteral feed.
2. Flush the enteral feeding tube with the recommended volume of water.
3. Draw medication solution into an appropriate size and type of syringe.
4. Flush the medication dose down the feeding tube.
5. Finally, flush with the recommended volume of water.
6. Re-start the feed.

Alternatively, at step (3) measure the medicine in a suitable container and then draw into an appropriate syringe. Ensure that the measure is rinsed and that this rinsing water is administered also to ensure that the total dose is given. **Do not** measure liquid medicines using a catheter-tipped syringe as this results in excessive dosing owing to the volume of the tip.

Intrajejunal administration

There are no specific data relating to the jejunal administration of loratadine. Administer using the above method. Consider further dilution of the liquid immediately prior to administration to reduce osmolarity. Monitor for loss of effect or increased side-effects.

References

1. *BNF 50*, September 2005.
2. Personal communication, Alpharma; 21 January 2003.
3. Dollery C. *Therapeutic Drugs*, 2nd edn. London: Churchill Livingstone; 1998.

Lorazepam

Formulations available[1]

Brand name (Manufacturer)	Formulation and strength	Product information/Administration information
Lorazepam (Genus, IVAX)	Tablets 1 mg, 2.5 mg	Tablets can be crushed. Tablets can also be administered sublingually.[2, 3]
Lorazepam (Wyeth)	Injection 4 mg/mL (1 mL)	Injection can be used sublingually.

Site of absorption (oral administration)

Specific site of absorption is not documented. Following oral administration, peak plasma concentration occurs after 2 hours.[4] Lorazepam is also absorbed sublingually.

Alternative routes available

Parenteral route is available. Injection and tablets can also be used sublingually.[2, 3]

Interactions

Specific interaction with food is not documented.

Health and safety

Standard precautions apply.

Suggestions/recommendations

- Use an alternative therapy available as a liquid preparation if clinically appropriate; both diazepam and temazepam are available in liquid formulation.
- Crush tablets and disperse in water immediately prior to administration.
- A prolonged break in feeding is not required.

Intragastric administration

1. Stop the enteral feed.
2. Flush the enteral feeding tube with the recommended volume of water.
3. Place the tablet in a mortar and crush to a fine powder using the pestle.
4. Add a few millilitres of water and mix to form a paste.
5. Add up to 15 mL of water and mix thoroughly, ensuring that there are no large particles of tablet.
6. Draw this into an appropriate size and type of syringe.
7. Flush the medication dose down the feeding tube.
8. Add another 15 mL of water to the mortar and stir to ensure that any remaining drug is rinsed from the container. Draw this water into the syringe and also flush this via the feeding tube (this will rinse the mortar and syringe and ensure that the total dose is administered).
9. Finally, flush the enteral feeding tube with the recommended volume of water.
10. Re-start the feed, unless a prolonged break is required.

Intrajejunal administration

There are no specific data on jejunal administration of lorazepam. Administer using the above method. Monitor for increased side-effects or loss of efficacy.

References

1. *BNF 50*, September 2005.
2. Ghanchi FD, Khan MY Sublingual lorazepam as premedication in peribulbar anesthesia. *J Cataract Refract Surg.* 1997; 23(10): 1581–1584.
3. Grennblatt DJ, Divoll M, Harmatz JS, Shader RI. Pharmacokinetic comparison of sublingual lorazepam with intravenous, intramuscular, and oral lorazepam. *J Pharm Sci.* 1982; 71(2): 248–252.
4. Dollery C. *Therapeutic Drugs*, 2nd edn. London: Churchill Livingstone; 1998.

Losartan potassium

Formulations available [1]

Brand name (Manufacturer)	Formulation and strength	Product information/Administration information
Cozaar (MSD)	Tablets 25 mg, 50 mg, 100 mg	Film-coated tablets [2] Tablets do not disperse readily in water, but crush easily and mix with 10 mL of water to form a fine suspension that flushes down an 8Fr NG tube without blockage. [3]
Cozaar-Comp (MSD)	Tablets Losartan 50 mg + hydrochlorothiazide 12.5 mg	Film-coated tablets [4] No specific data on enteral tube administration are available for this formulation.

Site of absorption (oral administration)

Specific site of absorption is not documented. Peak plasma concentrations of losartan are reached within 1 hour of oral dosing.[2]

Alternative routes available

No other routes of administration are available for any of the angiotensin II antagonists.

Interactions

Food does not affect absorption of losartan.[2]

Health and safety

Standard precautions apply.

Suggestions/recommendations

- If the route of administration is likely to be long term, consider changing to irbesartan (see monograph) owing to lack of data and poor dispersion characteristics.
- If continued therapy with losartan is indicated, the tablets can be crushed and mixed with water immediately prior to administration.
- A prolonged break in feeding is not required.

Intragastric administration

1. See notes above.
2. Stop the enteral feed.
3. Flush the enteral feeding tube with the recommended volume of water.
4. Place the tablet in a mortar and crush to a fine powder using the pestle.
5. Add a few millilitres of water and mix to form a paste.
6. Add up to 15 mL of water and mix thoroughly, ensuring that there are no large particles of tablet.
7. Draw this into an appropriate size and type of syringe.
8. Flush the medication dose down the feeding tube.
9. Add another 15 mL of water to the mortar and stir to ensure that any remaining drug is rinsed from the container. Draw this water into the syringe and also flush this via the feeding tube (this will rinse the mortar and syringe and ensure that the total dose is administered).
10. Finally, flush the enteral feeding tube with the recommended volume of water.
11. Re-start the feed, unless a prolonged break is required.

Intrajejunal administration

There are no specific data relating to the jejunal administration of losartan. Use the above method. Monitor for loss of efficacy or increased side-effects.

References

1. *BNF* 50, September 2005.
2. Cozaar (MSD), Summary of Product Characteristics; July 2003.
3. BPNG data on file, 2004.
4. Cozaar-Comp (MSD), Summary of Product Characteristics; October 2002.

Macrogols

Formulations available[1]

Brand name (Manufacturer)	Formulation and strength	Product information/Administration information
Idrolax (Schwarz)	Oral powder 10 g/sachet	Macrogol 4000. No specific data on enteral tube administration are available for this formulation.
Movicol (Norgine)	Oral powder 13.125 g/sachet	Macrogol 3350. The company has anecdotal reports of Movicol being administered via enteral feeding tubes, but does not have specific data.[2] Sachet dissolves in 125 mL of water to give a clear solution that draws up into easily but owing to its volume requires several manipulations to administer the dose. The solution flushes well via a fine-bore feeding tube.[3] When dissolved in 125 mL of water, the solution also contains 65 mmol/L sodium, 53 mmol/L chloride, 5.4 mmol/L potassium, 17 mmol/L bicarbonate.[5]
Movicol-Half (Norgine)	Oral powder 6.563 g/sachet	Macrogol 3350. Electrolyte profile as above.[6]
Movicol Paediatric Plain (Norgine)	Oral powder 6.563 g/sachet	Macrogol 3350. Electrolyte profile as above.[7]

Site of absorption (oral administration)

Macrogol 4000 and Macrogol 3350 are not absorbed or broken down in the GI tract; they act by decreasing intestinal fluid resorption.[4,5]

Alternative routes available

Not applicable.

Interactions

There is no significant interaction with food.

Health and safety

Standard precautions apply.

Suggestions/recommendations

- Dissolve the powder in water as directed and flush down the feeding tube. Flush well after dosing. No prolonged break in feeding is necessary.
- Not suitable for fluid-restricted patients owing to the large volume necessary to administer the dose.
- If chronic constipation is a problem, seek dietetic advice on the suitability of a fibre-enriched feed.

Intragastric administration

1. Stop the enteral feed.
2. Flush the enteral feeding tube with the recommended volume of water.
3. Measure the appropriate quantity of water into a suitable size container.
4. Add the contents of the sachet and allow to dissolve.
5. Draw into an appropriate size and type of syringe; owing to the large volume this will be several syringe volumes.
6. Flush the medication dose down the feeding tube.
7. Finally, flush with the recommended volume of water.
8. Re-start the feed, unless a prolonged break is required.

Intrajejunal administration

As the mechanism of action is local within the bowel, jejunal administration should not affect efficacy. Administer as above.

References

1. *BNF 50*, September 2005.
2. Personal communication, Norgine; 24 January 2003.
3. BPNG data on file, 2004.
4. Idrolax (Schwarz), Summary of Product Characteristics; November 2002.
5. Movicol (Norgine), Summary of Product Characteristics; August 2002.
6. Movicol-Half (Norgine), Summary of Product Characteristics; December 2002.
7. Movicol Paediatric Plain (Norgine), Summary of Product Characteristics; 30 March 2005.

Magnesium preparations

Formulations available [1]

Brand name (Manufacturer)	Formulation and strength	Product information/Administration information
Magnesium glycerophosphate (special, distributed by IDIS)	Tablets 4 mmol/tablet	Produced by a variety of specials manufacturers. Some will disperse in water.
Magnesium glycerophosphate (Special Products Ltd)	Oral liquid 1 mmol/mL	Unlicensed manufactured 'special'. The oral liquid can be administered undiluted via an enteral feeding tube. [3] pH is 8.
Magnesium sulphate (Auden McKenzie, Aurum, Celltech)	Injection 50% (2 mmol/mL)	Not suitable for enteral administration.
Magnesium sulphate (GSL – Epsom Salts)		Poorly absorbed orally, used as laxative.

Formulations available[1] (*continued*)

Brand name (Manufacturer)	Formulation and strength	Product information/Administration information
Magnesium oxide (specials manufacturers)	Capsules Various strengths	Converted to magnesium chloride by gastric acid.[2] No specific data on enteral tube administration are available for this formulation.
Magnesium Hydroxide Mixture BP (various manufacturers)		Poorly absorbed orally, used as laxative.

Site of absorption (oral administration)

The main site of absorption of magnesium is the distal small intestine.[2]

Alternative routes available

Magnesium sulphate injection available for parenteral use.

Interactions

No specific interaction with food.

Health and safety

Standard precautions apply.

Suggestions/recommendations

- Use manufactured special liquid.
- A prolonged break in feeding is not required.

Intragastric administration

1. Stop the enteral feed.
2. Flush the enteral feeding tube with the recommended volume of water.
3. Draw the medication solution into an appropriate size and type of syringe.
4. Flush the medication dose down the feeding tube.
5. Finally, flush with the recommended volume of water.
6. Re-start the feed, unless a prolonged break is required.

Alternatively, at step (3) measure the medicine in a suitable container and then draw into an appropriate syringe. Ensure that the measure is rinsed and that this rinsing water is administered also to ensure that the total dose is given. **Do not** measure liquid medicines using a catheter-tipped syringe as this results in excessive dosing owing to the volume of the tip.

Intrajejunal administration

Some magnesium salts such as the oxide, hydroxide and trisilicate are converted by gastric acid to the chloride salt. Therefore, these salts administered directly into the jejunum are likely to have a reduced bioavailability.

Use glycerophosphate solution, as above, and titrate dose to response.

References

1. *BNF* 50, September 2005.
2. Dollery C. *Therapeutic Drugs*, 2nd edn. London: Churchill Livingstone; 1998.
3. Personal communication, Special Products Ltd; 20 January 2003.

Mebendazole

Formulations available[1]

Brand name (Manufacturer)	Formulation and strength	Product information/Administration information
Mebendazole (OTC product)	Tablets 100 mg	Ovex (Janssen-Cilag) tablets can be chewed.[2] No specific data on enteral tube administration are available for this formulation.
Vermox (Janssen-Cilag)	Tablets 100 mg	No specific data on enteral tube administration are available for this formulation.
Vermox (Janssen-Cilag)	Suspension 100 mg/5 mL	The manufacturer has no specific data regarding the administration of the liquid via an enteral feeding tube.[2] Sucrose-based suspension; does not contain sorbitol.[3]

Site of absorption (oral administration)

Specific site of absorption is not documented.[3]

Alternative routes available

None available for mebendazole.

Interactions

No specific interaction with food is documented.[3]

Health and safety

Standard precautions apply.

Suggestions/recommendations

- Use the liquid preparation.
- A prolonged break in feeding is not required.

Intragastric administration

1. Stop the enteral feed.
2. Flush the enteral feeding tube with the recommended volume of water.
3. Shake the medication bottle thoroughly to ensure adequate mixing.
4. Draw the medication suspension into an appropriate size and type of syringe.
5. Flush the medication dose down the feeding tube.
6. Finally, flush with the recommended volume of water.
7. Re-start the feed, unless a prolonged break is required.

Alternatively, at step (4) measure the medicine in a suitable container. Draw this into an appropriate syringe. Ensure that the measure is rinsed and that this rinsing water is administered also to ensure that the total dose is given. **Do not** measure liquid medicines using a catheter-tipped syringe as this results in excessive dosing owing to the volume of the tip.

Intrajejunal administration

No specific data are available on jejunal administration of mebendazole. Administer using the above method. Monitor for loss of efficacy or increased side-effects.

References

1. *BNF* 50, September 2005.
2. Personal communication, Janssen-Cilag; 22 January 2003.
3. Vermox Suspension (Janssen-Cilag), Summary of Product Characteristics; June 2005.

Mebeverine hydrochloride

Formulations available [1]

Brand name (Manufacturer)	Formulation and strength	Product information/Administration information
Colofac (Solvay)	Tablets 135 mg	Tablets can be crushed. [2]
Colofac (Solvay)	Liquid 50 mg/5 mL	15 mL liquid = 1 tablet. Yellow, banana-flavoured, sugar-free suspension. [3] 2.5 mmol Na per 15 mL dose. [3]
Colofac MR (Solvay)	M/R capsules 200 mg	Do not crush. Not suitable for administration via enteral feeding tube.
Mebeverine (Alpharma, APS, Arrow, Generics, Hillcross, IVAX)	Tablets 135 mg	No specific data on enteral tube administration are available for this formulation.

Site of absorption (oral administration)

Specific site of absorption is not documented. Rapid and complete absorption occurs following oral administration. [3]

Alternative routes available

None for mebeverine. Hyoscine butylbromide (Buscopan) is available in parenteral formulation.

Interactions

There is no documented interaction with food; mebeverine is most effective when given 20 minutes before food.

Health and safety

Standard precautions apply.

Suggestions/recommendations

- Use the liquid preparation 20 minutes before feeds.

Intragastric administration

1. Best given 20 minutes before feed commences.
2. Flush the enteral feeding tube with the recommended volume of water.
3. Shake the medication bottle thoroughly to ensure adequate mixing.
4. Draw the medication suspension into an appropriate size and type of syringe.
5. Flush the medication dose down the feeding tube.
6. Finally, flush with the recommended volume of water.
7. Wait 20 minutes before starting the feed.

Alternatively, at step (4) measure the medicine in a suitable container. Draw this into an appropriate syringe. Ensure that the measure is rinsed and that this rinsing water is administered also to ensure that the total dose is given. **Do not** measure liquid medicines using a catheter-tipped syringe as this results in excessive dosing owing to the volume of the tip.

Intrajejunal administration

There are no specific data relating to jejunal administration of mebeverine. Use the above method and monitor for signs of loss of efficacy.

References

1. *BNF 50*, September 2005.
2. Personal Communication, Solvay; 19 February 2003.
3. Colofac (Solvay), Summary of Product Characteristics; September 2000.

Medroxyprogesterone

Formulations available[1]

Brand name (Manufacturer)	Formulation and strength	Product information/Administration information
Farlutal (Pharmacia)	Injection 200 mg/mL (2.5 mL)	No specific data on enteral tube administration are available for this formulation.

Formulations available[1] (continued)

Brand name (Manufacturer)	Formulation and strength	Product information/Administration information
Provera (Pharmacia)	Tablets 2.5 mg, 5 mg, 10 mg, 100 mg, 200 mg, 400 mg	The tablets can be crushed and dispersed in water; as there are no stability data, this should be done immediately prior to administration.[2] The 5 mg and 100 mg tablets (only strengths tested) disperse in 10 mL of water within 5 minutes. The 5 mg tablets give a fine dispersion, the 100 mg a slightly coarser dispersion; both flush via an 8Fr NG tube without blockage.[3]

Site of absorption (oral administration)

Specific site of absorption is not documented. Peak plasma concentration occurs 2–6 hours following oral dosing.[4]

Alternative routes available

Parenteral route is available.

Interactions

There is no documented interaction with food.[4]

Health and safety

Standard precautions apply.

Suggestions/recommendations

- Disperse the tablets in water immediately prior to administration.
- A prolonged break in feeding is not required.

Intragastric administration

1. Stop the enteral feed.
2. Flush the enteral feeding tube with the recommended volume of water.
3. Place the tablet in the barrel of an appropriate size and type of syringe.
4. Draw 10 mL of water into the syringe and allow the tablet to dissolve, shaking if necessary.
5. Flush the medication dose down the feeding tube.
6. Draw another 10 mL of water into the syringe and also flush this via the feeding tube (this will rinse the syringe and ensure that the total dose is administered).
7. Finally, flush with the recommended volume of water.
8. Re-start the feed, unless a prolonged break is required.

Alternatively, at step (3) place the tablet into a medicine pot, add 10 mL of water and allow the tablet to dissolve. Draw this into an appropriate syringe. Ensure that the measure is rinsed and that this rinsing water is administered also to ensure that the total dose is given.

Intrajejunal administration

There are no specific data on jejunal administration. Administer as above.

References

1. *BNF* 50, September 2005.
2. Personal communication, Pharmacia; March 11 2003.
3. BPNG data on file, 2004.
4. Provera (Pharmacia), Summary of Product Characteristics; August 2001.

Mefenamic acid

Formulations available[1]

Brand name (Manufacturer)	Formulation and strength	Product information/Administration information
Mefenamic acid (Arrow, Chemidex (Ponstan), IVAX, Sanofi-Synthelabo, Sterwin, Tarus)	Capsules 250 mg	No specific data on enteral tube administration are available for this formulation.
Mefenamic acid (Alpharma, APS, Ashbourne, Chemidex (Ponstan Forte), IVAX, Sanofi-Synthelabo, Sterwin, Tarus)	Tablets 500 mg	No specific data on enteral tube administration are available for this formulation.
Mefenamic acid (Chemidex)	Paediatric oral suspension 50 mg/5 mL	Very expensive, more than £70 per 125 mL bottle.[1] Strength inappropriate for adult dosing.

Site of absorption (oral administration)

Specific site of absorption is not documented. Mefenamic acid is well absorbed following oral absorption, with peak plasma concentrations occurring 2–4 hours post dose.[2]

Alternative routes available

None available for mefenamic acid. Other NSAIDs are available in rectal and parenteral formulations.

Interactions

No specific interaction with food is documented.

Health and safety

Standard precautions apply.

Suggestions/recommendations

- Owing to the lack of data, high cost of the liquid preparation and the high volume of the adult dose, consider changing to an alternative NSAID if clinically appropriate.

References

1. *BNF* 50, September 2005.
2. Dollery C. *Therapeutic Drugs*, 2nd edn. London: Churchill Livingstone; 1998.

Megestrol acetate

Formulations available[1]

Brand name (Manufacturer)	Formulation and strength	Product information/Administration information
Megace (Bristol-Myers Squibb)	Tablets 40 mg, 160 mg	Megestrol acetate is practically insoluble. Tablets disintegrate rapidly when placed in 10 mL of water to give a fine dispersion that settles quickly but flushes via an 8Fr NG tube without blockage.[2]

Site of absorption (oral administration)

Specific site of absorption is not documented. Peak plasma concentration occurs 1–3 hours following oral administration.[3]

Alternative routes available

None available for megestrol.

Interactions

No specific interaction with food is documented.[4]

Health and safety

Standard precautions apply.

Suggestions/recommendations

- Disperse the tablets in water immediately prior to administration.
- A prolonged break in feeding is not required.

Intragastric administration

1. Stop the enteral feed.
2. Flush the enteral feeding tube with the recommended volume of water.
3. Place the tablet in the barrel of an appropriate size and type of syringe.
4. Draw 10 mL of water into the syringe and allow the tablet to dissolve, shaking if necessary.
5. Flush the medication dose down the feeding tube.
6. Draw another 10 mL of water into the syringe and also flush this via the feeding tube (this will rinse the syringe and ensure that the total dose is administered).
7. Finally, flush with the recommended volume of water.
8. Re-start the feed, unless a prolonged break is required.

Alternatively, at step (3) place the tablet into a medicine pot, add 10 mL of water and allow the tablet to dissolve. Draw this into an appropriate syringe. Ensure that the measure is rinsed and that this rinsing water is administered also to ensure that the total dose is given.

Intrajejunal administration

There are no specific data available on jejunal administration. Administer using the above method. Monitor for increased side-effects or loss of efficacy.

References

1. *BNF* 50, September 2005.
2. BPNG data on file, 2005.
3. Megace (BMS), Summary of Product Characteristics; October 1998.
4. Dollery C. *Therapeutic Drugs*, 2nd edn. London: Churchill Livingstone; 1998.

Meloxicam

Formulations available [1]

Brand name (Manufacturer)	Formulation and strength	Product information/Administration information
Mobic (Boehringer Ingelheim)	Tablets 7.5 mg, 15 mg	Film-coated tablets. The tablets will disperse in water to give an almost clear suspension within a few minutes; virtually neutral taste. [2] Tablets disperse within 5 minutes when placed in 10 mL of water; [3] the dispersion flushes via an 8Fr NG tube without blockage.
Mobic (Boehringer Ingelheim)	Suppositories 7.5 mg, 15 mg	Tablets and suppositories are bioequivalent. [4]

Site of absorption (oral administration)

Specific site of absorption is not documented. [5]

Alternative routes available

Suppositories are available. The dose is considered clinically equivalent.

Interactions

There is no documented interaction with food. [5]

Health and safety

Standard precautions apply.

Suggestions/recommendations

- Doses of tablets and suppositories are considered clinically equivalent and therefore interchangeable; this may be appropriate for short-term use.
- Alternatively, tablets can be dispersed in water immediately prior to dosing.
- A prolonged break in feeding is not necessary.

Intragastric administration

1. Stop the enteral feed.
2. Flush the enteral feeding tube with the recommended volume of water.
3. Place the tablet in the barrel of an appropriate size and type of syringe.
4. Draw 10 mL of water into the syringe and allow the tablet to disperse, shaking if necessary.
5. Flush the medication dose down the feeding tube.
6. Draw another 10 mL of water into the syringe and also flush this via the feeding tube (this will rinse the syringe and ensure that the total dose is administered).
7. Finally, flush with the recommended volume of water.
8. Re-start the feed.

Alternatively, at step (3) place the tablet into a medicine pot, add 10 mL of water and allow the tablet to dissolve. Draw this into an appropriate syringe. Ensure that the measure is rinsed and that this rinsing water is administered also to ensure that the total dose is given.

Intrajejunal administration

There are no specific data relating to the jejunal administration of meloxicam. Use the above method and monitor for loss of efficacy.

References

1. *BNF* 50, September 2005.
2. Personal communication, Boehringer; 6 March 2003.
3. BPNG data on file, 2004.
4. Mobic Suppositories (Boehringer Ingelheim), Summary of Product Characteristics; August 2003.
5. Mobic Tablets (Boehringer Ingelheim), Summary of Product Characteristics; August 2003.

Memantine hydrochloride

Formulations available[1]

Brand name (Manufacturer)	Formulation and strength	Product information/Administration information
Ebixa (Lundbeck)	Tablets 10 mg	Scored, film-coated tablets. No specific data on enteral tube administration are available for this formulation.
Ebixa (Lundbeck)	Oral drops 10 mg/g	5 mg = 10 drops. Contains sorbitol;[2] however, the dose volume is so small that sorbitol dosing unlikely to be significant. Drops can be added to water for ease of administration.[3]

Site of absorption (oral administration)

Specific site of absorption is not documented. Peak plasma concentration occurs 3–8 hours following oral dosing.[2]

Alternative routes available

None available for memantine.

Interactions

Food does not affect memantine absorption.[2]

Health and safety

Standard precautions apply.

Suggestions/recommendations

- Use oral drops.
- A prolonged break in feeding is not required.

Intragastric administration

1. Stop the enteral feed.
2. Flush the enteral feeding tube with the recommended volume of water.
3. Measure the required number of drops of oral liquid into an appropriate container.
4. Add 10 mL of water to the drops.
5. Draw into an appropriate size and type of syringe.
6. Flush the medication dose down the feeding tube.
7. Rinse the measure and administer this also to ensure that the total dose is given.
8. Finally, flush with the recommended volume of water.
9. Re-start the feed, unless a prolonged break is required.

Intrajejunal administration

There is no specific information relating to the jejunal administration of memantine. Peak plasma concentration occur several hours after dosing, so the site of absorption is highly unlikely to be the stomach or duodenum; therefore, jejunal administration should not affect bioavailability. Administer using the above method.

References

1. *BNF* 50, September 2005.
2. Ebixa 10 mg/g oral drops (Lundbeck), Summary of Product Characteristics; September 2002.
3. Personal communication, Lundbeck; July 2005.

Mercaptopurine

Formulations available[1]

Brand name (Manufacturer)	Formulation and strength	Product information/Administration information
Puri-Nethol (GSK)	Tablets 50 mg	GSK has no information on the administration of Puri-Nethol via enteral feeding tube.[2]
Mercaptopurine	Tablets 10 mg	Manufactured 'special'. No specific data on enteral tube administration are available for this formulation.
Mercaptopurine (Nova Labs)	Suspension 10–100 mg/5 mL	Manufactured 'special'. 12-week expiry. Viscosity is suitable for administration via enteral feeding tubes.[3]

Site of absorption (oral administration)

Specific site of absorption is not documented. Peak plasma concentration occurs 0.5–4 hours following oral administration.[4]

Alternative routes available

No alternative available.

Interactions

No specific interaction with food is documented.[4]

Health and safety

Cytotoxic drug. Do not crush tablets. Used closed systems wherever possible. Protective clothing should be worn. Dispose of the syringe safely as cytotoxic waste.

Suggestions/recommendations

- Where practical, use a commercially prepared 'special' suspension. Alternatively, the tablets can be dispersed in water using a closed system, see below.
- A prolonged break in feeding is not required.

Intragastric administration

1. Stop the enteral feed.
2. Flush the enteral feeding tube with the recommended volume of water.
3. Shake the medication bottle thoroughly to ensure adequate mixing.
4. Draw the medication suspension into an appropriate size and type of syringe.
5. Flush the medication dose down the feeding tube.
6. Draw an equal volume of water into the syringe and also flush this via the feeding tube (this will rinse the syringe and ensure that the total dose is administered).
7. Finally, flush with the recommended volume of water.
8. Re-start the feed, unless a prolonged break is required.

Do not measure liquid medicines using a catheter-tipped syringe as this results in excessive dosing owing to the volume of the tip.

Tablet administration (closed system)

1. Stop the enteral feed.
2. Flush the enteral feeding tube with the recommended volume of water.
3. Place the tablet in the barrel of an appropriate size and type of syringe.
4. Draw 10 mL of water into the syringe and allow the tablet to dissolve, shaking if necessary.
5. Flush the medication dose down the feeding tube.
6. Draw another 10 mL of water into the syringe and also flush this via the feeding tube (this will rinse the syringe and ensure that the total dose is administered).
7. Finally, flush with the recommended volume of water.
8. Re-start the feed.

Intrajejunal administration

There is no specific information relating to jejunal administration of mercaptopurine. Administer using the above method

References

1. *BNF* 50, September 2005.
2. Personal communication, GSK; 22 January 2003.
3. Personal communication, Nova Labs; 24 March 2005.
4. Dollery C. *Therapeutic Drugs*, 2nd edn. London: Churchill Livingstone; 1998.

Mesalazine

Formulations available[1]

Brand name (Manufacturer)	Formulation and strength	Product information/Administration information
Asacol (Procter & Gamble)	Foam enema 1 g	Rectal administration. Local therapeutic action only.
Asacol (Procter & Gamble)	Suppositories 250 mg, 500 mg	Rectal administration. Local therapeutic action only.
Asacol MR (Procter & Gamble)	E/C tablets 400 mg	These tablets are enteric coated to release mesalazine in the terminal ileum; the tablets cannot be split or crushed.[2] Do not crush. Not suitable for enteral tube administration.
Ipocol (Sandoz)	E/C tablets 400 mg	Enteric coated tablets. Do not crush. Not suitable for enteral tube administration.
Mesren MR (IVAX)	E/C tablets 400 mg	Enteric coated tablets. Do not crush. Not suitable for enteral tube administration.
Pentasa (Ferring)	M/R tablets 500 mg M/R granules 1 g/sachet	M/R tablets disperse in water to give M/R granules. The M/R granules in the tablets are slightly smaller than those in the sachets[3] and therefore the tablets should be used in preference to the sachets; however, the tablet contents can only be drawn into a catheter tipped syringe owing to their size and will only flush down a 16Fr tube without blockage.[4]
Pentasa (Ferring)	Retention Enema 1 g	Rectal administration. Local therapeutic action only.
Pentasa (Ferring)	Suppositories 1 g	Rectal administration. Local therapeutic action only.
Salofalk (Dr Falk)	E/C tablets 250 mg M/R granules 500 mg/sachet, 1 g/sachet	Enteric coated pH-dependent tablets; must not be crushed.[5] Do not crush. Not suitable for enteral tube administration.

Formulations available[1] (*continued*)

Brand name (Manufacturer)	Formulation and strength	Product information/Administration information
Salofalk (Dr Falk)	Enema 2 g	Rectal administration. Local therapeutic action only.
Salofalk (Dr Falk)	Suppositories 500 mg	Rectal administration. Local therapeutic action only.
Salofalk (Dr Falk)	Rectal foam 1 g/application	Rectal administration. Local therapeutic action only.

Site of absorption (oral administration)

Mesalazine is absorbed in the small bowel but its action is locally in the terminal small bowel and colon; therefore, all preparations are formulated to release the mesalazine low down in the bowel.

Alternative routes available

Topical therapy using a rectal 5-ASA preparation should be used first-line in local rectal disease.

Interactions

There is no documented interaction with food.[6]

Health and safety

Standard precautions apply.

Suggestions/recommendations

- None of the oral preparations are suitable for enteral tube administration, as they cannot be crushed. Use topical preparations where clinically appropriate. Consider changing to sulfasalazine liquid preparation or using alternative therapy such as steroids.

References

1. *BNF* 50, September 2005.
2. Personal communication, Procter & Gamble; 22 January 2003.
3. Personal communication, Ferring Pharmaceuticals; 20 January 2003.
4. BPNG data on file, 2004.
5. Personal communication, Provalis Healthcare; 5 February 2003.
6. Asacol MR (Procter & Gamble), Summary of Product Characteristics; April 2003.

Metformin hydrochloride

Formulations available[1]

Brand name (Manufacturer)	Formulation and strength	Product information/Administration information
Glucophage (Merck)	Tablets 500 mg, 850 mg	Tablets are film-coated but can be crushed if required.[2] Tablets do not disperse well in water owing to the size of the tablet, but do crush easily and disperse well in water to form a fine suspension that flushes easily via an 8Fr NG tube.[3]
Metformin (Alpharma, APS, Arrow, Auden McKenzie, CP, Generics, Hillcross, IVAX, Kent, Sovereign, Sterwin, Taro, Zanza)	Tablets 500 mg, 850 mg	Alpharma and Zanza brand tablets do not disperse well in water but do crush easily and mix with water to form a fine suspension that flushes easily via an 8Fr NG tube.[3]
Metformin (Rosemont)	Oral solution 500 mg/5 mL	Unlicensed special – 9-month expiry.[4] Available on request only.

Site of absorption (oral administration)

Specific site of absorption is not documented. Peak plasma concentration occurs 2.5 hours after oral dosing.[5]

Alternative routes available

None available for metformin. Insulin can be used for parenteral therapy.

Interactions

Food decreases, delays and reduces the absorption of metformin; however, the dose should be taken with or after food.[5]

A decrease in vitamin B_{12} absorption has been observed in long-term treatment; this is considered to be clinically insignificant.[5]

Health and safety

Standard precautions apply.

Suggestions/recommendations

- Although tablets can be crushed and mixed with water, the quality of the suspension is operator-dependent and the risk of tube blockage is high owing to the bulk of the tablet. If crushing tablets is not considered appropriate, the liquid 'special' preparation should be used. The dose should be administered shortly after starting the feed.

Intragastric administration

Where possible use the liquid preparation to minimise the risk of tube blockage.

1. Stop the enteral feed.
2. Flush the enteral feeding tube with the recommended volume of water.
3. Shake the medication bottle thoroughly to ensure adequate mixing.
4. Draw the medication suspension into an appropriate size and type of syringe.
5. Flush the medication dose down the feeding tube.
6. Finally, flush with the recommended volume of water.
7. Re-start the feed immediately.

Alternatively, at step (4) measure the medicine in a suitable container and then add an equal volume of water and mix thoroughly. Draw this into an appropriate syringe. Ensure that the measure is rinsed and that this rinsing water is administered also to ensure that the total dose is given. **Do not** measure liquid medicines using a catheter-tipped syringe as this results in excessive dosing owing to the volume of the tip.

Tablet administration

1. Stop the enteral feed.
2. Flush the enteral feeding tube with the recommended volume of water.
3. Place the tablet in a mortar and crush to a fine powder using the pestle.
4. Add a few millilitres of water and mix to form a paste.
5. Add up to 15 mL of water and mix thoroughly, ensuring that there are no large particles of tablet.
6. Draw this into an appropriate syringe.
7. Flush the medication dose down the feeding tube.
8. Add another 15 mL of water to the mortar and stir to ensure that any remaining drug is rinsed from the container. Draw this water into the syringe and also flush this via the feeding tube (this will rinse the mortar and syringe and ensure total dose is administered).
9. Finally, flush the enteral feeding tube with the recommended volume of water.
10. Re-start the feed immediately.

Intrajejunal administration

There are no specific data relating to jejunal administration of metformin. Monitor blood sugar levels for loss of effect. Use the above method.

References

1. *BNF 50*, September 2005.
2. Personal communication, Merck; 23 January 2003.
3. BPNG data on file, 2004.
4. Personal communication, Rosemont; July 2004.
5. Glucophage (Merck), Summary of Product Characteristics; May 2003.

Methotrexate

Formulations available[1]

Brand name (Manufacturer)	Formulation and strength	Product information/Administration information
Methotrexate (Lederle, Mayne, Pharmacia (Matrex))	Tablets 2.5 mg, 10 mg	The tablets will disperse in water.[2, 3]
Methotrexate (Mayne, Goldshield)	Injection 2.5 mg/mL, 25 mg/mL, 100 mg/mL	The injection can be diluted with water and administered orally.[4] The absorption from the solution gives similar plasma concentration to tablet formulation.[4] An extended expiry can be given if a preservative is used.[2]
Methotrexate (Nova Labs)	Suspension 2.5–50 mg/5 mL	Manufactured 'special'. Shelf life 1–3 months. The viscosity is such that the product remains suspended on standing, but viscosity reduces on shaking to facilitate administration. This should be suitable for administration via a feeding tube and is unlikely to cause blockage, although Nova Labs has no specific data.[5]

Site of absorption (oral administration)

Methotrexate is well absorbed from the GI tract by an active transport mechanism utilised by dietary folate. Peak plasma concentration occurs 1–5 hours following oral administration. Methotrexate also undergoes enterohepatic circulation.[6]

Alternative routes available

Parenteral route is available. Subcutaneous injections once weekly have been used for rheumatoid arthritis and Crohn disease.

Interactions

No interaction with feed is documented.

Health and safety

Cytotoxic drug. Do not crush the tablets. Used closed systems wherever possible. Protective clothing should be worn. Dispose of any contaminated syringes safely as cytotoxic waste.

Suggestions/recommendations

- Where practical, use a commercially prepared 'special' suspension. Alternatively, the tablets can be dispersed in water, using a closed system.
- A prolonged break in feeding is not required.

Intragastric administration

1. Stop the enteral feed.
2. Flush the enteral feeding tube with the recommended volume of water.
3. Shake the medication bottle thoroughly to ensure adequate mixing.
4. Draw the medication suspension into an appropriate size and type of syringe.
5. Flush the medication dose down the feeding tube.
6. Finally, flush with the recommended volume of water.
7. Re-start the feed, unless a prolonged break is required.

Do not measure liquid medicines using a catheter-tipped syringe as this results in excessive dosing owing to the volume of the tip.

Tablet administration (closed system)

1. Stop the enteral feed.
2. Flush the enteral feeding tube with the recommended volume of water.
3. Place the tablet in the barrel of an appropriate size and type of syringe.
4. Draw 10 mL of water into the syringe and allow the tablet to dissolve, shaking if necessary.
5. Flush the medication dose down the feeding tube.
6. Draw another 10 mL of water into the syringe and also flush this via the feeding tube (this will rinse the syringe and ensure that the total dose is administered).
7. Finally, flush with the recommended volume of water.
8. Re-start the feed.

Intrajejunal administration

The absorption of methotrexate is unlikely to be reduced by jejunal administration. Administer using the above method.

References

1. *BNF 50*, September 2005.
2. Personal communication, Pharmacia; 11 March 2003.
3. BPNG data on file, 2004.
4. Personal communication, Mayne; 29 January 2003.
5. Personal communication, Nova Labs; 24 March 2005.
6. Dollery C. *Therapeutic Drugs*, 2nd edn. London: Churchill Livingstone; 1998.

Methyldopa

Formulations available[1]

Brand name (Manufacturer)	Formulation and strength	Product information/Administration information
Methyldopa (Alpharma, CP, Hillcross, IVAX, Sovereign)	Tablets 125 mg, 250 mg, 500 mg	Tablets can be crushed; however, the tablet coating may not dissolve and may block the tube.[2]

Formulations available[1] (continued)

Brand name (Manufacturer)	Formulation and strength	Product information/Administration information
Aldomet (MSD)	Tablets 250 mg, 500 mg	Film-coated. No specific data on enteral tube administration are available for this formulation.
Extemporaneous preparations		Formula for extemporaneous preparation are available. Contact Nova Labs for details and current stability data.

Site of absorption (oral administration)

Absorption occurs throughout the small bowel and is thought to be via the active transport system used by dietary amino acids.[4] Bioavailability is variable but approximately 25%. Peak plasma concentration occurs 2–3 hours after oral administration.[3]

Alternative routes available

No alternative routes available for methyldopa. Other antihypertensives are available in parenteral formulations.

Interactions

No specific interaction with food is documented. Absorption of methyldopa is reduced by iron salts.[3]

Health and safety

Standard precautions apply.

Suggestions/recommendations

- Where clinically appropriate, change to an alternative antihypertensive therapy.
- Alternatively, tablets could be crushed and dispersed in water immediately prior to administration.
- A prolonged break in feeding is not required.

Intragastric administration

See notes above.

1. Stop the enteral feed.
2. Flush the enteral feeding tube with the recommended volume of water.
3. Place the tablet in a mortar and crush to a fine powder using the pestle.
4. Add a few millilitres of water and mix to form a paste.
5. Add up to 15 mL of water and mix thoroughly, ensuring that there are no large particles of tablet.
6. Draw this into an appropriate syringe.
7. Flush the medication dose down the feeding tube.
8. Add another 15 mL of water to the mortar and stir to ensure that any remaining drug is rinsed from the container. Draw this water into the syringe and also flush this via the feeding tube (this will rinse the mortar and syringe and ensure total dose is administered).
9. Finally, flush the enteral feeding tube with the recommended volume of water.
10. Re-start the feed, unless a prolonged break is required.

Intrajejunal administration

Jejunal administration is unlikely to affect bioavailability.

References

1. *BNF* 50, September 2005.
2. Personal communication, Alpharma; 21 January 2003.
3. Aldomet (MSD), Summary of Product Characteristics; August 2001.
4. Dollery C. *Therapeutic Drugs*, 2nd edn. London: Churchill Livingstone; 1998.

Methylprednisolone

Formulations available[1]

Brand name (Manufacturer)	Formulation and strength	Product information/Administration information
Medrone (Pharmacia)	Tablets 2 mg, 4 mg, 16 mg, 100 mg	Scored. Tablets disperse in water.[2]
Solu-Medrone (Pharmacia)	Injection 40 mg, 125 mg, 500 mg, 1 g, 2 g	As sodium succinate. No specific data on enteral tube administration are available for this formulation.
Depo-Medrone (Pharmacia)	Injection 40 mg/mL	As acetate. Deep i.m. injection only.

Site of absorption (oral administration)

Specific site of absorption is not documented. Peak plasma concentration occurs 1–2 hours following oral dosing.[3]

Alternative routes available

Parenteral route is available.

Interactions

Specific interaction with food is not documented.[3]

Health and safety

Standard precautions apply.

Suggestions/recommendations

- Disperse the tablets in water immediately prior to administration.
- A prolonged break in feeding is not required.
- Parenteral route should be used if absorption is compromised.

Intragastric administration

1. Stop the enteral feed.
2. Flush the enteral feeding tube with the recommended volume of water.
3. Place the tablet in the barrel of an appropriate size and type of syringe.
4. Draw 10 mL of water into the syringe and allow the tablet to dissolve, shaking if necessary.
5. Flush the medication dose down the feeding tube.
6. Draw another 10 mL of water into the syringe and also flush this via the feeding tube (this will rinse the syringe and ensure that the total dose is administered).
7. Finally, flush with the recommended volume of water.
8. Re-start the feed, unless a prolonged break is required.

Alternatively, at step (3) place the tablet into a medicine pot, add 10 mL of water and allow the tablet to dissolve. Draw this into an appropriate syringe. Ensure that the measure is rinsed and that this rinsing water is administered also to ensure that the total dose is given.

Intrajejunal administration

There are no specific data relating to jejunal administration. Administer using the method above. Monitor for loss of efficacy or increased side-effects.

References

1. *BNF 50*, September 2005.
2. Personal communication, Pharmacia; 11 March 2003.
3. Dollery C. *Therapeutic Drugs*, 2nd edn. London: Churchill Livingstone; 1998.

Metoclopramide hydrochloride

Formulations available[1]

Brand name (Manufacturer)	Formulation and strength	Product information/Administration information
Metoclopramide (Alpharma, Antigen, APS, CP, IVAX)	Tablets 5 mg, 10 mg	Alpharma: Tablets can be crushed but use of a liquid formulation is recommended.[2]
Metoclopramide (Rosemont, Sandoz)	Syrup 5 mg/5 mL	Sugar-free Contains 0.23 g sorbitol/5 mL.[3] Clear, nonviscous liquid, flushes easily via fine-bore tube without further dilution.[5]
Metoclopramide (Antigen, Phoenix)	Injection 5 mg/mL (2 mL)	I.m. or i.v. injection. No specific data on enteral tube administration are available for this formulation.
Maxolon (Shire)	Tablets 5 mg, 10 mg	Tablets can be crushed, but liquid forms are available.[4]
Maxolon (Shire)	Syrup 5 mg/5 mL	Does not contain sorbitol. May be diluted to half strength with purified water but should be used within 1 month.[7]

Formulations available [1] (*continued*)

Brand name (Manufacturer)	Formulation and strength	Product information/Administration information
Maxolon (Shire)	Paediatric liquid 1 mg/mL	No specific data; however, this formulation is expected to be suitable for enteral tube administration.
Maxolon (Shire)	Injection 5 mg/mL (2 mL)	No specific data on enteral tube administration are available for this formulation.
Maxolon High Dose (Shire)	Injection 5 mg/mL (20 mL)	No specific data on enteral tube administration are available for this formulation.
Gastrobid Continuous (Napp)	M/R tablets 15 mg	Modified-released preparation; unsuitable for use via enteral feeding tube.
Maxolon SR (Shire)	M/R Capsules 15 mg	Modified-released preparation, unsuitable for use via enteral feeding tube. [4]

Site of absorption (oral administration)

No specific site is documented. Peak plasma concentration occurs 0.5–2 hours following oral dosing in fasted subjects. [6]

Alternative routes available

Parenteral route is available.

Interactions

No specific interaction with food is documented. [6]

Health and safety

Standard precautions apply.

Suggestions/recommendations

- Use a liquid preparation. No further dilution is necessary for intragastric administration. The liquid formulation can be diluted with at least an equal volume of water if administering into the jejunum to reduce osmolarity. A prolonged break in feeding is not required.
- Parenteral route can be used if absorption is compromised.

Intragastric administration

1. Stop the enteral feed.
2. Flush the enteral feeding tube with the recommended volume of water.
3. Draw the medication solution into an appropriate size and type of syringe.
4. Flush the medication dose down the feeding tube.
5. Finally, flush with the recommended volume of water.
6. Re-start the feed, unless a prolonged break is required.

Alternatively, at step (3) measure the medicine in a suitable container and then draw into an appropriate syringe. Ensure that the measure is rinsed and that this rinsing water is administered also to ensure that the total dose is given. **Do not** measure liquid medicines using a catheter-tipped syringe as this results in excessive dosing owing to the volume of the tip.

Intrajejunal administration

1. Stop the enteral feed.
2. Flush the enteral feeding tube with the recommended volume of water.
3. Draw the medication liquid into an appropriate size and type of syringe.
4. Draw an equal volume of water and a little air into the syringe and shake to mix thoroughly.
5. Flush the medication dose down the feeding tube.
6. Draw an equal volume of water into the syringe and also flush this via the feeding tube (this will rinse the syringe and ensure that the total dose is administered).
7. Finally, flush with the recommended volume of water.
8. Re-start the feed, unless a prolonged break is required.

Alternatively, at step (3) measure the medicine in a suitable container and then add an equal volume of water and mix thoroughly. Draw this into an appropriate syringe. Ensure that the measure is rinsed and that this rinsing water is administered also to ensure that the total dose is given. **Do not** measure liquid medicines using a catheter-tipped syringe as this results in excessive dosing owing to the volume of the tip.

References

1. *BNF* 50, September 2005.
2. Personal communication, Alpharma; 21 January 2003.
3. Personal communication, Rosemont; 20 January 2005.
4. Personal communication, Shire; 17 February 2003.
5. BPNG data on file, 2004.
6. Dollery C. *Therapeutic Drugs*, 2nd edn. London: Churchill Livingstone; 1998.
7. Maxolon Syrup (Shire), Summary of Product Characteristics; March 2001.

Metolazone

Formulations available[1]

Brand name (Manufacturer)	Formulation and strength	Product information/Administration information
Metenix 5 (Borg)	Tablet 5 mg	Tablets do not disperse readily, but will disintegrate if shaken in 10 mL of water for 5 minutes; the resulting pale blue, coarse dispersion flushes via an 8Fr NG tube without blockage.[2]

Site of absorption (oral administration)

Specific site of absorption is not documented; diuretic effect occurs within 1 hour of an oral dose.[3]

Alternative routes available

None available for metolazone. Furosemide and bumetanide available as parenteral formulations.

Interactions

There is no documented interaction with food.[3]

Health and safety

Standard precautions apply.

Suggestions/recommendations

- Disperse the tablet in water immediately prior to administration.
- A prolonged break in feeding is not required.

Intragastric administration

1. Stop the enteral feed.
2. Flush the enteral feeding tube with the recommended volume of water.
3. Place the tablet in the barrel of an appropriate size and type of syringe.
4. Draw 10 mL of water into the syringe and allow the tablet to dissolve, shaking if necessary.
5. Flush the medication dose down the feeding tube.
6. Draw another 10 mL of water into the syringe and also flush this via the feeding tube (this will rinse the syringe and ensure that the total dose is administered).
7. Finally, flush with the recommended volume of water.
8. Re-start the feed, unless a prolonged break is required.

Alternatively, at step (3) place the tablet into a medicine pot, add 10 mL of water and allow the tablet to dissolve. Draw this into an appropriate syringe. Ensure that the measure is rinsed and that this rinsing water is administered also to ensure that the total dose is given.

Intrajejunal administration

There are no specific data relating to the jejunal administration of metolazone. Administer using the above method. Monitor for increased side-effects of loss of efficacy.

References

1. *BNF* 50, September 2005.
2. BPNG data on file, 2004.
3. Metenix 5 (Aventis), Summary of Product Characteristics; November 2001.

Metoprolol tartrate

Formulations available[1]

Brand name (Manufacturer)	Formulation and strength	Product information/Administration information
Betaloc (AstraZeneca)	Tablets 50 mg, 100 mg	No specific data on enteral tube administration are available for this formulation.
Betaloc (AstraZeneca)	Injection 1 mg/mL (5 mL)	No specific data on enteral tube administration are available for this formulation.
Lopresor (Novartis)	Tablets 50 mg, 100 mg	No specific data on enteral tube administration are available for this formulation.
Metoprolol (Alpharma, APS, Hillcross, IVAX)	Tablets 50 mg, 100 mg	Tablets can be crushed.[3] Tablets do not disperse readily in water.

Formulations available [1] (continued)

Brand name (Manufacturer)	Formulation and strength	Product information/Administration information
Betaloc-SA (AstraZeneca)	M/R tablet 200 mg	Swallow whole, do not chew. [1] Modified-release preparation; do not crush.
Lopresor SR (Novartis)	M/R tablet 200 mg	Swallow whole, do not chew. [1] Modified-release preparation do not crush.
Metoprolol (Martindale)	Suspension 10 mg/5 mL	Manufactured 'special'. Viscous white suspension. Flushes with some resistance. Mixes with an equal volume of water to reduce viscosity.
Extemporaneous preparation	Suspension 10 mg/mL	*Extemporaneous metoprolol suspension 10 mg/mL:* Metoprolol 100 mg tablets 10 tablets Cherry syrup to 100 mL Store in a refrigerator or at room temperature. 60-day expiry. [4]

Site of absorption (oral administration)

Specific site of absorption is not documented. Metoprolol is absorbed rapidly with peak plasma concentrations occurring within 2 hours. [2]

Alternative routes available

Parenteral route is available; see SPC for dosing guidelines.

Interactions

Food may increase the bioavailability of metoprolol; [5] however, there is no comment on clinical significance therefore it may be assumed not to be clinically important.

Health and safety

Standard precautions apply.

Suggestions/recommendations

- Where clinically appropriate change to an alternative beta-blocker available as a liquid formulation.
- The 'special' or an extemporaneous suspension can be used if continuation with metoprolol is clinically appropriate. The tablet can be crushed and dispersed in water; however, this should be considered a last resort.
- Parenteral route may be considered appropriate where control of heart rate or blood pressure is critical or where enteral absorption is compromised.

Intragastric administration

For administration of suspension, special or extemporaneous

1. Stop the enteral feed.
2. Flush the enteral feeding tube with the recommended volume of water.
3. Shake the medication bottle thoroughly to ensure adequate mixing.
4. Draw the medication suspension into an appropriate size and type of syringe.
5. Draw an equal volume of water and a little air into the syringe and shake to mix thoroughly.
6. Flush the medication dose down the feeding tube.
7. Draw an equal volume of water into the syringe and also flush this via the feeding tube (this will rinse the syringe and ensure that the total dose is administered).
8. Finally, flush with the recommended volume of water.
9. Re-start the feed, unless a prolonged break is required.

Alternatively, at step (4) measure the medicine in a suitable container and then add an equal volume of water and mix thoroughly. Draw this into an appropriate syringe. Ensure that the measure is rinsed and that this rinsing water is administered also to ensure that the total dose is given. **Do not** measure liquid medicines using a catheter-tipped syringe as this results in excessive dosing owing to the volume of the tip.

Intrajejunal administration

There are no specific data relating to jejunal administration of metoprolol. Administer using the above method. Alternatively, administer using tablets using the method below (see notes above).

1. Stop the enteral feed.
2. Flush the enteral feeding tube with the recommended volume of water.
3. Place the tablet in a mortar and crush to a fine powder using the pestle.
4. Add a few millilitres of water and mix to form a paste.
5. Add up to 15 mL of water and mix thoroughly, ensuring that there are no large particles of tablet.
6. Draw into an appropriate size and type of syringe.
7. Flush the medication dose down the feeding tube.
8. Add another 15 mL of water to the mortar and stir to ensure that any remaining drug is rinsed from the container. Draw this water into the syringe and also flush this via the feeding tube (this will rinse the mortar and syringe and ensure total dose is administered).
9. Finally, flush the enteral feeding tube with the recommended volume of water.
10. Re-start the feed.

References

1. *BNF 50*, September 2005.
2. Betaloc (AstraZeneca), Summary of Product Characteristics; May 2002.
3. Personal communication, Alpharma; 21 January 2003.
4. Allen LV, Erickson MA. Stability of labetalol hydrochloride, metoprolol tartrate, verapamil hydrochloride and spironolactone with hydrochlorothiazide in extemporaneously compounded oral liquids. *Am J Health Syst Pharm.* 1996; 53: 2304–2309.
5. Dollery C. *Therapeutic Drugs*, 2nd edn. London: Churchill Livingstone; 1998.

Metronidazole

Formulations available

Brand name (Manufacturer)	Formulation and strength	Product information/Administration information
Flagyl (Hawgreen)	Tablets 200 mg, 400 mg Suppositories 500 mg, 1 g	Film-coated tablets.[1] Metronidazole is slightly soluble in water.[4] Metronidazole is rapidly absorbed from the rectal mucosa; peak plasma concentrations occur after approx. 1 hour.[2]
Flagyl S (Hawgreen)	Suspension 200 mg/5 mL	Benzoate salt.[1] Metronidazole benzoate is practically insoluble in water.[4] Creamy, nongranular suspension. Viscous suspension, requires significant pressure to flush down a feeding tube. Dilution with an equal volume of water immediately before dosing reduces flushing resistance to an acceptable level.[7]
Norzol (Rosemont)	Suspension 200 mg/5 mL	Benzoate salt.[6] Contains 0.57 g of sorbitol per 5 mL dose.[9] Cloudy white liquid. Very viscous and difficult to flush. Mixes easily with an equal volume of water.[7]
Metronidazole (Hillcross)	Suspension 200 mg/5 Ml	Benzoate salt.
Metrolyl (Sandoz)	Suppositories 500 mg, 1 g	Rectal administration.
Metronidazole (Alpharma)	Tablets 200 mg, 400 mg, 500 mg	400 mg tablets do not disperse readily in water. Tablets crush easily using pestle and mortar and mix easily with water to form a milky suspension that flushes easily via an 8Fr nasogastric tube.[7]
Vaginyl (DDSA)	Tablets 200 mg, 400 mg	No specific data on enteral tube administration are available for this formulation.
Metronidazole (Norton)	Tablets 200 mg, 400 mg	400 mg tablets will disintegrate within 5 minutes if agitated continuously in 10 mL of water to form a fine dispersion that will flush down an 8Fr nasogastric tube but requires frequent shaking as particles settle quickly in the syringe.[7]
Metronidazole (Arrow, APS, Kent, IVAX, Hillcross)	Tablets 200 mg, 400 mg	No specific data on enteral tube administration are available for this formulation.

Formulations available (*continued*)

Brand name (Manufacturer)	Formulation and strength	Product information/Administration information
Metronidazole (Ranbaxy)	Tablets 200 mg, 400 mg	Both 200 mg and 400 mg tablets disintegrate within 2–5 minutes when placed in 10 mL of water. Both form granular dispersions, the granules in the 200 mg tablet being slightly smaller; however, both strengths will block an 8Fr nasogastric tube.[7] When the tablets are crushed effectively using a pestle and mortar, the resulting powder mixes easily with water and flushes readily down a nasogastric tube.[7]
Extemporaneous preparation[8]	Suspension 50 mg/mL	Metronidazole (base) suspension 50 mg/5 mL: Metronidazole 200 mg tablet 25 tablets Cherry syrup to 100 mL Store at room temperature or refrigerate. 60-day expiry. Extemporaneous preparations using crushed tablets must be prepared in facilities with suitable containment equipment.

Site of absorption (oral administration)

Metronidazole (base) is readily absorbed; bioavailability approaches 100%. Peak plasma concentrations occur 1–2 hours post dose. Absorption is delayed but not reduced by food;[4] the recommendation to take after food is to reduce the incidence of gastrointestinal side-effects.[5]

Metronidazole benzoate is hydrolysed in the stomach[4] and has approximately 80% bioavailability, which is reduced by the presence of food; hence the recommendation to take before food.[5]

Alternative routes available

Rectal route is available: usual dose 1 g every 8 hours in adults, reduced to 12-hourly after 3 days.[1] Intravenous route is also available: 500 mg every 8 hours.

Interactions

Food reduces the bioavailability of metronidazole benzoate.[4]

Health and safety

COSHH suggest avoiding third-party contact with crushed tablets.[3]

Suggestions/recommendations

- When possible use the intravenous or rectal route. Use the liquid preparation for intragastric administration. In theory the tablet formulation should be used for jejunal administration; however, this should be considered a last resort and alternative antibiotic therapy should be considered.

Intragastric administration

Use the suspension for nasogastric or gastrostomy administration, diluting the suspension immediately prior to administration.

1. Stop the enteral feed.
2. Flush the enteral feeding tube with the recommended volume of water.
3. Allow a 1-hour break before dose administration, if possible.
4. Shake the medication bottle thoroughly to ensure adequate mixing.
5. Draw the medication suspension into an appropriate size and type of syringe.
6. Draw an equal volume of water and a little air into the syringe and shake to mix thoroughly.
7. Flush the medication dose down the feeding tube.
8. Draw an equal volume of water into the syringe and also flush this via the feeding tube (this will rinse the syringe and ensure that the total dose is administered).
9. Finally, flush with the recommended volume of water.
10. Re-start the feed, unless a prolonged break is required.

Alternatively, at step (5) measure the medicine in a suitable container and then add an equal volume of water and mix thoroughly. Draw this into an appropriate syringe. Ensure that the measure is rinsed and that this rinsing water is administered also to ensure that the total dose is given. **Do not** measure liquid medicines using a catheter-tipped syringe as this results in excessive dosing owing to the volume of the tip.

Intrajejunal administration

A suspension should be made using the tablets[8] (see notes above) if it is necessary to administer via a tube exiting in the jejunum.

1. Stop the enteral feed.
2. Flush the enteral feeding tube with the recommended volume of water.
3. Place the tablet in a mortar and crush to a fine powder using the pestle.
4. Add a few millilitres of water and mix to form a paste.
5. Add up to 15 mL of water and mix thoroughly, ensuring that there are no large particles of tablet.
6. Draw this into an appropriate size and type of syringe.
7. Flush the medication dose down the feeding tube.
8. Add another 15 mL of water to the mortar and stir to ensure that any remaining drug is rinsed from the container. Draw this water into the syringe and also flush this via the feeding tube (this will rinse the mortar and syringe and ensure total dose is administered).
9. Finally, flush the enteral feeding tube with the recommended volume of water.
10. Re-start the feed, unless a prolonged break is required.

References

1. Flagyl and Flagyl-S (Hawgreen), Summary of Product Characteristics; May 2001.
2. Flagyl Suppositories, Summary of Product Characteristics; May 2001.
3. Personal communication, Alpharma Ltd; 21 January 2003.
4. Sweetman SC, ed. *Martindale*, 34th edn. London: Pharmaceutical Press; 2005.
5. Personal communication, Hawgreen Ltd; 3 December 2004.
6. Norzol Metronidazole Suspension 200 mg/5 mL (Rosemont), Summary of Product Characteristics; 9 January 2002.
7. BPNG data on file, 2004/5.
8. Allen LV, Erickson MA. Stability of ketoconazole, metolazone, metronidazole, procainamide hydrochloride and spironolactone in extemporaneously compounded oral liquids. *Am J Health Syst Pharm*. 1996; 53: 2073–2078.
9. Personal communication, Rosemont; 20 January 2005.

Mexiletine hydrochloride

Formulations available[1]

Brand name (Manufacturer)	Formulation and strength	Product information/Administration information
Mexitil (Boehringer Ingelheim)	Capsules 50 mg, 200 mg	Capsules can be opened and the contents mixed with water and flushed via feeding tube.[2]
Mexitil (Boehringer Ingelheim)	Injection 25 mg/mL (10 mL)	Injection can be given orally. pH 5.0–6.0.[2]
Mexiletine (extemporaneous preparation)	Suspension 10 mg/mL	*Extemporaneous mexiletine suspension 10 mg/mL:* Mexiletine 200 mg capsules 5 capsules Sterile water for irrigation to 100 mL Stability data for 90-day expiry when stored in a refrigerator.[3] However, as the preparation does not contain a preservative, it may be appropriate to shorten the expiry on grounds of microbiological stability.

Site of absorption (oral administration)

Mexiletine is absorbed in the upper portion of the small intestine. Peak plasma concentration occurs 2–3 hours after oral administration.[4]

Alternative routes available

Parenteral formulation available.

Interactions

No specific interaction with food is documented.

Health and safety

Standard precautions apply.

Suggestions/recommendations

- Use alternative therapy where appropriate.
- When continued therapy with mexiletine is indicated, open the capsules and disperse in water immediately prior to administration.
- A prolonged break in feeding is not required.

Intragastric administration

1. Stop the enteral feed.
2. Flush the enteral feeding tube with the recommended volume of water.
3. Open the capsule and pour the contents into a medicine pot.
4. Add 15 mL of water.
5. Stir to disperse the powder.
6. Draw into an appropriate size and type of syringe and administer via the feeding tube.
7. Add a further 15 mL of water to the medicine pot; stir to ensure that any powder remaining in the pot is mixed with water.
8. Draw up this dispersion and flush down the tube. This will ensure that the whole dose is given.
9. Flush the tube with the recommended volume of water.
10. Restart feed, unless a prolonged break is required.

Intrajejunal administration

No specific data are available on jejunal administration. Monitor for increased side-effects or loss of efficacy. Administer using the above method.

References

1. *BNF 50*, September 2005.
2. Personal communication, Boehringer; 6 March 2003.
3. Nahata MC, Morosco RS, Hipple TF. Stability of mexiletine in two extemporaneous liquid formulations stored under refrigeration and at room temperature. *J Am Pharm Assoc.* 2000; 40: 257–259.
4. Mexitil Capsules (Boehringer), Summary of Product Characteristics; May 2003.

Minoxidil

Formulations available [1]

Brand name (Manufacturer)	Formulation and strength	Product information/Administration information
Loniten (Pharmacia)	Tablets 2.5 mg, 5 mg, 10 mg	Tablets can be crushed and mixed with water. [2] Tablets disperse in water within 2 minutes to give a fine dispersion that settles quickly but flushes via an 8Ff NG tube without blockage. [3]

Site of absorption (oral administration)

Specific site is not documented. Minoxidil appears in the blood within 30 minutes of administration. [4] Peak hypotensive effect occurs after 2–3 hours. [5]

Alternative routes available

None available for minoxidil.

Interactions

No specific interaction with food is documented. [5]

Health and safety

Standard precautions apply.

Suggestions/recommendations

- Disperse the tablets in water immediately prior to administration.
- A prolonged break in feeding is not required.

Intragastric administration

1. Stop the enteral feed.
2. Flush the enteral feeding tube with the recommended volume of water.
3. Place the tablet in the barrel of an appropriate size and type of syringe.
4. Draw 10 mL of water into the syringe and allow the tablet to disperse, shaking if necessary.
5. Flush the medication dose down the feeding tube.
6. Draw another 10 mL of water into the syringe and also flush this via the feeding tube (this will rinse the syringe and ensure that the total dose is administered).
7. Finally, flush with the recommended volume of water.
8. Re-start the feed, unless a prolonged break is required.

Alternatively, at step (3) place the tablet into a medicine pot, add 10 mL of water and allow the tablet to disperse. Draw this into an appropriate syringe. Ensure that the measure is rinsed and that this rinsing water is administered also to ensure that the total dose is given.

Intrajejunal administration

There are no specific data relating to jejunal administration. Administer using the above method. Monitor for increased side-effects or loss of efficacy.

References

1. *BNF* 50, September 2005.
2. Personal communication, Pharmacia; 11 March 2003.
3. BPNG data on file, 2005.
4. Dollery C. *Therapeutic Drugs*, 2nd edn. London: Churchill Livingstone; 1998.
5. Loniten (Pharmacia), Summary of Product Characteristics; April 2001.

Mirtazapine

Formulations available[1]

Brand name (Manufacturer)	Formulation and strength	Product information/Administration information
Zispin SolTab (Organon)	Tablets 500 mg	When place in 10 mL of water, microgranules float to top of dispersion and cling to the side of the pot and syringe; they settle quickly and there is risk of tube blockage if they are not redispersed in the syringe prior to administration. It is difficult to give the full dose.[2]
Mirtazapine (Rosemont)	Oral solution 15 mg/mL	Sugar-free oral solution. 66 mL bottle.

Formulations available[1] (continued)

Brand name (Manufacturer)	Formulation and strength	Product information/Administration information
Mirtazapine (nonproprietary)	Tablets 30 mg	No specific data on enteral tube administration of this formulation.

Site of absorption (oral administration)

Specific site of absorption is not documented. Peak plasma concentration occurs 2 hours after oral dosing.[3]

Alternative routes available

None available for mirtazapine.

Interactions

Food has no effect on the pharmacokinetics of mitazapine.[3]

Health and safety

Standard precautions apply.

Suggestions/recommendations

- Use the oral liquid preparation; no further dilution is necessary.
- A prolonged break in feeding is not necessary.

Intragastric administration

1. Stop the enteral feed.
2. Flush the enteral feeding tube with the recommended volume of water.
3. Draw the medication solution into an appropriate size and type of syringe.
4. Flush the medication dose down the feeding tube.
5. Finally, flush with the recommended volume of water.
6. Re-start the feed, unless a prolonged break is required.

Alternatively, at step (3) measure the medicine in a suitable container and then draw into an appropriate syringe. Ensure that the measure is rinsed and that this rinsing water is administered also to ensure that the total dose is given. **Do not** measure liquid medicines using a catheter-tipped syringe as this results in excessive dosing owing to the volume of the tip.

Intrajejunal administration

Administer using the above method. Monitor for increased side-effects or loss of efficacy.

References

1. *BNF 50*, September 2005.
2. BPNG data on file, 2004.
3. Zispin (Organon), Summary of Product Characteristics; June 2003.

Misoprostol

Formulations available [1]

Brand name (Manufacturer)	Formulation and strength	Product information/Administration information
Cytotec (Pharmacia)	Tablets 200 microgram	Dose two to four times daily. The manufacturer recommends that tablets are not crushed owing to the unstable nature of the drug, but is aware of anecdotal reports of nasogastric administration. [3]

Site of absorption (oral administration)

Absorption is rapid, with peak plasma concentrations occurring after 30 minutes. [2]

Alternative routes available

None available for misoprostol. Parenteral formulations are available for other anti-ulcer therapy.

Interactions

There is no documented interaction with food. Recommended to be taken with food to minimise incidence of diarrhoea. [2]

Health and safety

Because of the exposure risks from inhalation of crushed tablets, they should not be handled by women of childbearing age. Protective clothing should be worn.

Suggestions/recommendations

- Owing to poor stability, an alternative therapy such as a histamine receptor antagonist (ranitidine) or a proton pump inhibitor (lansoprazole) should be considered if clinically appropriate.
- If continued therapy with misoprostol is indicated, the tablets can be crushed and mixed with water immediately prior to administration (see notes above); this should be considered a last resort.

Intragastric administration

1. Stop the enteral feed.
2. Flush the enteral feeding tube with the recommended volume of water.
3. Place the tablet in a mortar and crush to a fine powder using the pestle.
4. Add a few millilitres of water and mix to form a paste.
5. Add up to 15 mL of water and mix thoroughly, ensuring that there are no large particles of tablet.
6. Draw this into an appropriate syringe.
7. Flush the medication dose down the feeding tube.
8. Add another 15 mL of water to the mortar and stir to ensure that any remaining drug is rinsed from the container. Draw this water into the syringe and also flush this via the feeding tube (this will rinse the mortar and syringe and ensure total dose is administered).
9. Finally, flush the enteral feeding tube with the recommended volume of water.
10. Re-start the feed immediately.

Intrajejunal administration

There are no specific data on the jejunal administration of misoprostol. An alternative therapy known to be absorbed from the jejunum should be used.

References

1. *BNF* 50, September 2005.
2. Cytotec (Pharmacia), Summary of Product Characteristics; March 2003.
3. Personal communication, Pharmacia; 11 March 2003.

Moclobemide

Formulations available[1]

Brand name (Manufacturer)	Formulation and strength	Product information/Administration information
Moclobemide (APS, Generics, PLIVA, Ratiopharm, Sandoz)	Tablets 150 mg, 300 mg	APS brand tablets do not disintegrate readily in water but will disperse in water if shaken for 5 minutes. The resulting fine white dispersion flushes via an 8Fr NG tube without blockage.[2]
Manerix (Roche)	Tablets 150 mg, 300 mg	Film-coated. Scored.[3] No specific data on enteral tube administration are available for this formulation.

Site of absorption (oral administration)

Specific site of absorption is not documented. Peak plasma concentration occurs 1–2 hours post oral dose.[4]

Alternative routes available

None available for moclobemide.

Interactions

The rate but not the extent of moclobemide absorption is reduced by food; this is not clinically significant.[4]

Health and safety

Standard precautions apply.

Suggestions/recommendations

- Consider changing to an alternative antidepressant available as a liquid preparation. Alternatively, disperse the tablets in water immediately prior to administration.
- A prolonged break is feeding is not necessary.

Intragastric administration

1. Stop the enteral feed.
2. Flush the enteral feeding tube with the recommended volume of water.
3. Place the tablet in the barrel of an appropriate size and type of syringe.
4. Draw 10 mL of water into the syringe and allow the tablet to disperse, shaking if necessary.
5. Flush the medication dose down the feeding tube.
6. Draw another 10 mL of water into the syringe and also flush this via the feeding tube (this will rinse the syringe and ensure that the total dose is administered).
7. Finally, flush with the recommended volume of water.
8. Re-start the feed, unless a prolonged break is required.

Alternatively, at step (3) place the tablet into a medicine pot, add 10 mL of water and allow the tablet to disperse. Draw this into an appropriate syringe. Ensure that the measure is rinsed and that this rinsing water is administered also to ensure that the total dose is given.

Intrajejunal administration

There is no specific information on the jejunal administration of moclobemide. Administer using the above method. Monitor for loss of efficacy or increased side-effects.

References

1. *BNF* 50, September 2005.
2. BPNG data on file, 2005.
3. Manerix (Roche), Summary of Product Characteristics; August 2004.
4. Dollery C. *Therapeutic Drugs*, 2nd edn. London: Churchill Livingstone; 1998.

Modafinil

Formulations available[1]

Brand name (Manufacturer)	Formulation and strength	Product information/Administration information
Provigil (Cephalon)	Tablets 100 mg, 200 mg	The bioavailability of Provigil tablets is approximately that of an aqueous suspension. Provigil could theoretically be crushed and mixed with water. As there are no stability data to support the storage of such a suspension it should be used immediately.[2]

Site of absorption (oral administration)

Specific site of absorption is not documented. Peak plasma concentration occurs 2–4 hours following oral administration.[3]

Alternative routes available

None available for modafinil.

Interactions

Food may delay the peak level of modafinil by approximately 1 hour,[3] but does not affect overall bioavailability.[3]

Health and safety

Standard precautions apply.

Suggestions/recommendations

- Crush the tablets and disperse in water immediately prior to administration.
- A prolonged break in feeding is not required.

Intragastric administration

1. Stop the enteral feed.
2. Flush the enteral feeding tube with the recommended volume of water.
3. Place the tablet in a mortar and crush to a fine powder using the pestle.
4. Add a few millilitres of water and mix to form a paste.
5. Add up to 15 mL of water and mix thoroughly, ensuring that there are no large particles of tablet.
6. Draw this into an appropriate syringe.
7. Flush the medication dose down the feeding tube.
8. Add another 15 mL of water to the mortar and stir to ensure that any remaining drug is rinsed from the container. Draw this water into the syringe and also flush this via the feeding tube (this will rinse the mortar and syringe and ensure total dose is administered).
9. Finally, flush the enteral feeding tube with the recommended volume of water.
10. Re-start the feed, unless a prolonged break is required.

Intrajejunal administration

There is no specific information relating to jejunal administration of modafinil. Administer using the above method. Monitor for loss of efficacy or increased side-effects.

References

1. *BNF 50*, September 2005.
2. Personal communication, Cephalon; 21 January 2003.
3. Provigil (Cephalon), Summary of Product Characteristics; December 2003.

Moexipril hydrochloride

Formulations available[1]

Brand name (Manufacturer)	Formulation and strength	Product information/Administration information
Perdix (Schwarz)	Tablets 7.5 mg, 15 mg	Film-coated, scored tablets.[2] No specific data on enteral tube administration are available for this formulation.

Site of absorption (oral administration)

Specific site of absorption is not documented.

Alternative routes available

No alternative routes available for any of the ACE inhibitors.

Interactions

There is no documented interaction with food.[2]

Health and safety

Standard precautions apply.

Suggestions/recommendations

- As no data are available for moexipril, conversion to an alternative ACEI should be considered.

References

1. *BNF 50*, September 2005.
2. Perdix 7.5 mg (Schwarz), Summary of Product Characteristics; November 2001.

Morphine sulfate

Formulations available[1]

Brand name (Manufacturer)	Formulation and strength	Product information/Administration information
Immediate-release preparations		
Oromorph (Boehringer Ingelheim)	Solution 10 mg/5 mL	Although no specific data are available, the liquid can be administered via the feeding tube.[2] Contains corn syrup and sucrose.
Oromorph Concentrated oral solution (Boehringer Ingelheim)	Solution 100 mg/5 mL	Also available as unit-dose-vials presentation. Although no specific data are available, the liquid can be administered via the feeding tube.[2]
Oromorph Unit Dose Vials (Boehringer Ingelheim)	Oral solution Unit dose vials 10 mg/5 mL, 30 mg/5 mL, 100 mg/5 mL	Does not contain sorbitol or sucrose.[3]
Sevredol (Napp)	Tablets 10 mg, 20 mg, 50 mg	Immediate-release tablets. Napp recommends that Sevredol tablets should not be crushed.[4]
Morphine (Aurum, Martindale)	Suppositories 10 mg, 15 mg, 20 mg, 30 mg	Morphine sulfate or morphine hydrochloride. Doses are equivalent to oral administration.
Morphine Sulphate (Aurum, Celltech)	Injection 10 mg/mL, 15 mg/mL, 20 mg/mL, 30 mg/mL	No specific data on enteral tube administration are available for this formulation.

Formulations available[1] (continued)

Brand name (Manufacturer)	Formulation and strength	Product information/Administration information
Modified-release preparations Morcap SR (Mayne)	Capsules 20 mg, 50 mg, 100 mg	Hard gelatin capsule containing modified-release pellets. No specific data on tube administration.
Morphgesic MR (Amdipharm)	Tablets 10 mg, 30 mg, 60 mg, 100 mg	Modified-release tablets. Do not crush. Not suitable for enteral tube administration.
MST Continuous (Napp)	Tablets 5 mg, 10 mg, 15 mg, 30 mg, 60 mg, 100 mg, 200 mg	Modified-release tablets. Do not crush. Not suitable for enteral tube administration.
MST Continuous (Napp)	Suspension 20 mg, 30 mg, 60 mg, 100 mg, 200 mg	Modified-release granules to mix with water to form a suspension. In an in-house study the granules were mixed with 10 mL of water and passed through 8Fr and 6Fr NG tubes successfully. When the suspensions are given by this route, do not administer with oral rehydration therapies, concentrated lactate solutions or similar treatments.[4]
MXL (Napp)	Capsules 30 mg, 60 mg, 90 mg, 120 mg, 150 mg, 200 mg	Modified-release capsules. Napp advises not to disperse the capsule contents in water as they are lipophilic, clump together and risk blocking the tube.[4]
Zomorph (Link)	Capsules 10 mg, 30 mg, 60 mg, 100 mg, 200 mg	Modified-release granules in hard gelatin capsule. Granules pour easily from the capsule and do not clump together when mixed with water. They can be drawn up into the syringe and flushed via an 8Fr NG tube without blockage; however, the granules settle quickly in the syringe and care must be taken to deliver the complete dose.[5] Link recommends that the tube diameter should be more then 16Fr with an open distal end or lateral pores.[6]

Site of absorption (oral administration)

Morphine is absorbed in the proximal small bowel.[2]

Alternative routes available

Formulations for parenteral (i.v., i.m. and s.c) and rectal routes are available.

Interactions

There is no significant interaction with food.

Health and safety

Standard precautions apply.

Suggestions/recommendations

- For immediate pain relief use oral solution; no further dilution is necessary.
- The tube must be flushed well following dosing to ensure that the total dose is delivered.
- For sustained pain relief, use MST Continuous sachets, dispersed in at least 10 mL of water. Flush the tube well following dosing to ensure that the total dose is delivered. Note that any granules left in the tube will break down over a period of time and a bolus of morphine will be delivered when the tube is next flushed; this has resulted in a reported fatality.
- For high maintenance doses or for patient with very fine-bore tubes, consider changing to a fentanyl transdermal patch (consult product literature for dose conversion).

Intragastric administration

Immediate-release morphine

1. Stop the enteral feed.
2. Flush the enteral feeding tube with the recommended volume of water.
3. Draw the medication solution into an appropriate size and type of syringe.
4. Flush the medication dose down the feeding tube.
5. Finally, flush with the recommended volume of water.
6. Re-start the feed, unless a prolonged break is required.

Alternatively, at step (3) measure the medicine in a suitable container and then draw into an appropriate syringe. Ensure that the measure is rinsed and that this rinsing water is administered also to ensure that the total dose is given. **Do not** measure liquid medicines using a catheter-tipped syringe as this results in excessive dosing owing to the volume of the tip.

Modified-release morphine

1. Stop the enteral feed.
2. Flush the enteral feeding tube with the recommended volume of water.
3. Measure a suitable quantity of water into a measuring pot.
4. Add the contents of the sachet and allow to disperse.
5. Draw into an appropriate size and type of syringe.
6. Flush the medication dose down the feeding tube.
7. Rinse the measure and administer this also to ensure that the total dose is given.
8. Finally, flush with the recommended volume of water.
9. Re-start the feed, unless a prolonged break is required.

Intrajejunal administration

For intrajejunal administration use the unit-dose vials when possible; alternatively, dilute the oral liquid with an equal volume of water immediately prior to administration, following the method outlined above.

References

1. *BNF* 50, September 2005.
2. Personal communication, Boehringer Ingelheim; 6 March 2003.
3. Oramorph Unit Dose Vials (BI), Summary of Product Characteristics; July 2002.
4. Personal communication, Napp; 29 January 2003.
5. BPNG data on file, 2004.
6. Personal communication, Link; 4 February 2003.

Moxonidine

Formulations available[1]

Brand name (Manufacturer)	Formulation and strength	Product information/Administration information
Physiotens (Solvay)	Tablets 200 microgram, 300 microgram, 400 microgram	Tablets will disintegrate in water at room temperature within 2 minutes.[2] Tablets disintegrate within 2 minutes when placed in 10 mL of water; the resulting dispersion flushes via an 8Fr NG tube without blockage.[3]

Site of absorption (oral administration)

Specific site of absorption is not documented. Peak plasma concentration occurs 30–180 minutes following oral dosing.[4]

Alternative routes available

None available for moxonidine.

Interactions

Food reduces and delays peak concentrations slightly; this is not clinically significant.[2]

Health and safety

Standard precautions apply.

Suggestions/recommendations

- Disperse tablet in water immediately prior to administration.
- A prolonged break in feeding is not required.

Intragastric administration

1. Stop the enteral feed.
2. Flush the enteral feeding tube with the recommended volume of water.
3. Place the tablet in the barrel of an appropriate size and type of syringe.
4. Draw 10 mL of water into the syringe and allow the tablet to disperse, shaking if necessary.
5. Flush the medication dose down the feeding tube.
6. Draw another 10 mL of water into the syringe and also flush this via the feeding tube (this will rinse the syringe and ensure that the total dose is administered).
7. Finally, flush with the recommended volume of water.
8. Re-start the feed, unless a prolonged break is required.

Alternatively, at step (3) place the tablet into a medicine pot, add 10 mL of water and allow the tablet to disperse. Draw this into an appropriate syringe. Ensure that the measure is rinsed and that this rinsing water is administered also to ensure that the total dose is given.

Intrajejunal administration

There are no specific data relating to the jejunal administration of moxonidine. Administer using the above method and monitor for loss of efficacy or increased side-effects.

References

1. *BNF* 50, September 2005.
2. Personal communication, Solvay; 19 February 2003.
3. BPNG data on file, 2005.
4. Physiotens (Solvay), Summary of Product Characteristics; March 2002.

Mycophenolate mofetil

Formulations available[1]

Brand name (Manufacturer)	Formulation and strength	Product information/Administration information
CellCept (Roche)	Capsules 250 mg	Mycophenolate is teratogenic, so the capsules should not be opened owing to the risk of operator exposure.[2]
CellCept (Roche)	Tablets 500 mg	Mycophenolate is teratogenic, so the tablets should not be crushed owing to the risk of operator exposure.[2]
CellCept (Roche)	Oral suspension 1 g/5 mL	If required, CellCept 1 g/5 mL powder for oral suspension can be administered via a nasogastric tube with a minimum size of 8F (minimum 1.7 mm interior diameter.[4] Contains sorbitol.[4]
CellCept (Roche)	Intravenous infusion 500 mg	No specific data on enteral tube administration are available for this formulation.
Myfortic (Novartis)	Tablet 180 mg, 360 mg	Enteric coated tablet. Not suitable for administration via enteral feeding tube.

Site of absorption (oral administration)

Mycophenolate mofetil dissolves rapidly in the stomach. Absorption may occur through the gastric mucosa, but the main site of absorption is the duodenum and jejunum. Enterohepatic circulation implies that further reabsorption occurs in the third part of the duodenum and the large bowel after the action of the intestinal flora in converting inactive mycophenolate acid glucuronide back into active mycophenolic acid.[2] Although not quantified, it is expected that a substantial proportion of the dose would be absorbed following jejunal administration.[3]

Alternative routes available

Parenteral route is available and should be used if enteral absorption is compromised.

Interactions

Food decreases peak plasma concentration of mycophenolate; however, total bioavailability is unaffected.[4]

Health and safety

Standard precautions apply when handling the liquid preparation. The tablets should not be crushed and the capsules should not be opened owing to the risks of occupational exposure.

Suggestions/recommendations

- Administer the dose using the liquid preparation; do not dilute further.
- A prolonged break in feeding is not required.

Intragastric administration

1. Stop the enteral feed.
2. Flush the enteral feeding tube with the recommended volume of water.
3. Draw the medication solution into an appropriate size and type of syringe.
4. Flush the medication dose down the feeding tube.
5. Draw an equal volume of water into the syringe and also flush this via the feeding tube (this will rinse the syringe and ensure that the total dose is administered).
6. Finally, flush with the recommended volume of water.
7. Re-start the feed, unless a prolonged break is required.

Alternatively, at step (3) measure the medicine in a suitable container and then draw into an appropriate syringe. Ensure that the measure is rinsed and that this rinsing water is administered also to ensure that the total dose is given. **Do not** measure liquid medicines using a catheter-tipped syringe as this results in excessive dosing owing to the volume of the tip.

Intrajejunal administration

See notes above. Administer using the above method.

References

1. *BNF 50*, September 2005.
2. Personal communication, Roche; 6 February 2003.
3. Personal communication, Roche; 15 January 2003.
4. CellCept Suspension (Roche), Summary of Product Characteristics; October 2002.

Nabumetone

Formulations available[1]

Brand name (Manufacturer)	Formulation and strength	Product information/Administration information
Relifex (Meda)	Tablets 500 mg	No specific data on enteral tube administration are available for this formulation.
Relifex (Meda)	Suspension 500 mg/5 mL	Contains sorbitol[2] 1.25 mg/5 mL.[3] pH 3.5–4.5.[3]
Nabumetone (Alpharma, APS, Generics)	Tablets 500 mg	Alpharma advises against crushing tablets as they are film-coated and irritant.[5]

Site of absorption (oral administration)

Nabumetone is absorbed intact through the small intestine and undergoes extensive first-pass metabolism.[3]

Alternative routes available

No alternative route is available for nabumetone. Nabumetone is similar in efficacy to diclofenac, which is available as injection and suppositories.

Interactions

Absorption is not affected by food but is increased when nabumetone is taken with milk;[4] therefore, there is a possibility that enteral feed may increase absorption of nabumetone.

Health and safety

Standard precautions apply.

Suggestions/recommendations

- Use a liquid formulation. There is a possibility that absorption may be increased by enteral feed, so side-effects should be monitored.

Intragastric administration

1. Stop the enteral feed.
2. Flush the enteral feeding tube with the recommended volume of water.
3. Shake the medication bottle thoroughly to ensure adequate mixing.
4. Draw up liquid preparation into an appropriate size and type of syringe.
5. Flush the medication dose down the feeding tube.
6. Finally, flush with the recommended volume of water.
7. Re-start the feed, unless a prolonged break is required.

Alternatively, at step (4) measure required dose in a suitable container. Draw this into an appropriate syringe. Ensure that the measure is rinsed and that this rinsing water is administered also to ensure that the total dose is given. **Do not** measure liquid preparations using a catheter-tipped syringe as this results in excessive dosing owing to the volume of the tip.

Intrajejunal administration

There are no specific data relating to the jejunal administration of nabumetone. Administer following the method above and monitor for loss of effect or increased side-effects.

References

1. *BNF 50*, September 2005.
2. Relifex Suspension (Meda), Summary of Product Characteristics; May 2002.
3. Personal communication, Meda Pharmaceuticals; 31 January 2005.
4. Dollery C. *Therapeutic Drugs*, 2nd edn. London: Churchill Livingstone; 1998.
5. Personal communication, Alpharma Ltd; 21 January 2003.

Nadolol

Formulations available[1]

Brand name (Manufacturer)	Formulation and strength	Product information/Administration information
Corgard (Sanofi-Synthelabo)	Tablets 80 mg	Tablets may be crushed.[2] Tablets do not disperse readily but disperse when shaken in 10 mL of water for 5 minutes give a fine suspension that flushes down an 8Fr tube[4] without blockage.

Site of absorption (oral administration)

Specific site of absorption is not documented. Peak plasma concentration occurs 3–4 hours after oral dosing.[3]

Alternative routes available

None available for nadolol, other beta-blockers available as parenteral formulations.

Interactions

Rate and extent of absorption of nadolol are not affected by food.[3]

Health and safety

Standard precautions apply.

Suggestions/recommendations

- Change to an alternative beta-blocker available in liquid formulation where clinically appropriate. Alternatively, disperse tablets in water immediately prior to administration.
- A prolonged break in feeding is not necessary.

Intragastric administration

1. Stop the enteral feed.
2. Flush the enteral feeding tube with the recommended volume of water.
3. Place the tablet in the barrel of an appropriate size and type of syringe.
4. Draw 10 mL of water into the syringe and allow the tablet to disperse, shaking as required.
5. Flush the medication dose down the feeding tube.
6. Draw another 10 mL of water into the syringe and also flush this via the feeding tube (this will rinse the syringe and ensure that the total dose is administered).
7. Finally, flush with the recommended volume of water.
8. Re-start the feed, unless a prolonged break is required.

Alternatively, at step (3) place the tablet into a medicine pot, add 10 mL of water and allow the tablet to disperse. Draw this into an appropriate syringe. Ensure that the measure is rinsed and that this rinsing water is administered also to ensure that the total dose is given.

Intrajejunal administration

There are no specific data relating to the jejunal administration of nadolol. Monitor for lack of efficacy or increased side-effects. Follow the above method.

References

1. *BNF* 50, September 2005.
2. Personal communication, Sanofi-Synthelabo; 3 February 2003.
3. Corgard (Sanofi-Synthelabo), Summary of Product Characteristics; March 2003.
4. BPNG data on file, 2005.

Naftidrofuryl oxalate

Formulations available[1]

Brand name (Manufacturer)	Formulation and strength	Product information/Administration information
Naftidrofuryl (Alpharma)	Capsules 100 mg	Capsule contents can be used.[2]
Praxilene (Merck)	Capsules 100 mg	Opening capsules and swallowing contents can cause irritation to the oesophagus. Contents can be administered via an enteral tube.[3] Sufficient fluid should be taken during treatment to maintain adequate level of diuresis.[4]

Site of absorption (oral administration)

Specific site of absorption is not documented. Peak plasma concentration occurs 30 minutes following oral dosing.[4]

Alternative routes available

None available for naftidrofuryl oxalate.

Interactions

No specific interaction with food is documented.[4]

Health and safety

Standard precautions apply.

Suggestions/recommendations

- Disperse capsule contents in water immediately prior to administration. Flush the tube well before and after dosing to ensure adequate hydration.
- A prolonged break in feeding is not required.

Intragastric administration

1. Stop the enteral feed.
2. Flush the enteral feeding tube with the recommended volume of water.
3. Open the capsule and pour the contents into a medicine pot.
4. Add 15 mL of water.
5. Stir to disperse the powder.
6. Draw into an appropriate size and type of syringe and administer via the feeding tube.
7. Add a further 15 mL of water to the medicine pot; stir to ensure that any powder remaining in the pot is mixed with water.
8. Draw up this dispersion and flush down the tube. This will ensure that the whole dose is given.
9. Flush the tube with the recommended volume of water.
10. Re-start feed, unless a prolonged break is required.

Intrajejunal administration

There are no specific data relating to jejunal administration of naftidrofuryl. Administer using the above method. Monitor for loss of efficacy or increased side-effects.

References

1. *BNF 50*, September 2005.
2. Personal communication, Alpharma; 21 January 2003.
3. Personal communication, Merck; 23 January 2003.
4. Praxilene (Merck), Summary of Product Characteristics; June 1999.

Naproxen

Formulations available[1]

Brand name (Manufacturer)	Formulation and strength	Product information/Administration information
Naprosyn (Roche)	Tablets 250 mg, 500 mg	Crushing the standard tablet preparation prior to administration will not affect efficacy. It can be mixed with water. Naproxen is virtually insoluble at low pH, but increasingly soluble with increasing pH.[2]
Naprosyn EC (Roche)	Tablets 250 mg, 375 mg, 500 mg	Enteric coated tablets; do not crush.
Synflex (Roche)	Tablets 275 mg	275 mg naproxen sodium = 250 mg naproxen. Naproxen sodium dissolves rapidly in gastric juice, producing finer particles than on dissolution of plain naproxen and leading to a more rapid absorption.[3]
Naproxen (Alpharma, APS, Arrow, Ashbourne, CP, Hillcross, IVAX, Sterwin)	Tablets 250 mg, 500 mg	No specific data on enteral tube administration are available for this formulation.

Formulations available[1] (continued)

Brand name (Manufacturer)	Formulation and strength	Product information/Administration information
Naproxen (Alpharma, Arden, APS, Arrow, Ashbourne, Berk, Cox, Generics, IVAX)	Tablets 250 mg, 375 mg, 500 mg	Enteric coated tablets, do not crush. Not suitable for enteral tube administration.

Site of absorption (oral administration)

Absorption is in the upper small bowel. Naproxen sodium peak plasma concentration occurs 1 hour after oral dosing, Naproxen peak plasma concentration occur 2 hours after oral administration in fasted subjects.[3]

Alternative routes available

No alternative routes of administration available for naproxen (suppository and suspension formulation discontinued). Diclofenac possesses similar analgesic properties and is available as suppositories and injection.

Interactions

Absorption is delayed but not reduced by food.[3]

Health and safety

Standard precautions apply.

Suggestions/recommendations

- Consider changing to diclofenac dispersible tablets to facilitate enteral administration. If necessary, uncoated tablets can be crushed and dispersed in water immediately prior to administration; this should be considered a last resort.
- A prolonged break in feeding is not required.

Intragastric administration

1. Stop the enteral feed.
2. Flush the enteral feeding tube with the recommended volume of water.
3. Place the tablet in the mortar and crush to a fine powder using the pestle.
4. Add a few millilitres of water and mix to form a paste.
5. Add up to 15 mL of water and mix thoroughly, ensuring that there are no large particles of tablet.
6. Draw this into an appropriate size and type of syringe.
7. Flush the medication dose down the feeding tube.
8. Add another 15 mL of water to the mortar and stir to ensure that any remaining drug is rinsed from the container. Draw this water into the syringe and also flush this via the feeding tube (this will rinse the mortar and syringe and ensure total dose is administered).
9. Finally, flush the enteral feeding tube with the recommended volume of water.
10. Re-start the feed, unless a prolonged break is required.

Intrajejunal administration

Jejunal administration is not expected to effect bioavailability as enteric coated tablets are available. Administer using the above method.

References

1. *BNF* 50, September 2005.
2. Personal communication, Roche; 6 February 2003.
3. Dollery C. *Therapeutic Drugs*, 2nd edn. London: Churchill Livingstone; 1998.

Nebivolol

Formulations available[1]

Brand name (Manufacturer)	Formulation and strength	Product information/Administration information
Nebilet (Menarini)	Tablets 5 mg	Nebivolol hydrochloride. No specific data on enteral tube administration are available for this formulation.

Site of absorption (oral administration)

Site of absorption is not documented; rapid absorption occurs following oral intake.[2]

Alternative routes available

None available for nebivolol; other beta-blockers are available as parenteral formulations.

Interactions

Absorption is unaffected by food.[2]

Health and safety

Standard precautions apply.

Suggestions/recommendations

- Change to an alternative beta-blocker available as liquid formulation such as atenolol (see monograph).

References

1. *BNF* 50, September 2005.
2. Nebilet (Menarini), Summary of Product Characteristics; July 2001.

Nefopam hydrochloride

Formulations available[1]

Brand name (Manufacturer)	Formulation and strength	Product information/Administration information
Acupan (3M)	Tablets 30 mg	Film-coated tablets. Tablets disperse if shaken in 10 mL of water for 3–4 minutes. Dispersion settles very quickly but flushes via tube without blockage, though there is risk of leaving some of the dose in the container if it is not adequately rinsed.[2]
Acupan (3M)	Injection 20 mg/mL	For i.m. injection. No specific data on enteral tube administration are available for this formulation.

Site of absorption (oral administration)

Specific site of absorption is not documented. Peak plasma concentration occurs 1–3 hours following oral administration.[3]

Alternative routes available

Parenteral formulation is available. 20 mg i.m. = 60 mg orally.[1]

Interactions

There are no specific documented interaction with food.

Health and safety

Standard precautions apply.

Suggestions/recommendations

- Use tablets dispersed in water immediately prior to administration. Consider changing to an alternative opiate available in more suitable formulation.
- A prolonged break in feeding is not required.

Intragastric administration

1. Stop the enteral feed.
2. Flush the enteral feeding tube with the recommended volume of water.
3. Place the tablet in the barrel of an appropriate size and type of syringe.
4. Draw 10 mL of water into the syringe and allow the tablet to disperse, shaking if necessary.
5. Flush the medication dose down the feeding tube.
6. Draw another 10 mL of water into the syringe and also flush this via the feeding tube (this will rinse the syringe and ensure that the total dose is administered).
7. Finally, flush with the recommended volume of water.
8. Re-start the feed, unless a prolonged break is required.

Alternatively, at step (3) place the tablet into a medicine pot, add 10 mL of water and allow the tablet to disperse. Draw this into an appropriate syringe. Ensure that the measure is rinsed and that this rinsing water is administered also to ensure that the total dose is given.

Intrajejunal administration

Follow the guidance above. There are no specific data relating to the administration of nefopam via the jejunum. Monitor for loss of efficacy or increased side-effects.

References

1. *BNF* 50, September 2005.
2. BPNG data on file, 2005.
3. Acupan Tablets (3M), Summary of Product Characteristics; November 2000.

Nelfinavir

Formulations available[1]

Brand name (Manufacturer)	Formulation and strength	Product information/Administration information
Viracept (Roche)	Tablets 250 mg	*US data sheet*: Patients may place the whole tablets or crushed tablets in a small amount of water to dissolve before ingestion. Once mixed with water the entire contents must be consumed in order to obtain the full dose. If not consumed immediately the mixture must be stored under refrigeration for no more than 6 hours.[2] Tablets disintegrate within 2 minutes when placed in 10 mL of water to give dispersion of large blue granules that can be drawn up into the syringe. There is high risk of blockage of fine-bore tubes. Responds to flushing.[4]
Viracept (Roche)	Powder 50 mg/g	Provided with 1 g and 5 g scoop. Powder may be mixed with water, milk, formula feeds or pudding. It should not be mixed with acidic foods or juices owing to its taste.[3] The powder can be mixed with dietary supplements.[2]

Site of absorption (oral administration)

Specific site is not documented. Peak plasma concentration occurs 2–4 hours following oral dose with food.[3]

Alternative routes available

None available.

Interactions

Administration of nelfinavir with food increases bioavailability and AUC compared with those in fasting subjects. Nelfinavir should be taken with food.[2]

Health and safety

Standard precautions apply.

Suggestions/recommendations

- Disperse the tablets in water prior to administration. Administer the dose with or directly after feed.
- Alternatively, use powder dissolved in sufficient water.

Intragastric administration

1. Stop the enteral feed.
2. Flush the enteral feeding tube with the recommended volume of water.
3. Place the tablet in the barrel of an appropriate size and type of syringe.
4. Draw 10 mL of water into the syringe and allow the tablet to disperse, shaking if necessary.
5. Flush the medication dose down the feeding tube.
6. Draw another 10 mL of water into the syringe and also flush this via the feeding tube (this will rinse the syringe and ensure that the total dose is administered).
7. Finally, flush with the recommended volume of water.
8. Re-start the feed, unless a prolonged break is required.

Alternatively, at step (3) place the tablet into a medicine pot, add 10 mL of water and allow the tablet to disperse. Draw this into an appropriate syringe. Ensure that the measure is rinsed and that this rinsing water is administered also to ensure that the total dose is given.

Intrajejunal administration

There are no specific data relating to jejunal administration of nelfinavir. Administer using the above method. Monitor for loss of efficacy and side-effects.

References

1. *BNF* 50, September 2005.
2. Personal communication, Alpharma; 21 January 2003.
3. Viracept Oral Powder (Roche), Summary of Product Characteristics; February 2003.
4. BPNG data on file, 2005.

Neomycin sulphate

Formulations available[1]

Brand name (Manufacturer)	Formulation and strength	Product information/Administration information
Neomycin (APS, Biorex Sovereign)	Tablets 500 mg	Tablets disintegrate when shaken in 10 mL of water for 5 minutes to give a very fine dispersion that flushes via an 8Fr NG tube without blockage.[2]

Site of absorption (oral administration)

Absorption of neomycin is minimal following oral dosing. See SPC for further details.

Alternative routes available

Not applicable. Neomycin is too toxic for systemic use.

Interactions

No interaction with food is documented.[3] There is no evidence to suggest that food reduces the efficacy of neomycin locally in the bowel.

Health and safety

Standard precautions apply.

Suggestions/recommendations

- Disperse in water immediately prior to administration.
- A prolonged break in feeding is not required.

Intragastric administration

1. Stop the enteral feed.
2. Flush the enteral feeding tube with the recommended volume of water.
3. Place the tablet in the barrel of an appropriate size and type of syringe.
4. Draw 10 mL of water into the syringe and allow the tablet to disperse, shaking if necessary.
5. Flush the medication dose down the feeding tube.
6. Draw another 10 mL of water into the syringe and also flush this via the feeding tube (this will rinse the syringe and ensure that the total dose is administered).
7. Finally, flush with the recommended volume of water.
8. Re-start the feed, unless a prolonged break is required.

Alternatively, at step (3) place the tablet into a medicine pot, add 10 mL of water and allow the tablet to disperse. Draw this into an appropriate syringe. Ensure that the measure is rinsed and that this rinsing water is administered also to ensure that the total dose is given.

Intrajejunal administration

Therapeutic effect is topical only. Action will only be from point of administration.

References

1. *BNF* 50, September 2005.
2. BPNG data on file, 2005.
3. Nivemycin (Sovereign), Summary of Product Characteristics; January 1999.

Nevirapine

Formulations available[1]

Brand name (Manufacturer)	Formulation and strength	Product information/Administration information
Viramune (Boehringer Ingelheim)	Tablets 200 mg	Tablets can be crushed but produce a 'slurry' if mixed with water; use of the suspension is likely to be preferable.[2]
Viramune (Boehringer Ingelheim)	Suspension 50 mg/5 mL	Off-white homogenous suspension. Contains sorbitol[3] 1.156 g/5 mL dose.[4]

Site of absorption (oral administration)

Specific site is not documented. Nevirapine is well absorbed following oral administration, with peak plasma concentration occurring 4 hours post dose.[3]

Alternative routes available

None available for nevirapine.

Interactions

The absorption of nevirapine is not affected by food, antacids or alkaline-buffered formulations (e.g., didanosine).[3]

Health and safety

Standard precautions apply.

Suggestions/recommendations

- Use liquid formulation.
- A prolonged break in feeding is not required.

Intragastric administration

1. Stop the enteral feed.
2. Flush the enteral feeding tube with the recommended volume of water.
3. Draw the medication solution into an appropriate size and type of syringe.
4. Flush the medication dose down the feeding tube.
5. Finally, flush with the recommended volume of water.
6. Re-start the feed, unless a prolonged break is required.

Alternatively, at step (4) measure the medicine in a suitable container and then draw into an appropriate syringe. Ensure that the measure is rinsed and that this rinsing water is administered also to ensure that the total dose is given. **Do not** measure liquid medicines using a catheter-tipped syringe as this results in excessive dosing owing to the volume of the tip.

Intrajejunal administration

There is no specific information on jejunal administration. Administer using the above method. Plasma concentration can be measured (see www.hiv-druginteractions.org).

References

1. *BNF* 50, September 2005.
2. Personal communication, Boehringer Ingelheim; 6 March 2003.
3. Viramune Suspension (Boehringer Ingelheim), Summary of Product Characteristics; March 2003.
4. Personal communication, Boehringer Ingelheim; August 2005.

Nicardipine hydrochloride

Formulations available[1]

Brand name (Manufacturer)	Formulation and strength	Product information/Administration information
Cardene (Yamanouchi)	Capsules 20 mg, 30 mg	No specific data on enteral tube administration are available for this formulation.
Nicardipine (Generics)	Capsules 20 mg, 30 mg	No specific data on enteral tube administration are available for this formulation.
Cardene SR (Yamanouchi)	Capsules 30 mg, 45 mg	Modified-release capsules, not suitable for administration via feeding tube.

Site of absorption (oral administration)

Specific site of absorption is not documented. Plasma levels are detectable within 20 minutes, peak plasma concentration occurs 0.5–2 hours post dose.[2]

Alternative routes available

None available for nicardipine.

Interactions

When given with a high-fat meal peak plasma concentrations are reduced by 30%.[2]

Health and safety

Standard precautions apply.

Suggestions/recommendations

- It may be possible to administer the immediate-release capsules, but specific data are lacking; the three-times daily dosing is a disadvantage.
- Consider changing to once-daily amlodipine (see monograph) if clinically appropriate.

References

1. *BNF* 50, September 2005.
2. Cardene (Yamanouchi), Summary of Product Characteristics; July 2002.

Nicorandil

Formulations available[1]

Brand name (Manufacturer)	Formulation and strength	Product information/Administration information
Ikorel (Rhône-Poulenc Rorer)	Tablets 10 mg, 20 mg	Ikorel tablets are hygroscopic and readily absorb water. The manufacturer has anecdotal reports of the tablets being crushed and administered via feeding tubes.[2] Tablets disperse within 5 minutes when placed in 10 mL of water. This results in a fine suspension that flushes via an 8Fr NG tube without blockage.[3]

Site of absorption (oral administration)

Nicorandil is absorbed well from the small intestine, with the peak plasma concentration occurring 30–60 minutes following oral dosing.[4]

Alternative routes available

None available for nicorandil.

Interactions

Food decreases the rate but not the extent of absorption.[2]

Health and safety

Standard precautions apply.

Suggestions/recommendations

- Disperse the tablets in water immediately prior to administration.
- A prolonged break in feeding is not necessary.

Intragastric administration

1. Stop the enteral feed.
2. Flush the enteral feeding tube with the recommended volume of water.
3. Place the tablet in the barrel of an appropriate size and type of syringe.
4. Draw 10 mL of water into the syringe and allow the tablet to disperse, shaking if necessary.
5. Flush the medication dose down the feeding tube.
6. Draw another 10 mL of water into the syringe and also flush this via the feeding tube (this will rinse the syringe and ensure that the total dose is administered).
7. Finally, flush with the recommended volume of water.
8. Re-start the feed, unless a prolonged break is required.

Alternatively, at step (3) place the tablet into a medicine pot, add 10 mL of water and allow the tablet to disperse. Draw this into an appropriate syringe. Ensure that the measure is rinsed and that this rinsing water is administered also to ensure that the total dose is given.

Intrajejunal administration

There are no specific reports relating to jejunal administration of nicorandil; however, nicorandil is well absorbed from the small intestine. Administer using the above method.

References

1. *BNF* 50, September 2005.
2. Personal communication, Aventis; 13 February 2003.
3. BPNG data on file, 2004.
4. Ikorel (Rhône-Poulenc Rorer), Summary of Product Characteristics; August 2002.

Nifedipine

Formulations available[1]

Brand name (Manufacturer)	Formulation and strength	Product information/Administration information
Nifedipine (Alpharma, APS, CP, Hillcross, IVAX)	Capsules 5 mg, 10 mg	Alpharma does not recommend extraction of the contents of the capsule owing to light sensitivity.[2] Internal volumes and therefore concentrations of extracted liquid vary between manufacturers; accurate dosing of paediatric doses is problematic. Consult the manufacturer at time of use for clarification of internal volume, as generic suppliers change manufacturer.
Adalat (Bayer)	Capsules 5 mg, 10 mg	5 mg capsule = 0.17 mL.[3] 10 mg capsule = 0.34 mL.[3]
Adalat LA (Bayer)	M/R tablets 20 mg, 30 mg, 60 mg	Once-daily dosed M/R tablets. Tablets should not be crushed and are unsuitable for enteral tube administration.[7]
Adalat Retard (Bayer)	M/R tablets 10 mg, 20 mg	Licensed recommendation is to swallow whole; the tablets can be crushed and dispersed in water, but the modified-release properties will be lost and dose frequency will need to be adjusted to reflect this. The tablets should be crushed immediately prior to administration, as nifedipine is light-sensitive.[3] Although crushing the M/R tablets results in statistically significant differences in AUC and C_{max}, there was no statistical or clinical difference in blood pressure reduction.[4]
Adipine MR (Trinity)	M/R tablets 10 mg, 20 mg	Modified-release preparation, do not crush. Not suitable for enteral tube administration.
Cardilate MR (IVAX)	M/R tablets 10 mg, 20 mg	Modified-release preparation, do not crush. Not suitable for enteral tube administration.
Coracten SR (Celltech)	M/R capsules 10 mg, 20 mg	The capsules contain mini-tablets. These should not be crushed.
Coracten XL (Celltech)	M/R capsules 30 mg, 60 mg	The capsules contain mini-tablets. 30 mg contains 4 mini-tablets; 60 mg contains 8 mini-tablets. These mini-tablets must not be crushed.[6]

Formulations available[1] (continued)

Brand name (Manufacturer)	Formulation and strength	Product information/Administration information
Fortipine LA (Goldshield)	M/R tablets 40 mg	Modified-release preparation, do not crush. Not suitable for enteral tube administration.
Hypolar Retard 20 (Sandoz)	M/R tablets 20 mg	Modified-release preparation, do not crush. Not suitable for enteral tube administration.
Nifedipress MR (Dexcel)	M/R tablets 10 mg	Modified-release preparation, do not crush. Not suitable for enteral tube administration.
Nifopress Retard (Goldshield)	M/R tablets 20 mg	Modified-release preparation, do not crush. Not suitable for enteral tube administration.
Slofedipine (Sterwin)	M/R tablets 20 mg	Modified-release preparation, do not crush. Not suitable for enteral tube administration.
Slofedipine XL (Sterwin)	M/R tablets 30 mg, 60 mg	Modified-release preparation, do not crush. Not suitable for enteral tube administration.
Tensipine MR (Genus)	M/R tablets 10 mg, 20 mg	Modified-release preparation, do not crush. Not suitable for enteral tube administration.

Site of absorption (oral administration)

Nifedipine is absorbed primarily via the gastric mucosa.[3] It is poorly absorbed by the buccal mucosa, and absorption from 'sublingual' administration is likely to be the result of swallowing the contents of the nifedipine capsules.[5]

Alternative routes available

None available for nifedipine.

Interactions

Absorption is not significantly affected by food.

Health and safety

Standard precautions apply.

Suggestions/recommendations

- The most practical solution is to consider changing to once-daily amlodipine (see monograph) if clinically appropriate.
- Extraction of the contents of the capsules requires a degree of manual dexterity and complete dosing cannot be guaranteed.
- Adalat Retard tablets can be crushed and dispersed in water and must be given immediately.
- Immediate-release nifedipine should be administered three times a day. Rapid drops in blood pressure and rebound tachycardia can occur when the immediate-release preparations are used.

Intragastric administration

Administration of Adalat Retard tablets (see notes above)

1. Stop the enteral feed.
2. Flush the enteral feeding tube with the recommended volume of water.
3. Place the tablet in a mortar and crush to a fine powder using the pestle.
4. Add a few millilitres of water and mix to form a paste.
5. Add up to 15 mL of water and mix thoroughly, ensuring that there are no large particles of tablet.
6. Draw this into an appropriate size and type of syringe.
7. Flush the medication dose down the feeding tube.
8. Add another 15 mL of water to the mortar and stir to ensure that any remaining drug is rinsed from the container. Draw this water into the syringe and also flush this via the feeding tube (this will rinse the mortar and syringe and ensure total dose is administered).
9. Finally, flush the enteral feeding tube with the recommended volume of water.
10. Re-start the feed, unless a prolonged break is required.

Intrajejunal administration

There is no information relating to the jejunal administration of nifedipine via a jejunostomy tube; as the primary site of nifedipine absorption is the gastric mucosa, the amount absorbed in the jejunum is unknown. See notes above.

References

1. *BNF* 50, September 2005.
2. Personal communication, Alpharma; 21 January 2003.
3. Personal communication, Bayer Plc; 28 November 2002.
4. Lepage R, *et al.* Pharmacokinetics and pharmacodynamics of intact and crushed nifedipine prolonged action (PA) tablets. *Can J Cardiol.* 2000; 16(Suppl F): 106F [Abstract 56].
5. van Harten J, Burggraaf K, Danhof M, van Brummelen P, Breimer DD. Negligible sublingual absorption of nifedipine. *Lancet.* 1987; 12(2;8572): 1363–1365.
6. Personal communication, Celltech; 31 March 2003.
7. Adalat LA (Bayer), Summary of Product Characteristics; June 2002.

Nimodipine

Formulations available[1]

Brand name (Manufacturer)	Formulation and strength	Product information/Administration information
Nimotop (Bayer)	Tablets 30 mg	Film-coated tablets.[2] Nimodipine is extremely light-sensitive.[3] Nimotop tablets have been crushed and administered via enteral feeding tubes as part of clinical trials; the subgroup of patients receiving their dose via this route were not analysed separately.[4]
Nimotop (Bayer)	I.v. infusion 200 microgram/mL	No specific data on enteral tube administration are available for this formulation.

Site of absorption (oral administration)

Specific site of absorption is not documented. Peak plasma concentration occurs 30–60 minutes after oral dosing.[2]

Alternative routes available

Parenteral route is available.

Interactions

There is no documented interaction with food.[2, 5]

Health and safety

Standard precautions apply.

Suggestions/recommendations

- Tablets should be crushed at the bedside and administered immediately.
- A prolonged break in feeding is not required.

Intragastric administration

1. Stop the enteral feed.
2. Flush the enteral feeding tube with the recommended volume of water.
3. Place the tablet in a mortar and crush to a fine powder using the pestle.
4. Add a few millilitres of water and mix to form a paste.
5. Add up to 15 mL of water and mix thoroughly, ensuring that there are no large particles of tablet.
6. Draw this into an appropriate size and type of syringe.
7. Flush the medication dose down the feeding tube.
8. Add another 15 mL of water to the mortar and stir to ensure that any remaining drug is rinsed from the container. Draw this water into the syringe and also flush this via the feeding tube (this will rinse the mortar and syringe and ensure total dose is administered).
9. Finally, flush the enteral feeding tube with the recommended volume of water.
10. Re-start the feed, unless a prolonged break is required.

Intrajejunal administration

If using a jejunal tube, consider using the parenteral route owing to the lack of data relating to jejunal administration.

References

1. *BNF* 50, September 2005.
2. Nimotop (Bayer), Summary of Product Characteristics; June 2002.
3. Personal communication, Bayer plc; 28 November 2002.
4. Pickard JD, Murray GD, Illingworth R, *et al*. Effect of oral nimodipine on cerebral infarction and outcome after subarachnoid haemorrhage: British Aneurysm Nimodipine Trial. *BMJ* 1989; 298: 636–642.
5. Dollery C. *Therapeutic Drugs*, 2nd edn. London: Churchill Livingstone; 1998.

Nisoldipine

Formulations available[1]

Brand name (Manufacturer)	Formulation and strength	Product information/Administration information
Syscor MR (Forest)	M/R tablet 10 mg, 20 mg, 30 mg	Under no circumstances should the tablets be bitten, chewed or broken up.[2]

Site of absorption (oral administration)

Nonmetabolised nisoldipine can be detected in the plasma 15–30 minutes after oral dosing of a solution,[2] suggesting gastric or upper GI absorption.

Alternative routes available

None available for nisoldipine.

Interactions

Food increases peak concentrations and decreases AUC; it is therefore recommended that Syscor be taken before food.[2]

Health and safety

Standard precautions apply.

Suggestions/recommendations

- Syscor MR is unsuitable for administration via an enteral feeding tube; consider changing to once-daily amlodipine (see monograph).

References

1. *BNF* 50, September 2005.
2. Syscor (Forest), Summary of Product Characteristics; August 1998.

Nitrazepam

Formulations available[1]

Brand name (Manufacturer)	Formulation and strength	Product information/Administration information
Nitrazepam (Alpharma, APS, CP, DDSA, Generics, ICN, IVAX)	Tablets 5 mg	Tablets can be crushed.[2]

Formulations available[1] (continued)

Brand name (Manufacturer)	Formulation and strength	Product information/Administration information
Nitrazepam (Norgine)	Oral suspension 2.5 mg/5 mL	Sucrose based syrup.[3]
Nitrazepam (Rosemont)	Oral suspension 5 mg/5 mL	Manufactured 'special'. Contains 0.45 g sorbitol/5 mL.[4]

Site of absorption (oral administration)

Specific site of absorption is not documented. Peak plasma concentration occurs 2–3 hours following oral dose.[3]

Alternative routes available

None available.

Interactions

No specific interaction with food is documented.[3]

Health and safety

Standard precautions apply.

Suggestions/recommendations

- Use a liquid formulation. Consider diluting the liquid formulation immediately prior to jejunal administration to reduce the osmolarity.
- A prolonged break in feeding is not required.

Intragastric administration

1. Stop the enteral feed.
2. Flush the enteral feeding tube with the recommended volume of water.
3. Shake the medication bottle thoroughly to ensure adequate mixing.
4. Draw the medication suspension into an appropriate size and type of syringe.
5. Flush the medication dose down the feeding tube.
6. Finally, flush with the recommended volume of water.
7. Re-start the feed, unless a prolonged break is required.

Alternatively, at step (4) measure the medicine in a suitable container and then add an equal volume of water and mix thoroughly. Draw this into an appropriate syringe. Ensure that the measure is rinsed and that this rinsing water is administered also to ensure that the total dose is given. **Do not** measure liquid medicines using a catheter-tipped syringe as this results in excessive dosing owing to the volume of the tip.

Intrajejunal administration

1. Stop the enteral feed.
2. Flush the enteral feeding tube with the recommended volume of water.
3. Shake the medication bottle thoroughly to ensure adequate mixing.
4. Draw the medication suspension into an appropriate size and type of syringe.
5. Draw twice the dose volume of water and a little air into the syringe and shake to mix thoroughly.
6. Flush the medication dose down the feeding tube.
7. Draw an equal volume of water into the syringe and also flush this via the feeding tube (this will rinse the syringe and ensure that the total dose is administered).
8. Finally, flush with the recommended volume of water.
9. Re-start the feed, unless a prolonged break is required.

Alternatively, at step (4) measure the medicine in a suitable container and then add an equal volume of water and mix thoroughly. Draw this into an appropriate syringe. Ensure that the measure is rinsed and that this rinsing water is administered also to ensure that the total dose is given. **Do not** measure liquid medicines using a catheter-tipped syringe as this results in excessive dosing owing to the volume of the tip.

References

1. *BNF* 50, September 2005.
2. Personal communication, Alpharma; 21 January 2003.
3. Somnite (Norgine), Summary of Product Characteristics; July 1997.
4. Personal communication, Rosemont; 20 January 2005.

Nitrofurantoin

Formulations available[1]

Brand name (Manufacturer)	Formulation and strength	Product information/Administration information
Nitrofurantoin (Alpharma, APS)	Tablets 50 mg, 100 mg	Tablets do not disperse readily but will disintegrate if shaken in 10 mL of water for 5 minutes to give a bright yellow, fine dispersion that flushes easily without blockage.[2]
Nitrofurantoin (Goldshield)	Oral suspension 25 mg/5 mL	Bright yellow, slightly viscous liquid, resistant to flushing via an 8Fr NG tube. Mixes well with an equal volume of water, which reduces resistance to flushing.[2]
Furadantin (Goldshield)	Tablets 50 mg, 100 mg	No specific data on enteral tube administration are available for this formulation.
Macrobid (Goldshield)	Capsules 100 mg	Modified-release capsule. Not suitable for administration via the feeding tube.
Macrodantin (Goldshield)	Capsules 50 mg, 100 mg	Capsule can be opened and contents mixed with water. There are some larger granules, which settle quickly and may block finer tubes.[2]

Site of absorption (oral administration)

Specific site of absorption is not documented. Peak plasma concentration occurs 1–4 hours following oral dosing in fasted subjects. [3]

Alternative routes available

None available.

Interactions

No specific interaction with food is documented.

Health and safety

Standard precautions apply.

Suggestions/recommendations

- Use a liquid preparation.
- A prolonged break in feeding is not required.

Intragastric administration

1. Stop the enteral feed.
2. Flush the enteral feeding tube with the recommended volume of water.
3. Draw the medication suspension into an appropriate size and type of syringe.
4. Draw an equal volume of water and a little air into the syringe and shake to mix thoroughly.
5. Flush the medication dose down the feeding tube.
6. Finally, flush with the recommended volume of water.
7. Re-start the feed, unless a prolonged break is required.

Alternatively, at step (3) measure the medicine in a suitable container and then add an equal volume of water and mix thoroughly. Draw this into an appropriate syringe. Ensure that the measure is rinsed and that this rinsing water is administered also to ensure that the total dose is given. **Do not** measure liquid medicines using a catheter-tipped syringe as this results in excessive dosing owing to the volume of the tip.

Intrajejunal administration

Administer using the above method. Monitor for increased side-effects or loss of efficacy.

References

1. *BNF* 50, September 2005.
2. BPNG data on file, 2004/05
3. Dollery C. *Therapeutic Drugs*, 2nd edn. London: Churchill Livingstone; 1998.

Nizatidine

Formulations available[1]

Brand name (Manufacturer)	Formulation and strength	Product information/Administration information
Axid (Flynn)	Capsules 150 mg, 300 mg	No specific data on enteral tube administration are available for this formulation.
Axid (Flynn)	Injection 25 mg/mL	No specific data on enteral tube administration are available for this formulation.
Nizatidine (APS, Generics, Niche)	Capsules 150 mg, 300 mg	No specific data on enteral tube administration are available for this formulation.

Site of absorption (oral administration)

Specific site of absorption is not documented. Peak plasma concentration occurs within 2 hours of oral administration.[2]

Alternative routes available

Parenteral route is available.

Interactions

No interaction with food is documented.[2]

Health and safety

Standard precautions apply

Suggestions/recommendations

- As no liquid formulation of nizatidine is available, use ranitidine (see monograph); oral doses are identical.

References

1. *BNF* 50, September 2005.
2. Axid (Lilly), Summary of Product Characteristics; April 2001.

Norethisterone

Formulations available [1]

Brand name (Manufacturer)	Formulation and strength	Product information/Administration information
Norethisterone (Alpharma, CP, Sandoz)	Tablets 5 mg	Tablets can be crushed, although precautions should be taken to avoid operator exposure. [2] CP brand tablets disperse when shaken in 10 mL of water for 5 minutes to give a fine dispersion, with some visible particles, that flushes via an 8Fr NG tube without blockage. [3]
Primulut N (Schering Health)	Tablets 5 mg	No specific data on enteral tube administration are available for this formulation.
Utovlan (Pharmacia)	Tablets 5 mg	Tablets can be crushed; owing to lack of stability data, this should be done immediately prior to administration. [4]
Micronor HRT (Janssen-Cilag)	Tablets 1 mg	No specific data on enteral tube administration are available for this formulation.

Site of absorption (oral administration)

Specific site is not documented. Peak plasma concentration occurs 1–3 hours following oral dosing. [5]

Alternative routes available

None available.

Interactions

No specific interaction with food is documented. [5, 6]

Health and safety

Standard precautions apply.

Suggestions/recommendations

- Disperse the tablets in water immediately prior to administration.
- A prolonged break in feeding is not required.

Intragastric administration

1. Stop the enteral feed.
2. Flush the enteral feeding tube with the recommended volume of water.
3. Place the tablet in the barrel of an appropriate size and type of syringe.
4. Draw 10 mL of water into the syringe and allow the tablet to disperse, shaking if necessary.
5. Flush the medication dose down the feeding tube.
6. Draw another 10 mL of water into the syringe and also flush this via the feeding tube (this will rinse the syringe and ensure that the total dose is administered).
7. Finally, flush with the recommended volume of water.
8. Re-start the feed, unless a prolonged break is required.

Alternatively, at step (4) place the tablet into a medicine pot, add 10 mL of water and allow the tablet to disperse. Draw this into an appropriate syringe. Ensure that the measure is rinsed and that this rinsing water is administered also to ensure that the total dose is given.

Intrajejunal administration

There are no specific data relating to jejunal administration of norethisterone. Administer using the above method. Monitor for loss of efficacy or increased side-effects.

References

1. *BNF 50*, September 2005.
2. Personal communication, Alpharma; 21 January 2003.
3. BPNG data on file, 2005.
4. Personal communication, Pharmacia; March 11 2003.
5. Dollery C. *Therapeutic Drugs*, 2nd edn. London: Churchill Livingstone; 1998.
6. Sweetman SC, ed. *Martindale*, 34th edn. London: Pharmaceutical Press; 2005.

Ofloxacin

Formulations available[1]

Brand name (Manufacturer)	Formulation and strength	Product information/Administration information
Ofloxacin (APS, Dexcel, Generics)	Tablets 200 mg, 400 mg	No specific data on enteral tube administration are available for this formulation.
Tarivid (Aventis)	Tablets 200 mg, 400 mg	Film-coated tablets. Tablets do not disperse readily in water. The tablet can be crushed, but the flaky coating makes crushing difficult. When mixed with water the coating takes a few minutes to dissolve; then the contents form a milky dispersion that flushes via an 8Fr NG tube without blockage.[2]
Tarivid (Aventis)	Injection 2 mg/mL (50 mL, 100 mL)	Ofloxacin hydrochloride. No specific data on enteral tube administration are available for this formulation.

Site of absorption (oral administration)

Specific site of absorption is not documented. Peak plasma concentration occurs 1–3 hours following oral dosing.[3]

Alternative routes available

Parenteral route is available.

Interactions

There is a significant interaction when ofloxacin is mixed directly with Ensure.[4] Reducing the available concentration by 46%; co-administration in patients reduced bioavailability by 10%, although peak plasma concentration was reduced by 36%; however, this was not substantiated by another study using a similar method.[5] The absorption of ofloxacin is not affected by food and the mechanism of the interaction with enteral feed is unknown.

Health and safety

Standard precautions apply.

Suggestions/recommendations

- For serious infections use the parenteral formulation.
- As tablets do not disperse readily in water, consider changing to an alternative antibiotic available in a liquid or dispersible tablet formulation.
- When oral therapy with ofloxacin is indicated, consider using the higher end of the dose range.
- Stop feed 1 hour pre-dose and restart feed 2 hours post dose.

Intragastric administration

See notes above.

1. Stop the enteral feed.
2. Flush the enteral feeding tube with the recommended volume of water.
3. Wait for at least 1 hour.
4. Place the tablet in a mortar and crush to a fine powder using the pestle.
5. Add a few millilitres of water and mix to form a paste.
6. Add up to 15 mL of water and mix thoroughly, ensuring that there are no large particles of tablet.
7. Draw this into an appropriate size and type of syringe.
8. Flush the medication dose down the feeding tube.
9. Add another 15 mL of water to the mortar and stir to ensure that any remaining drug is rinsed from the container. Draw this water into the syringe and also flush this via the feeding tube (this will rinse the mortar and syringe and ensure that the total dose is administered).
10. Finally, flush the enteral feeding tube with the recommended volume of water.
11. Wait for at least 2 hours before re-starting the feed.

Intrajejunal administration

There are no specific data on jejunal administration of ofloxacin. Consider an alternative antibiotic. Administer using the above method; use the higher end of the dose range. Monitor for increased side-effects or loss of efficacy.

References

1. *BNF 50*, September 2005.
2. BPNG data on file, 2005.
3. Tarivid (Aventis), Summary of Product Characteristics; April 2002.
4. Wright DH, Pietz SL, Konstantinides FN, Rotschafer JC. Decreased in vitro fluoroquinolone concentrations after admixture with an enteral feeding formulation. *JPEN J Parenter Enteral Nutr.* 2000; 24(1): 42–48.
5. Stockley IH. *Drug Interactions*, 4th edn. London: Pharmaceutical Press; 1996.

Olanzapine

Formulations available[1]

Brand name (Manufacturer)	Formulation and strength	Product information/Administration information
Zyprexa (Lilly)	Tablets 2.5 mg, 5 mg, 7.5 mg, 10 mg, 15 mg	No specific data on enteral tube administration are available for this formulation.
Zyprexa Velotab (Lilly)	Orodispersible tablets 5 mg, 10 mg, 15 mg	Tablet can be dispersed in water.[2]
Zyprexa (Lilly)	Injection 5 mg/mL (10 mg)	Licensed for maximum of 3 days treatment.

Site of absorption (oral administration)

Specific site of absorption is not documented. Peak plasma concentration occurs 5–8 hours following oral dosing.[2]

Alternative routes available

Parenteral formulation can be used for acute treatment. Licensed for a maximum of 3 days' treatment.

Interactions

Absorption is not affected by food.[2]

Health and safety

Standard precautions apply.

Suggestions/recommendations

- Disperse Zyprexa Velotab in water immediately prior to administration.
- A prolonged break in feeding is not required.

Intragastric administration

1. Stop the enteral feed.
2. Flush the enteral feeding tube with the recommended volume of water.
3. Measure a suitable quantity of water into a measuring pot.
4. Add the tablet and allow to disperse.
5. Draw into an appropriate size and type of syringe.
6. Flush the medication dose down the feeding tube.
7. Rinse the measure and administer this also to ensure that the total dose is given.
8. Finally, flush with the recommended volume of water.
9. Re-start the feed, unless a prolonged break is required.

Intrajejunal administration

There are no specific reports of jejunal administration of olanzapine. Administer using the above method. Monitor for loss of efficacy or increased side-effects.

References

1. *BNF* 50, September 2005.
2. Zyprexa (Lilly), Summary of Product Characteristics; September 2002.

Olmesartan medoxomil

Formulations available [1]

Brand name (Manufacturer)	Formulation and strength	Product information/Administration information
Olmetec (Sankyo)	Tablets 10 mg, 20 mg, 40 mg	Film-coated. [2] Olmesartan medoxomil. No specific data on enteral tube administration are available for this formulation.

Site of absorption (oral administration)

Specific site of absorption is unknown. Olmesartan is a prodrug; it is rapidly converted to the pharmacologically active metabolite by esterases in the gut mucosa and in portal blood during absorption from the GI tract. [2] Peak plasma concentrations of the active drug occur in the plasma within 2 hours of oral dosing. [2]

Alternative routes available

No other routes of administration are available for any of the angiotensin II antagonists.

Interactions

Food has minimal effect on absorption of olmesartan medoxomil. [2]

Health and safety

Standard precautions apply.

Suggestions/recommendations

- Owing to lack of data, consider changing to irbesartan (see monograph)

References

1. *BNF* 50, September 2005.
2. Olmetec (Sankyo), Summary of Product Characteristics; May 2003.

Olsalazine sodium

Formulations available[1]

Brand name (Manufacturer)	Formulation and strength	Product information/Administration information
Dipentum (Celltech)	Capsules 250 mg Tablets 500 mg	Tablets will disperse in 10 mL of water if shaken for at least 8 minutes. The dispersion is bright orange and will stain, but flushes down 8Fr NG tube without blockage.[2]

Site of absorption (oral administration)

Olsalazine is not absorbed; the azo bond is cleaved in the colon, releasing the mesalazine as the active component.[3]

Alternative routes available

No alternative routes are available for olsalazine; other 5-ASA preparations are available as suppositories and enemas.

Interactions

There is no documented interaction with food. Manufacturers recommend taking with food.[3]

Health and safety

Standard precautions apply. Capsule contents and dispersed tablets will stain.

Suggestions/recommendations

- Tablets can be dispersed in water in the barrel of a syringe to minimise exposure to the dispersion, which stains porous surfaces orange. Use alternative topical preparations where clinically appropriate.
- Consider changing to sulfasalazine liquid preparation or using alternative therapy such as steroids.

Intragastric administration

1. Stop the enteral feed.
2. Flush the enteral feeding tube with the recommended volume of water.
3. Place the tablet in the barrel of an appropriate size and type of syringe.
4. Draw 10 mL of water into the syringe and allow the tablet to disperse, shaking as required.
5. Flush the medication dose down the feeding tube.
6. Draw another 10 mL of water into the oral syringe and also flush this via the feeding tube (this will rinse the syringe and ensure that the total dose is administered).
7. Finally, flush with the recommended volume of water.
8. Re-start the feed, unless a prolonged break is required.

Alternatively, at step (3) place the tablet into a medicine pot, add 10 mL of water and allow the tablet to disperse. Draw this into an appropriate syringe. Ensure that the measure is rinsed and that this rinsing water is administered also to ensure that the total dose is given.

Intrajejunal administration

Jejunal administration will not affect the efficacy of the drug as the active compound in released in the colon. Administer as above.

References

1. *BNF* 50, September 2005.
2. BPNG data on file, 2004.
3. Dipentum (Celltech), Summary of Product Characteristics; October 2002.

Omeprazole

Formulations available[1]

Brand name (Manufacturer)	Formulation and strength	Product information/Administration information
Losec (AstraZeneca)	MUPS (dispersible tablets) 10 mg, 20 mg, 40 mg	Tablet disintegrates to give a dispersion of small granules. The granules settle quickly and have a tendency to block fine-bore feeding tubes (less than 8Fr).[2] The tablets may be dispersed in water or suspended in a small amount of fruit juice or yogurt after gentle mixing. It is important that the tablets should not be crushed or chewed.[7]
Losec (AstraZeneca)	Capsules 10 mg, 20 mg, 40 mg	Enteric coated granules within hard gelatin capsule. *Extemporaneous preparation:* 20 mg capsule contents can be dissolved in 10 mL of 8.4% sodium bicarbonate to give a 2 mg/mL solution; this is stable for 14 days at room temperature and for 45 days when refrigerated.[3, 4] This solution can be administered via nasogastric, duodenal or jejunal tube without risk of blockage or reduced efficacy.[5, 6]

Formulations available[1] (continued)

Brand name (Manufacturer)	Formulation and strength	Product information/Administration information
Losec (AstraZeneca)	Intravenous infusion 40 mg	Sodium salt. Injection can be administered via gastrostomy or jejunostomy tube; further information can be obtained from AstraZeneca.
Losec (AstraZeneca)	Intravenous injection 40 mg	Sodium salt. See above.
Omeprazole (Alpharma, APS, Generics, Kent, PLIVA, Ratiopharm)	Capsules 10 mg, 20 mg, 40 mg	See as for Losec capsules. Alpharma confirms that the capsule contents can be sprinkled on food or jam but must not be crushed.[8]
Omeprazole (Alpharma, Dexcel)	Tablets 10 mg, 20 mg, 40 mg	Both Alpharma and Dexcel brand are manufactured by Dexcel. The tablets disintegrate within 5 minutes when agitated in 10 mL of water to form a pink, milky dispersion that flushes down an 8Fr NG tube without blockage.[2]

Site of absorption (oral administration)

Absorption takes place in the small intestine and is usually complete within 3–6 hours.[7]
Bioavailability of omeprazole is increased from 40–50% to 65% by enteric coating; this reflects the instability of the drug in gastric acid.[9]

Alternative routes available

Parenteral route is available.[4]

Interactions

Food may delay peak plasma concentration but does not affect the total absorption of omeprazole.[7, 9]

Health and safety

Standard precautions apply.

Suggestions/recommendations

- The extemporaneous preparation detailed above should be used for fine-bore tubes (less than 12Fr).
- For large-bore tubes the Losec MUPS can be dispersed in water and administered according to the method detailed in the SPC.
- If excessive sodium bicarbonate intake is clinically inappropriate, the Dexcel brand tablets can be dispersed in water. The clinical effectiveness of the dispersed Dexcel brand tablets is unknown; however, as the entero-resistant coating has been removed, slightly larger doses may need to be given intragastrically to compensate for the reduced bioavailability.
- For jejunal administration, the extemporaneous solution or dispersed Dexcel brand tablets can be used.
- If intestinal absorptive capacity is unknown, consider using injection or infusion.

•

Intragastric administration

Extemporaneous omeprazole solution

1. Stop the enteral feed.
2. Flush the enteral feeding tube with the recommended volume of water.
3. Draw the medication solution into an appropriate size and type of syringe.
4. Flush the medication dose down the feeding tube.
5. Draw an equal volume of water into the syringe and also flush this via the feeding tube (this will rinse the syringe and ensure that the total dose is administered).
6. Finally, flush with the recommended volume of water.
7. Re-start the feed, unless a prolonged break is required.

Alternatively, at step (3) measure the medicine in a suitable container and then draw into an appropriate syringe. Ensure that the measure is rinsed and that this rinsing water is administered also to ensure that the total dose is given. **Do not** measure liquid medicines using a catheter-tipped syringe as this results in excessive dosing owing to the volume of the tip.

Dexcel tablets

1. Stop the enteral feed.
2. Flush the enteral feeding tube with the recommended volume of water.
3. Place the tablet in the barrel of an appropriate size and type of syringe.
4. Draw 10 mL of water into the syringe and allow the tablet to disperse, shaking as required.
5. Flush the medication dose down the feeding tube.
6. Draw another 10 mL of water into the syringe and also flush this via the feeding tube (this will rinse the syringe and ensure that the total dose is administered).
7. Finally, flush with the recommended volume of water.
8. Re-start the feed, unless a prolonged break is required.

Alternatively, at step (3) place the tablet into a medicine pot, add 10 mL of water and allow the tablet to disperse. Draw this into an appropriate syringe. Ensure that the measure is rinsed and that this rinsing water is administered also to ensure that the total dose is given.

Intrajejunal administration

Omeprazole is absorbed when administered into the jejunum with no reduction in bioavailability. Choice of formulation depends on the size of tube. See notes above.

References

1. *BNF 50*, September 2005.
2. BPNG data on file, 2004.
3. DiGiacinto JL, Olsen KM, Bergman KL, *et al*. Stability of suspension formulations of lansoprazole and omeprazole stored in amber-coloured plastic oral syringes. *Ann Pharmacother*. 2000; 34: 600–604.
4. Quercia RA, Fan C, Liu X, *et al*. Stability of omeprazole in an extemporaneously prepared oral liquid. *Am J Health Syst Pharm*. 1997; 54: 1833–1836.
5. Phillips JP, Metzler MH, Palmieri TL, *et al*. A prospective study of simplified omeprazole suspension for the prophylaxis of stress-related mucosal damage. *Crit Care Med*. 1996; 24(11): 1793–1800.
6. Phillips JP, Olsen KM, Rebuck JA, *et al*. A randomised, pharmacokinetic and pharmacodynamic, cross-over study of duodenal or jejunal administration compared to nasogastric administration of omeprazole suspension in patients at risk for stress ulcers. *Am J Gastroenterol*. 2001; 96(2): 367–372.
7. Losec MUPS (AstraZeneca), Summary of Product Characteristics; March 2005.
8. Personal communication, Alpharma; 21 January 2001.
9. Dollery C. *Therapeutic Drugs*, 2nd edn. London: Churchill Livingstone; 1998.

Ondansetron

Formulations available[1]

Brand name (Manufacturer)	Formulation and strength	Product information/Administration information
Zofran (GSK)	Tablets 4 mg, 8 mg	Ondansetron hydrochloride. No specific data on enteral tube administration are available for this formulation.
Zofran Melt (GSK)	Oral lyophilisates 4 mg, 8 mg	No specific data on enteral tube administration are available for this formulation.
Zofran (GSK)	Syrup 4 mg/5 mL	Ondansetron hydrochloride. Sugar-free. Contains sorbitol[3] 3 g/5 mL dose.[5]
Zofran (GSK)	Injection 2 mg/mL (2 mL, 4 mL)	Ondansetron hydrochloride. No specific data on enteral tube administration are available for this formulation.
Zofran (GSK)	Suppositories 16 mg	Rectal administration. Plasma levels are detectable 15–60 minutes following administration; peak plasma concentration occurs at 6 hours.[4]

Site of absorption (oral administration)

Specific site of absorption is not documented. Peak plasma concentrations occur 1–1.5 hours following oral dosing.[2]

Alternative routes available

Parenteral formulation is available. Can be administered by i.v. or i.m. injection.
Rectal formulation is available; once-daily dosing.

Interactions

Bioavailability of ondansetron is slightly enhanced by food.[3]

Health and safety

Standard precautions apply.

Suggestions/recommendations

- Consider suppository formulation for rectal administration.
- Use a liquid formulation for administration via the feeding tube; consider the total sorbitol dose administered for high-dose regimens.
- A prolonged break in feeding is not required.

Intragastric administration

1. Stop the enteral feed.
2. Flush the enteral feeding tube with the recommended volume of water.
3. Draw the medication solution into an appropriate size and type of syringe.
4. Flush the medication dose down the feeding tube.
5. Finally, flush with the recommended volume of water.
6. Re-start the feed, unless a prolonged break is required.

Alternatively, at step (3) measure the medicine in a suitable container and then draw into an appropriate syringe. Ensure that the measure is rinsed and that this rinsing water is administered also to ensure that the total dose is given. **Do not** measure liquid medicines using a catheter-tipped syringe as this results in excessive dosing owing to the volume of the tip.

Intrajejunal administration

There are no specific data on jejunal administration. Administer using the above method. Monitor for loss of efficacy or increased side-effects.

References

1. *BNF* 50, September 2005.
2. Dollery C. *Therapeutic Drugs*, 2nd edn. London: Churchill Livingstone; 1998.
3. Zofran Syrup (GSK), Summary of Product Characteristics; January 2003.
4. Zofran Suppositories (GSK), Summary of Product Characteristics; January 2003.
5. Personal communication, GlaxoSmithKline; February 2005.

Orciprenaline sulphate

Formulations available[1]

Brand name (Manufacturer)	Formulation and strength	Product information/Administration information
Alupent (Boehringer Ingelheim)	Syrup 10 mg/5 mL	Contains sorbitol.[2]

Site of absorption (oral administration)

Specific site of absorption is not documented. Onset of action is usually seen within 30 minutes of oral dosing.[2]

Alternative routes available

None for orciprenaline.

Interactions

No documented interaction with food.

Health and safety

Standard precautions apply.

Suggestions/recommendations

- Use the liquid preparation. Dilute with an equal volume of water immediately prior to administration.
- A prolonged break in feeding is not required.

Intragastric administration

1. Stop the enteral feed.
2. Flush the enteral feeding tube with the recommended volume of water.
3. Shake the medication bottle thoroughly to ensure adequate mixing.
4. Draw the medication suspension into an appropriate size and type of syringe.
5. Flush the medication dose down the feeding tube.
6. Finally, flush with the recommended volume of water.
7. Re-start the feed, unless a prolonged break is required.

Alternatively, at step (4) measure the medicine in a suitable container. Draw this into an appropriate syringe. Ensure that the measure is rinsed and that this rinsing water is administered also to ensure that the total dose is given. **Do not** measure liquid medicines using a catheter-tipped syringe as this results in excessive dosing owing to the volume of the tip.

Intrajejunal administration

There is no specific information relating to jejunal administration. Administer using the above method and monitor for loss of efficacy or increased side-effects.

References

1. *BNF 50*, September 2005.
2. Alupent Syrup (Boehringer Ingelheim), Summary of Product Characteristics, February 2003.

Orlistat

Formulations available[1]		
Brand name (Manufacturer)	**Formulation and strength**	**Product information/Administration information**
Xenical (Roche)	Capsules 120 mg	No specific data on enteral tube administration are available for this formulation.

Site of absorption (oral administration)

Olistat is not absorbed. It inhibits gut lipases to reduce fat absorption.[2]

Alternative routes available

None.

Interactions

Reduces absorption of fat and fat-soluble vitamins.[2]

Health and safety

Standard precautions apply.

Suggestions/recommendations

- Not appropriate for use in patients on enteral feed as calorie and fat content of intake can be controlled through manipulation and alteration of feed type and quantity. Seek specialist dietetic advice.

References

1. *BNF 50*, September 2005.
2. Xenical (Roche), Summary of Product Characteristics; March 2003.

Orphenadrine

Formulations available[1]

Brand name (Manufacturer)	Formulation and strength	Product information/Administration information
Orphenadrine (Rosemont)	Oral solution 50 mg/5 mL	Contains 0.45 g sorbitol/5 mL.[2]
Biorphen (Alliance)	Elixir 25 mg/5 mL	Alliance has no data to support the administration of Biorphen via enteral feeding tubes; however, no problems are anticipated with this route of administration.[3] Contains sorbitol[4] 1.75 g/5 mL dose.[6]
Disipal (Yamanouchi)	Tablets 50 mg	Sugar-coated tablets.[5] No specific data on enteral tube administration are available for this formulation.

Site of absorption (oral administration)

Specific site of absorption is unknown.[3]

Alternative routes available

None.

Interactions

There is no documented interaction with food.[4, 5]

Health and safety

Standard precautions apply.

Suggestions/recommendations

- Use a liquid preparation; if using Biorphen consider the sorbitol content.
- A prolonged break in feeding is not required.

Intragastric administration

1. Stop the enteral feed.
2. Flush the enteral feeding tube with the recommended volume of water.
3. Draw the medication solution into an appropriate size and type of syringe.
4. Flush the medication dose down the feeding tube.
5. Finally, flush with the recommended volume of water.
6. Re-start the feed, unless a prolonged break is required.

Alternatively, at step (3) measure the medicine in a suitable container and then draw into an appropriate syringe. Ensure that the measure is rinsed and that this rinsing water is administered also to ensure that the total dose is given. **Do not** measure liquid medicines using a catheter-tipped syringe as this results in excessive dosing owing to the volume of the tip.

Intrajejunal administration

There is no specific information on the jejunal administration of orphenadrine. Administer using the above method. Monitor for increased side-effects or loss of efficacy.

References

1. *BNF 50*, September 2005.
2. Personal communication, Rosemont; 20 January 2005.
3. Personal communication, Alliance; January 2003.
4. Biorphen (Alliance), Summary of Product Characteristics; April 2002.
5. Disipal (Yamanouchi), Summary of Product Characteristics; April 2002.
6. Personal communication, Alliance; July 2005.

Oxazepam

Formulations available[1]

Brand name (Manufacturer)	Formulation and strength	Product information/Administration information
Oxazepam (available from most generic manufacturers)	Tablets 10 mg, 15 mg, 30 mg	Alpharma brand tablets can be crushed.[2] They disperse rapidly in 10 mL of water to give a fine dispersion that flushes via an 8Fr NG tube without blockage.[3]

Site of absorption (oral administration)

Specific site of absorption is not documented. Peak plasma concentration occurs 1–5 hours following oral dosing.[4]

Alternative routes available

None available for oxazepam. Rectal route is available for diazepam; parenteral route is available for lorazepam.

Interactions

Food intake has no effect on bioavailability.[4]

Health and safety

Standard precautions apply.

Suggestions/recommendations

- Consider changing to an alternative therapy available in liquid formulation.
- If continued therapy with oxazepam is indicated, disperse the tablets in water immediately prior to administration. Alpharma brand are known to disperse in water; if using other brands, check for sizable particulates before administration.
- A prolonged break in feeding is not required.

Intragastric administration

1. Stop the enteral feed.
2. Flush the enteral feeding tube with the recommended volume of water.
3. Place the tablet in the barrel of an appropriate size and type of syringe.
4. Draw 10 mL of water into the syringe and allow the tablet to disperse, shaking if necessary.
5. Flush the medication dose down the feeding tube.
6. Draw another 10 mL of water into the syringe and also flush this via the feeding tube (this will rinse the syringe and ensure that the total dose is administered).
7. Finally, flush with the recommended volume of water.
8. Re-start the feed, unless a prolonged break is required.

Alternatively, at step (3) place the tablet into a medicine pot, add 10 mL of water and allow the tablet to disperse. Draw this into an appropriate syringe. Ensure that the measure is rinsed and that this rinsing water is administered also to ensure that the total dose is given.

Intrajejunal administration

There are no specific data relating to the jejunal administration of oxazepam. Administer using the above method. Monitor for increased side-effects or loss of efficacy.

References

1. *BNF* 50, September 2005.
2. Personal communication, Alpharma; 21 January 2003.
3. BPNG data on file, 2004.
4. Dollery C. *Therapeutic Drugs*, 2nd edn. London: Churchill Livingstone; 1998.

Oxprenolol hydrochloride

Formulations available[1]

Brand name (Manufacturer)	Formulation and strength	Product information/Administration information
Trasicor (Amdipharm)	Tablets 20 mg, 40 mg, 80 mg	Film-coated. 20 mg and 40 mg tablets will disperse in 10 mL of water if shaken for 5 minutes; this results in a very fine dispersion that flushes via an 8Fr NG tube without blockage.[2]

Formulations available[1] (continued)

Brand name (Manufacturer)	Formulation and strength	Product information/Administration information
Oxprenolol (Hillcross, IVAX)	Tablets 20 mg, 40 mg, 80 mg, 160 mg	Coated tablets. No specific data on enteral tube administration are available for this formulation.
Slow-Trasicor (Amdipharm)	M/R tablets 160 mg	Do not crush. Not suitable for enteral tube administration.

Site of absorption (oral administration)

Peak plasma concentration occurs 0.5–1.5 post oral dose.[3] There are data demonstrating oxprenolol is also absorbed in the colon and therefore jejunal administration would be expected to produce a similar bioavailability to oral administration.[4]

Alternative routes available

None available for oxprenolol; other beta-blockers are available as parenteral formulations.

Interactions

There is no documented interaction with food.[3]

Health and safety

Standard precautions apply.

Suggestions/recommendations

- Conventional release tablet requires two to three times daily dosing.
- Consider changing to an alternative once-daily beta-blocker such as atenolol (see monograph). If changing therapy is not appropriate, tablets can be dispersed in water immediately prior to administration, and can be administered via a gastrostomy or jejunostomy. A prolonged break in feeding is not required.

Intragastric administration

1. Stop the enteral feed.
2. Flush the enteral feeding tube with the recommended volume of water.
3. Place the tablet in the barrel of an appropriate size and type of syringe.
4. Draw 10 mL of water into the syringe and allow the tablet to disperse, shaking as required.
5. Flush the medication dose down the feeding tube.
6. Draw another 10 mL of water into the syringe and also flush this via the feeding tube (this will rinse the syringe and ensure that the total dose is administered).
7. Finally, flush with the recommended volume of water.
8. Re-start the feed, unless a prolonged break is required.

Alternatively, at step (3) place the tablet into a medicine pot, add 10 mL of water and allow the tablet to dissolve. Draw this into an appropriate syringe. Ensure that the measure is rinsed and that this rinsing water is administered also to ensure that the total dose is given.

Intrajejunal administration

The bioavailability of oxprenolol is unlikely to be affected by jejunal administration. The above method of administration can be followed.

References

1. *BNF 50*, September 2005.
2. BPNG data on file, 2005.
3. Dollery C. *Therapeutic Drugs*, 2nd edn. London: Churchill Livingstone; 1998.
4. Adams D. Administration of drugs through a jejunostomy tube. *Br J Intensive Care*. 1994; 4(1): 10–17.

Oxybutynin hydrochloride

Formulations available[1]

Brand name (Manufacturer)	Formulation and strength	Product information/Administration information
Oxybutynin (various manufacturers)	Tablets 2.5 mg, 3 mg, 5 mg	Tillomed brand tablets disperse readily when placed in 10 mL of water to give a fine dispersion that flushes easily via an 8Fr tube without blockage.[2]
Cystrin (Sanofi-Synthelabo)	Tablets 3 mg	Tablets do not disperse readily in water but will disintegrate if shaken in water for 5 minutes; this gives a fine dispersion with some visible particles that stick to side of syringe; ensure that the syringe is rinsed well. Does not block tube.[2] Tablets may be crushed.[3]
Ditropan (Sanofi-Synthelabo)	Tablets 2.5 mg, 5 mg	Tablets can be crushed.[3]
Ditropan (Sanofi-Synthelabo)	Elixir 2.5 mg/5 mL	Contains sucrose (1.3 g/5 mL) and sorbitol.[4]
Lyrinel XL (Janssen-Cilag)	M/R tablets 5 mg, 10 mg	Do not crush; unsuitable for administration via the feeding tubes.
Oxybutynin (Rosemont)	Oral solution 5 mg/5 mL	Manufactured 'special' preparation. Contains 1.36 g sorbitol/5 mL.[5] Sugar-free.
Kentera (UCB Pharma)	Patch 36 mg	One patch to be applied twice weekly.

Site of absorption (oral administration)

Specific site of absorption is not documented. However, the availability of modified-release products would indicate that oxybutynin is absorbed throughout the small bowel. Oxybutynin is poorly absorbed from the GI tract. Peak plasma concentration occurs 0.5–1 hour following oral administration.[4]

Alternative routes available

Transdermal patches are available. Intravesical installation is available on a named-patient basis.

Interactions

There are no documented interaction with food. [4]

Health and safety

Standard precautions apply.

Suggestions/recommendations

- Use transdermal patch where clinically appropriate. Use a liquid preparation for use via enteral feeding tube.
- A prolonged break in feeding is not required.

Intragastric administration

1. Stop the enteral feed.
2. Flush the enteral feeding tube with the recommended volume of water.
3. Shake the medication bottle thoroughly to ensure adequate mixing.
4. Draw the medication suspension into an appropriate size and type of syringe.
5. Flush the medication dose down the feeding tube.
6. Finally, flush with the recommended volume of water.
7. Re-start the feed, unless a prolonged break is required.

Alternatively, at step (4) measure the medicine in a suitable container and then add an equal volume of water and mix thoroughly. Draw this into the syringe with an appropriate adapter for the tube connector. Ensure that the measure is rinsed and that this rinsing water is administered also to ensure that the total dose is given. **Do not** measure liquid medicines using a catheter-tipped syringe as this results in excessive dosing owing to the volume of the tip.

Intrajejunal administration

There are no specific data relating to jejunal administration of oxybutynin. Administer as above. Monitor for loss of efficacy or increased side-effects.

References

1. *BNF* 50, September 2005.
2. BPNG data on file, 2004.
3. Personal communication, Sanofi-Synthelabo; 3 February 2004.
4. Ditropan Elixir (Sanofi-Synthelabo), Summary of Product Characteristics; November 2001.
5. Personal communication, Rosemont Pharma; 20 January 2005.

Oxycodone hydrochloride

Formulations available [1]

Brand name (Manufacturer)	Formulation and strength	Product information/Administration information
OxyNorm (Napp)	Capsules 5 mg, 10 mg, 20 mg	No specific data on enteral tube administration are available for this formulation.

Formulations available [1] (continued)

Brand name (Manufacturer)	Formulation and strength	Product information/Administration information
OxyNorm (Napp)	Liquid 5 mg/5 mL	There is no theoretical reason why OxyNorm should not be administered via an enteral feeding tube, although the manufacturer has no data to support this. [2] Does not contain sorbitol. [3]
OxyNorm Concentrate (Napp)	Oral solution 10 mg/mL	Can be mixed with a soft drink to increase palatability. [3] Does not contain sorbitol. [3]
OxyNorm (Napp)	Injection 10 mg/mL (1 mL, 2 mL)	No specific data on enteral tube administration are available for this formulation.
OxyContin (Napp)	Tablets 5 mg, 10 mg, 20 mg, 40 mg, 80 mg	Modified-release tablets. Cannot be crushed; not suitable for administration via enteral feeding tubes.

Site of absorption (oral administration)

Specific site is not documented. Peak plasma concentration occurs within 1 hour following oral dosing using liquid formulations. [3]

Alternative routes available

Parenteral formulation is available for oxycodone. Rectal, transdermal and parenteral formulations are available for alternative opiates.

Interactions

There is no documented interaction with food. [3]

Health and safety

Standard precautions apply.

Suggestions/recommendations

- Use the liquid formulation for administration via the feeding tube. When transferring from sustained-release preparation, divide the total daily dose by 6 and give 4-hourly using the liquid preparation.
- A prolonged break in feeding is not required.
- If a sustained opiate effect is required and 4-hourly dosing is not practical, consider using fentanyl or buprenorphine patches; seek advice for dose conversion.

Intragastric administration

1. Stop the enteral feed.
2. Flush the enteral feeding tube with the recommended volume of water.
3. Shake the medication bottle thoroughly to ensure adequate mixing.
4. Draw the medication liquid into an appropriate size and type of syringe.
5. Flush the medication dose down the feeding tube.
6. Finally, flush with the recommended volume of water.
7. Re-start the feed, unless a prolonged break is required.

Alternatively, at step (4) measure the medicine in a suitable container. Draw this into an appropriate syringe. Ensure that the measure is rinsed and that this rinsing water is administered also to ensure that the total dose is given. **Do not** measure liquid medicines using a catheter-tipped syringe as this results in excessive dosing owing to the volume of the tip.

Intrajejunal administration

There are no specific data relating to jejunal administration. Administer using the above method. Monitor for lack of efficacy or side-effects.

References

1. *BNF* 50, September 2005.
2. Personal communication, Napp; 29 January 2003.
3. Oxynorm Liquid (Napp), Summary of Product Characteristics; January 2002.

Oxytetracycline

Formulations available[1]

Brand name (Manufacturer)	Formulation and strength	Product information/Administration information
Oxytetracycline (Alpharma, APS, Ashbourne, DDSA, IVAX)	Tablets 250 mg	Oxytetracycline dehydrate. Coated tablets. Crushing of tablets is not recommended.[2]

Site of absorption (oral administration)

Absorption of oxytetracycline occurs in the stomach and duodenum.[3]

Alternative routes available

None available for oxytetracycline.

Interactions

Food, milk and some dairy products reduce absorption. Tetracyclines should be given 1 hour before or 2 hours after meals.[3]

Health and safety

Standard precautions apply.

Suggestions/recommendations

- Owing to the necessary break in feeding, the frequency of dosing and a lack of suitable formulation, consider changing to once-daily doxycycline (see monograph). Seek microbiological advice.

References

1. *BNF* 50, September 2005.
2. Personal communication, Alpharma; 21 January 2003.
3. Personal communication, Pfizer; 23 June 2003.

Pancreatic enzyme supplements

Formulations available [1]

Brand name (Manufacturer)	Formulation and strength	Product information/Administration information
Creon 10,000 (Solvay)	Capsules	Protease 600 units, lipase 10 000 units, amylase 8000 units. Capsules containing enteric-coated granules. Capsules can be opened, but the granules must not be crushed.
Creon 25,000 (Solvay)	Capsules	Protease 1000 units, lipase 25 000 units, amylase 18 000 units. Capsules containing enteric-coated granules. Capsules can be opened, but the granules must not be crushed.
Creon 40,000 (Solvay)	Capsules	Protease 1600 units, lipase 40 000 units, amylase 25 000 units Capsules containing enteric-coated granules. Capsules can be opened, but the granules must not be crushed.
Creon Micro (Solvay)	Gastro resistant granules	Protease 2000 units, lipase 50 000 units, amylase 36 000 units/g of granules. Granules may be mixed with food and swallowed whole. Not suitable for enteral tube administration.
Nutrizym 10 (Merck)	Capsules	Protease 500 units, lipase 10 000 units, amylase 9000 units. The pellets within the capsules are enteric coated, and can be swallowed with water. They may get stuck within the tube, especially smaller-sized tubes. [2]
Nutrizym 22 (Merck)	Capsules	Protease 1100 units, lipase 22 000 units, amylase 19 800 units. The pellets within the capsules are enteric coated, and can be swallowed with water. They may get stuck within the tube, especially smaller-sized tubes. [2]

Formulations available[1] (continued)

Brand name (Manufacturer)	Formulation and strength	Product information/Administration information
Pancrease (Janssen-Cilag)	Capsules	Protease 330 units, lipase 5000 units, amylase 2900 units. The intact beads can be administered via an NG tube in water or in milk.[3] There is no comment on the risk of tube blockage.
Pancrease HL (Janssen-Cilag)	Capsules	Protease 1250 units, lipase 25 000 units, amylase 22 500 units. The intact beads can be administered via an NG tube in water or in milk.[3] There is no comment on the risk of tube blockage.
Pancrex (Paynes & Byrne)	Granules	Protease 300 units, lipase 5000 units, amylase 4000 units/g. Granules can be mixed with milk or water.[4]
Pancrex V Paines & Byrne)	Capsules	Protease 430 units, lipase 8000 units, amylase 9000 units. The capsules contents can be mixed with feeds. The resulting mixture should be used within 1 hour.[5]
Pancrex V '125' Paines & Byrne)	Capsules	Protease 160 units, lipase 2950 units, amylase 3300 units. The capsules contents can be mixed with feeds. The resulting mixture should be used within 1 hour.[6]
Pancrex V Tablets Paines & Byrne)	Tablets	Protease 110 units, lipase 1900 units, amylase 1700 units. Enteric coated, sugar-coated tablets; must be swallowed whole.[7]
Pancrex V Tablets Forte Paines & Byrne)	Tablets	Protease 330 units, lipase 5600 units, amylase 5000 units. Enteric coated, sugar-coated tablets; must be swallowed whole.[8]
Pancrex V Paines & Byrne)	Powder	Protease 1400 units, lipase 25 000 units, amylase 30 000 units/g. Mix appropriate quantity of powder with water or milk prior to administration.[9]

Site of absorption (oral administration)

Pancreatic enzymes are not absorbed; they act locally in the proximal small bowel.

Alternative routes available

Alternative routes of administration are not appropriate.

Interactions

The pharmacological response is based on the interaction with food.

Health and safety

Standard precautions apply. Avoid handling or inhaling the capsule contents and dry powder preparations. Allergic reactions have been reported.[6]

Suggestions/recommendations [10]

Feed type	Enzyme dose
Standard whole-protein feed	Equivalent to that required for a similar volume of full-cream milk.
Peptide feed	50% of that required for a similar volume of full-cream milk.
Elemental feed	25% or less of that required for a similar volume of full-cream milk (dependent on percentage of MCT fat in feed).

- If transferring from oral diet and pancreatic enzyme supplements to complete enteral feed, consider a trial without supplements, especially if on a low dose of enzyme supplements. If the patient does not tolerate standard feed, consider a trial of peptide-based feed.
- For patients with wide-bore enteral feeding tubes, the granules can be used, dispersed in water immediately prior to administration. A dose should be given before and immediately after each feed if bolus feeding. If on a continuous feed, a dose should be given at the start of the feed and then at regular intervals throughout; these doses should be titrated to response and practicality.
- For fine-bore feeding tubes the capsules containing powder or the loose powder can be used. The dose of powder can be mixed with a small volume of water (10–20 mL) immediately prior to administration. The timing of doses can be given as above.

Intragastric administration

1. Stop the enteral feed.
2. Flush the enteral feeding tube with the recommended volume of water.
3. Open the capsule and pour the contents into a medicine pot.
4. Add 15 mL of water.
5. Stir to disperse the powder or granules (depending on bore size of tube).
6. Draw into an appropriate type and size of syringe and administer via the feeding tube.
7. Add a further 15 mL of water to the medicine pot; stir to ensure that any powder remaining in the pot is mixed with water.
8. Draw up this dispersion and flush down the tube. This will ensure that the whole dose is given.
9. Flush the tube with water.
10. Re-start feed immediately.

Intrajejunal administration

There are no specific data relating to jejunal administration of pancreatic supplements. There is no theoretical reason why the enzymes should be ineffective. Administer using the above method.

References

1. *BNF 50*, September 2005.
2. Personal communication, Merck; 23 January 2003.
3. Personal communication, Janssen-Cilag; 22 January 2003.
4. Pancrex Granules, Patient information leaflet; July 2001.
5. Pancrex V Capsules, Patient information leaflet; March 2001.
6. Pancrex V Capsules 125 mg, Patient information leaflet; March 2001.
7. Pancrex V Tablets (Paines & Byrne), Summary of Product Characteristics; July 2002.
8. Pancrex V Forte Tablets (Paines & Byrne), Summary of Product Characteristics; July 2002.
9. Pancrex V Powder, Patient information leaflet; March 2001.
10. Personal communication, Solvay; 19 February 2003.

Pantoprazole

Formulations available[1]

Brand name (Manufacturer)	Formulation and strength	Product information/Administration information
Protium (Altana)	Tablet 20 mg, 40 mg	Gastro-resistant coated tablet.[2] Tablet can be crushed and dissolved in 10 mL of 8.4% sodium bicarbonate for administration via NG tube; this solution is stable for 2 weeks at 5 °C. The peak plasma concentration is the same as the tablet administered orally, but bioavailability is reduced to 75% of oral equivalent.[3]
Protium (Altana)	Injection 40 mg	Reconstituted injection has pH of 9–10.[4] No data on enteral administration of this formulation.

Site of absorption (oral administration)

Peak concentrations occur after 2–2.5 hours. Pantoprazole is absorbed in the small bowel; the formulation is enteric-coated.[2]

Alternative routes available

Parenteral route is available.[4]

Interactions

Absorption is unaffected by food.[2]

Health and safety

Standard precautions apply.

Suggestions/recommendations

- Although it is possible to administer pantoprazole via NG tube following the method above, it would be appropriate to consider using the parenteral route or changing therapy to lansoprazole or omeprazole for ease of administration (see monographs). Alternatively, ranitidine may be used if a step-down approach is appropriate (see monograph).

References

1. *BNF 50*, September 2005.
2. Protium 20 mg tablet (Altana), Summary of Product Characteristics; March 2003.
3. Ferron GM, Ku S, Abell M, *et al.* (2003) Oral bioavailability of pantoprazole suspended in sodium bicarbonate solution. *Am J Health Syst Pharm.* 2003; 60(13): 1324–1329.
4. Protium 40 mg i.v. (Altana), Summary of Product Characteristics; April 2003.

Paracetamol

Formulations available[1]

(Owing to the large number of formulations available, only those that might be considered suitable are included below)

Brand name (Manufacturer)	Formulation and strength	Product information/Administration information
Paracetamol (various manufacturers)	Dispersible tablets 500 mg	Sterwin brand contains 388 mg sodium (17 mmol) per tablet.[2] Sterwin brand tablets effervesce in 10 mL of water to give a milky dispersion that flushes via an 8Fr NG tube without blockage.[3] Sterling Health brand contains 427 mg sodium (18.6 mmol) per tablet.[4]
Paracetamol (various manufacturers)	Paediatric soluble tablets 120 mg	No specific data on enteral tube administration are available for this formulation.
Paracetamol (various manufacturers)	Oral suspension 120 mg/5 mL	Rosemont suspension contains 0.68 g sorbitol/5 mL dose.[5]
Paracetamol (various manufacturers)	Oral suspension 250 mg/5 mL	Rosemont suspension contains 0.68 g sorbitol/5 mL dose.[6]
Paracetamol (AstraZeneca, Arum)	Suppositories 60 mg, 120 mg, 125 mg, 240 mg, 250 mg, 500 mg	Rectal use only. Bioavailability 40–60%. Time to peak plasma concentration is 2–3 hours.
Perfalgan (Bristol-Myers Squibb)	Infusion 10 mg/mL (100 mL)	Not suitable for enteral administration.

Site of absorption (oral administration)

Paracetamol is absorbed rapidly following oral administration. Administration into the jejunum achieves similar plasma concentration to oral administration.[6]

Alternative routes available

Rectal and parenteral routes are available.

Interactions

No interaction with food or enteral feed is documented.

Health and safety

Standard precautions apply.

Suggestions/recommendations

- Use tablets dispersed in 50 mL of water (for adults) for intragastric or intrajejunal administration. If the sodium content is problematic, use the liquid formulation. This can be used undiluted for intragastric administration; if administering intrajejunally, dilute with at least an equal quantity of water to reduce osmolarity and viscosity.
- Suppositories or injection can be considered useful alternatives.

Intragastric administration

1. Stop the enteral feed.
2. Flush the enteral feeding tube with the recommended volume of water.
3. Measure 50 mL of water into a measuring pot.
4. Add the effervescent tablet and allow to dissolve.
5. Draw into an appropriate size and type of syringe.
6. Flush the medication dose down the feeding tube.
7. Rinse the measure with 10–20 mL of water and administer this also to ensure that the total dose is given.
8. Finally, flush with the recommended volume of water.
9. Re-start the feed, unless a prolonged break is required.

Intrajejunal administration

Administration into the jejunum does not affect bioavailability. Administer using the above method.

References

1. *BNF* 50, September 2005.
2. Personal communication, Sterwin; July 2005.
3. BPNG data on file, 2005.
4. Personal communication, Sterling Health; July 2005.
5. Personal communication, Rosemont Pharma; 20 January 2005.
6. Adams D. Administration of drugs through a jejunostomy tube. *Br J Intensive Care*. 1994; 4(1): 10–17.

Paroxetine hydrochloride

Formulations available[1]

Brand name (Manufacturer)	Formulation and strength	Product information/Administration information
Paroxetine (Alpharma, Generics, Norton, Sandoz)	Tablets 20 mg	No specific data on enteral tube administration are available for this formulation.
Seroxat (GSK)	Tablets 20 mg, 30 mg	Film-coated, scored tablets. No specific data on enteral tube administration are available for this formulation.

Formulations available [1] (*continued*)

Brand name (Manufacturer)	Formulation and strength	Product information/Administration information
Seroxat (GSK)	Liquid 10 mg/5 mL	Orange liquid; viscous but flushes with only a slight resistance. Mixes with an equal volume of water, which reduces resistance to flushing. [2] Sugar-free, contains sorbitol. [3]

Site of absorption (oral administration)

Specific site of absorption is not documented.

Alternative routes available

Not applicable.

Interactions

The absorption of paroxetine is not affected by food or antacids. [3]

Health and safety

Standard precautions apply.

Suggestions/recommendations

- Use liquid preparation.
- A prolonged break in feeding is not required.

Intragastric administration

1. Stop the enteral feed.
2. Flush the enteral feeding tube with the recommended volume of water.
3. Draw the medication solution into an appropriate size and type of syringe.
4. Flush the medication dose down the feeding tube.
5. Finally, flush with the recommended volume of water.
6. Re-start the feed.

Alternatively, at step (3) measure the medicine in a suitable container and then draw into an appropriate syringe. Ensure that the measure is rinsed and that this rinsing water is administered also to ensure that the total dose is given. **Do not** measure liquid medicines using a catheter-tipped syringe as this results in excessive dosing owing to the volume of the tip.

Intrajejunal administration

There are no specific data relating to jejunal administration of paroxetine. Administer using the method above. Consider dilution of the dose immediately prior to administration to reduce osmolarity. Monitor for side-effects and loss of efficacy.

References

1. *BNF 50*, September 2005.
2. BPNG data on file, 2004.
3. Seroxat (GSK), Summary of Product Characteristics; April 2005.

Perindopril erbumine

Formulations available [1]

Brand name (Manufacturer)	Formulation and strength	Product information/Administration information
Coversyl (Servier)	Tablets 2 mg, 4 mg, 8 mg	2 mg and 4 mg tablets were crushed and suspended in 100 mL water; there was no decrease in concentration over 7 days when stored at 4–8 °C. No data are available for the 8 mg tablets, but as the composition is directly proportional to other strengths, the tablets can be crushed in water and the resulting suspension used immediately. [2] Both 2 mg and 4 mg disperse in 10 mL of water within 2–5 minutes to form a very fine dispersion that settles quickly but flushes down an 8Fr NG tube without blockage. [3]
Coversyl Plus (Servier)	Tablets Perindopril 4 mg, Indapamide 1.25 mg	Coversyl plus is an immediate-release product; the tablets can be crushed in water, but as there are no stability data the suspension should be used immediately. [2]

Site of absorption (oral administration)

Specific site of absorption is not documented. Peak plasma concentration occurs within 1 hour of oral dosing. [4]

Alternative routes available

No alternative route is available for any of the ACE inhibitors.

Interactions

Conversion of perindopril to perindoprilat, and thereby bioavailability, is reduced by the ingestion of food; therefore, perindopril should be taken before food. [4]

Health and safety

Standard precautions apply.

Suggestions/recommendations

- Feed should be stopped and the tube flushed with water 1–2 hours before administration.
- Tablets should be dispersed in water immediately prior to administration.
- If on continuous feeding, an ACE inhibitor unaffected by food and available as a liquid formulation, such as lisinopril (see monograph), could be substituted.

Intragastric administration

1. Stop the enteral feed.
2. Flush the enteral feeding tube with the recommended volume of water.
3. Wait for 2 hours before administering the dose.
4. Place the tablet in the barrel of an appropriate size and type of syringe.
5. Draw 10 mL of water into the syringe and allow the tablet to disperse, shaking if necessary.
6. Flush the medication dose down the feeding tube.
7. Draw another 10 mL of water into the syringe and also flush this via the feeding tube (this will rinse the syringe and ensure that the total dose is administered).
8. Finally, flush with the recommended volume of water.
9. Allow at least an hour before restarting feed.

Alternatively, at step (4) place the tablet into a medicine pot, add 10 mL of water and allow the tablet to disperse. Draw this into an appropriate syringe. Ensure that the measure is rinsed and that this rinsing water is administered also to ensure that the total dose is given.

Intrajejunal administration

No specific data are available. Monitor for signs of reduced efficacy. Administer as above.

References

1. *BNF* 50, September 2005.
2. Personal communication, Servier Laboratories Ltd; 3 March 2003.
3. BPNG data on file, 2004.
4. Coversyl 8 mg (Servier), Summary of Product Characteristics; February 2003.

Phenelzine

Formulations available[1]

Brand name (Manufacturer)	Formulation and strength	Product information/Administration information
Nardil (Hansam)	Tablets 15 mg	Film-coated tablets. Phenelzine sulfate No specific data on enteral tube administration are available for this formulation.

Site of absorption (oral administration)

Specific site is not documented. Peak plasma concentration occurs 2 hours following oral dosing.[2]

Alternative routes available

None available.

Interactions

Phenelzine causes an increased sensitivity to foods high in tryptophan; however, there is no specific pharmacokinetic interaction with food documented.[2] Enteral feed does not contain tryptophan.

Health and safety

Standard precautions apply.

Suggestions/recommendations

- Owing to lack of specific data, consider changing to an alternative antidepressant. Seek specialist advice.
- If alternative therapy is not appropriate, crush the tablets and disperse in water immediately prior to administration; this should be considered a last resort.
- A prolonged break in feeding is not required.

Intragastric administration

1. Stop the enteral feed.
2. Flush the enteral feeding tube with the recommended volume of water.
3. Place the tablet in a mortar and crush to a fine powder using the pestle.
4. Add a few millilitres of water and mix to form a paste.
5. Add up to 15 mL of water and mix thoroughly ensuring that there are no large particles of tablet.
6. Draw this into an appropriate size and type of syringe.
7. Flush the medication dose down the feeding tube.
8. Add another 15 mL of water to the mortar and stir to ensure that any remaining drug is rinsed from the container. Draw this water into the syringe and also flush this via the feeding tube (this will rinse the mortar and syringe and ensure that the total dose is administered).
9. Finally, flush the enteral feeding tube with the recommended volume of water.
10. Re-start the feed, unless a prolonged break is required.

Intrajejunal administration

There are no specific data relating to jejunal administration of phenelzine. Administer using the above method. Monitor for loss of efficacy or increased side-effects.

References

1. *BNF 50*, September 2005.
2. Dollery C. *Therapeutic Drugs*, 2nd edn. London: Churchill Livingstone; 1998.

Phenobarbital (Phenobarbitone)

Formulations available[1]

Brand name (Manufacturer)	Formulation and strength	Product information/Administration information
Phenobarbital (various manufacturers)	Tablets 15 mg, 30 mg, 60 mg	No specific data on enteral tube administration are available for this formulation.
Phenobarbital (various manufacturers)	Elixir 15 mg/5 mL	Contains alcohol 38%.

Formulations available[1] (continued)

Brand name (Manufacturer)	Formulation and strength	Product information/Administration information
Phenobarbital (Concord, Martindale)	Injection 200 mg/mL (1 mL)	I.m. route used for control of acute seizures. I.v. route used for status epilepticus.
Specials (various specials manufacturers)	Oral liquid Various strengths	Alcohol-free liquid. Available on request only.

Site of absorption (oral administration)

No specific site of absorption is documented. Peak plasma concentration occurs 6–18 hours following oral intake; peak plasma concentration occur 2–3 hours after i.m. dosing.[2]

Alternative routes available

Parenteral route is available, although usually reserved for acute treatment.

Interactions

There is no documented interaction with food.[2]

Health and safety

Standard precautions apply.

Suggestions/recommendations

- Use the liquid preparation.
- Note the very high alcohol concentration.
- A prolonged break in feeding is not necessary.

Intragastric administration

1. Stop the enteral feed.
2. Flush the enteral feeding tube with the recommended volume of water.
3. Shake the medication bottle thoroughly to ensure adequate mixing.
4. Draw the medication suspension into an appropriate size and type of syringe.
5. Flush the medication dose down the feeding tube.
6. Finally, flush with the recommended volume of water.
7. Re-start the feed, unless a prolonged break is required.

Alternatively, at step (4) measure the medicine in a suitable container. Draw this into an appropriate syringe. Ensure that the measure is rinsed and that this rinsing water is administered also to ensure that the total dose is given. **Do not** measure liquid medicines using a catheter-tipped syringe as this results in excessive dosing owing to the volume of the tip.

Intrajejunal administration

There are no specific data relating to jejunal administration. Administer as above; consider diluting the liquid formulation immediately prior to administration to reduce osmolarity. Monitor for loss of efficacy.

References

1. *BNF 50*, September 2005.
2. Dollery C. *Therapeutic Drugs*, 2nd edn. London: Churchill Livingstone; 1998.

Phenoxymethylpenicillin

Formulations available[1]

Brand name (Manufacturer)	Formulation and strength	Product information/Administration information
Phenoxymethylpeni-cillin (Alpharma, APS, Arrow, Berk, Generics, Kent, Sovereign)	Tablets 250 mg	Potassium salt. Avoid crushing the tablets owing to the risk of sensitisation to penicillin.
Phenoxymethylpeni-cillin (Alpharma, APS, Arrow, Generics, Kent, Sandoz, Sovereign)	Oral solution 125 mg/5 mL, 250 mg/5 mL	Potassium salt. Oral solution draws up easily and flushes via fine-bore tube without resistance or blockage.[2]
Benzylpenicillin Crystapen (Britannia)	Injection 600 mg, 1.2 g	Sodium salt. Not suitable for enteral administration. Salt form is acid labile.

Site of absorption (oral administration)

Specific site is not documented. Peak plasma concentration occurs within 30 minutes of oral dosing.[3]

Alternative routes available

Benzylpenicillin available in injection only. See SPC for dosing information.

Interactions

Phenoxymethylpenicillin is affected by food and gastric acid (although less than benzylpenicillin). To optimise absorption, it is recommended that oral doses be taken 1 hour before food or on an empty stomach.[3]

Health and safety

Do not crush the tablets owing to the risk of contact sensitisation.

Suggestions/recommendations

- Consider using an alternative antibiotic unaffected by food, to avoid interruptions in the feeding regimen.
- If continuing therapy with phenoxymethylpenicillin, use the liquid formulation for enteral administration.
- Stop feed at least 2 hours before the dose; do not restart feed for 1 hour after dose.
- Parenteral therapy with benzylpenicillin should be considered for serious infections.

Intragastric administration

1. Stop the enteral feed.
2. Flush the enteral feeding tube with the recommended volume of water.
3. Wait for 2 hours.
4. Draw the medication solution into an appropriate size and type of syringe.
5. Flush the medication dose down the feeding tube.
6. Finally, flush with the recommended volume of water.
7. Wait for at least 1 hour before re-starting the feed.

Alternatively, at step (4) measure the medicine in a suitable container and then draw into an appropriate syringe. Ensure that the measure is rinsed and that this rinsing water is administered also to ensure that the total dose is given. **Do not** measure liquid medicines using a catheter-tipped syringe as this results in excessive dosing owing to the volume of the tip.

Intrajejunal administration

There is no specific information on jejunal administration of phenoxymethylpenicillin. In theory, bioavailability would be increased, as the drug is not exposed to gastric acid. Administer using the above method.

References

1. *BNF 50*, September 2005.
2. BPNG data on file, 2005.
3. Dollery C. *Therapeutic Drugs*, 2nd edn. London: Churchill Livingstone; 1998.

Phenytoin

Formulations available[1]

Brand name (Manufacturer)	Formulation and strength	Product information/Administration information
Epanutin (Parke-Davis)	Capsules 25 mg, 50 mg, 100 mg, 300 mg	Phenytoin sodium. The powder can be poured from the capsules and mixed with 10 mL of water. The powder does not mix initially but if left for 5 minutes and then stirred it forms a fine dispersion that flushes down an 8Fr NG tube without blockage.[2]
Epanutin (Parke-Davis)	Infatabs 50 mg	Phenytoin base. Chewable tablets. No specific data on enteral tube administration are available for this formulation.
Epanutin (Parke-Davis)	Suspension 30 mg/5 mL	Phenytoin base. 90 mg/15 mL of suspension is approximately equivalent to 100 mg of phenytoin sodium. Viscous, thixotropic suspension.

Formulations available[1] (continued)

Brand name (Manufacturer)	Formulation and strength	Product information/Administration information
Epanutin (Parke-Davis)	Injection 50 mg/mL (5 mL)	Phenytoin sodium. Intravenous doses are given 6–8 hourly, as the half-life varies from 7 to 42 hours.[9] Epanutin can be given i.m. for short periods, but absorption is variable. See SPC for further guidance.
Phenytoin (Antigen, Mayne)	Injection 50 mg/mL (5 mL)	Phenytoin sodium. No specific data on enteral tube administration are available for this formulation.
Phenytoin (APS)	Capsules 50 mg, 100 mg	Phenytoin sodium. No specific data on enteral tube administration are available for this formulation.
Phenytoin (APS)	Tablets 50 mg, 100 mg	Phenytoin sodium. Tablets do not disperse readily in water, and are difficult to crush owing to the coating.[10]
Phenytoin (Rosemont)	Suspension 90 mg/5 mL	Phenytoin base. Sugar-free: unlicensed product.

Site of absorption (oral administration)

Phenytoin is absorbed from the small intestine after oral administration.[10] Peak plasma concentration occurs 2–4 hours and 10–12 hours post oral dosing.[3]

Alternative routes available

Parenteral route is available for phenytoin. See dosing guidance above.

Interactions

Bauer[4] established the interaction between phenytoin and enteral feeding, demonstrating that concurrent administration of enteral feed to patients established on phenytoin caused a significant drop in phenytoin plasma concentration. This paper was also the first to suggest that a 2-hour break either side of the dose could minimise this interaction; however, even when this method was used, doses of up to 1600 mg/day were required to achieve therapeutic concentrations. Ozuna and Friel demonstrated that allowing a break in feeding did not significantly improve phenytoin absorption.[5] Doak et al.[6] compared nasogastric administration of phenytoin base with the phenytoin salt and found no difference in total bioavailability, although there was a difference in pharmacokinetic profile, with the sodium salt giving an earlier peak.

Rodman[7] reports a dramatic drop in phenytoin plasma concentration when a patient was transferred from i.v. phenytoin to an equivalent dose of suspension given via the jejunostomy tube, and suggests that jejunal administration may further reduce the absorption of phenytoin.

The data are reviewed by Stockley[8] and recommendations for management are made. Although the data are inconclusive, a general recommendation of a 2-hour break either side of the dose is made.

Health and safety

Standard precautions apply.

Suggestions/recommendations

- Convert the dose from the usual preparation using the formula:

  100 mg phenytoin sodium = 90 mg of phenytoin base.

- Stop the enteral feed and flush the tube 2 hours before dosing.[10, 11, 12]
- Do not restart feed for at least two hours after dosing.[10, 11, 12]
- Phenytoin plasma concentration should be checked and the dose adjusted until therapeutic plasma concentration are achieved; this may require very high doses.
- Steps should be taken to ensure that the same protocol and timetable are followed each day to optimise dosing consistency. Plasma concentration should be checked if the feeding schedule is changed or stopped.
- If the volume of the suspension or dilution is too large, a concentrated suspension is available from Rosemont as a special product (unlicensed).

Intragastric administration

1. Stop the enteral feed.
2. Flush the enteral feeding tube with recommended volume of water.
3. Allow a 2 hour break without feed.
4. Shake the medication bottle thoroughly to ensure adequate mixing.
5. Measure the required volume of suspension and mix with an equal volume of water (this may be a large volume)
6. Draw the medication into an appropriate size and type of syringe (may need to dose in aliquots owing to the large volume).
7. Finally, flush the tube with the recommended volume of water.
8. Do not restart feed for at least 2 hours.

Jejunal administration

Absorption is exceptionally poor via the jejunal route; plasma concentration should be monitored closely if this route is used.

Follow the procedure above for administration; dilution of the suspension is important as phenytoin suspension is hyperosmolar and may cause diarrhoea when administered into the jejunum.

References

1. *BNF 50*, September 2005.
2. BPNG data on file, 2004.
3. Dollery C. *Therapeutic Drugs*, 2nd edn. London: Churchill Livingstone; 1998.
4. Bauer LA Interference of oral phenytoin absorption by continuous nasogastric feedings. *Neurology*. 1982; 32: 570–572.
5. Ozuna J, Friel P. Effect of enteral tube feeding on serum phenytoin levels. *Neurosurg Nursing*. 1984; 16(6): 289–291.
6. Doak KK, Haas CE, Dunnigan KJ, *et al.* Bioavailability of phenytoin acid and phenytoin sodium with enteral feedings. *Pharmacotherapy*. 1998; 18(31): 637–645.
7. Rodman DP, Stevenson TL, Ray TR. Phenytoin malabsorption after jejunostomy tube delivery. *Pharmacotherapy*. 1995; 15(6): 801–805.
8. Stockley IH. *Drug Interactions*, 4th edn. London: Pharmaceutical Press; 1996.
9. Epanutin Ready Mixed Parenteral (Parke-Davis), Summary of Product Characteristics; November 2001.
10. Epanutin Suspension (Parke-Davis), Summary of Product Characteristics; June 2003.
11. BPNG data on file, 2005.
12. Boullata JI, Armenti VT, eds. *Handbook of Drug–Nutrient Interactions*. Totowa, NJ: Humana Press; 2004.

Piroxicam

Formulations available[1]

Brand name (Manufacturer)	Formulation and strength	Product information/Administration information
Feldene (Pfizer)	Capsules 10 mg, 20 mg	No specific data on enteral tube administration are available for this formulation.
Feldene Melt (Pfizer)	Orodispersible tablet 20 mg	No specific data on enteral tube administration are available for this formulation.
Feldene (Pfizer)	Dispersible tablets 10 mg, 20 mg	Recommended to be dispersed in 50 mL of water.[2]
Feldene (Pfizer)	Injection 20 mg/mL (1 mL)	I.m. injection. Piroxicam betadex. No specific data on enteral tube administration are available for this formulation.
Brexidol (Trinity)	Tablets 20 mg	No specific data on enteral tube administration are available for this formulation.
Piroxicam (various manufacturers)	Capsules 10 mg, 20 mg	Alpharma recommends that the capsules are not opened.[3]
Piroxicam (Generics)	Dispersible tablets 10 mg	No specific data on enteral tube administration are available for this formulation.

Site of absorption (oral administration)

Specific site of absorption is not documented. Piroxicam is readily absorbed following oral or rectal absorption.[4]

Alternative routes available

Parenteral route is available.

Interactions

Absorption is unaffected by food.[4]

Health and safety

Standard precautions apply.

Suggestions/recommendations

- Use dispersible tablets for enteral administration. If a change in therapy is required, consider using diclofenac. Administering the dose as recommended will require a significant quantity of water.
- A prolonged break in feeding is not required.

Intragastric administration

1. Stop the enteral feed.
2. Flush the enteral feeding tube with the recommended volume of water.
3. Place the tablet in the barrel of an appropriate type of 50 mL syringe.
4. Draw 50 mL of water into the syringe and allow the tablet to disperse.
5. Flush the medication dose down the feeding tube.
6. Finally, flush with the recommended volume of water.
7. Re-start the feed, unless a prolonged break is required.

Alternatively, at step (3) place the tablet into a medicine pot, add 10 mL of water and allow the tablet to disperse. Draw this into an appropriate syringe. Ensure that the measure is rinsed and that this rinsing water is administered also to ensure that the total dose is given.

Intrajejunal administration

There are no specific data relating to the jejunal administration of piroxicam. Administer the dose as above. Monitor for loss of efficacy or side-effects.

References

1. *BNF* 50, September 2005.
2. Personal communication, Pfizer Ltd; 23 June 2003.
3. Personal communication, Alpharma; 21 January 2003.
4. Dollery C. *Therapeutic Drugs*, 2nd edn. London: Churchill Livingstone; 1998.

Pizotifen

Formulations available[1]

Brand name (Manufacturer)	Formulation and strength	Product information/Administration information
Pizotifen (Alpharma, APS, IVAX)	Tablets 500 microgram, 1.5 mg	As the hydrogen malate. Sugar-coated to mask taste; liquid preparation recommended.[2]
Sanomigran (Novartis)	Tablets 500 microgram, 1.5 mg	As the hydrogen malate. Sugar-coated tablets. No specific data on enteral tube administration are available for this formulation.
Sanomigran (Novartis)	Elixir 250 microgram/5 mL	As the hydrogen malate. Does not contain sorbitol.[3]

Site of absorption (oral administration)

Specific site of absorption is not documented. Absorption following oral administration is rapid.[3]

Alternative routes available

None available for pizotifen.

Interactions

There is no documented interaction with food.[3]

Health and safety

Standard precautions apply.

Suggestions/recommendations

- Use a liquid preparation via enteral feeding tube.
- A prolonged break in feeding is not required.

Intragastric administration

1. Stop the enteral feed.
2. Flush the enteral feeding tube with the recommended volume of water.
3. Draw the medication solution into an appropriate size and type of syringe.
4. Flush the medication dose down the feeding tube.
5. Finally, flush with the recommended volume of water.
6. Re-start the feed, unless a prolonged break is required.

Alternatively, at step (3) measure the medicine in a suitable container and then draw into an appropriate syringe. Ensure that the measure is rinsed and that this rinsing water is administered also to ensure that the total dose is given. **Do not** measure liquid medicines using a catheter-tipped syringe as this results in excessive dosing owing to the volume of the tip.

Intrajejunal administration

There is no specific information on jejunal administration. Administer as above and monitor for loss of efficacy or increased side-effects.

References

1. *BNF* 50, September 2005.
2. Personal communication, Alpharma; 21 January 2003.
3. Sanomigran (Novartis), Summary of Product Characteristics; November 2003.

Potassium

Formulations available[1]

Brand name (Manufacturer)	Formulation and strength	Product information/Administration information
Kay-Cee-L (Geistlich)	Syrup 1 mmol/mL	Potassium chloride. Jejunal administration of Kay-Cee-L has been reported to cause diarrhoea.[2] Contains sorbitol[3] 2 g/5 mL dose.
Kloref (Alpharma)	Tablets 6.7 mmol	Effervescent tablets. Tablets can be dispersed in water for administration via feeding tube but the volume may be too large.[4]

Formulations available[1] (*continued*)

Brand name (Manufacturer)	Formulation and strength	Product information/Administration information
Sando K (HK Pharma)	Tablets 12 mmol	Effervescent tablets. 12 mmol potassium; 8 mmol chloride.
Slow-K (Alliance)	Tablets 8 mmol	Modified-release preparation. Do not crush. Not suitable for administration via enteral feeding tube.

Site of absorption (oral administration)

Potassium chloride is readily absorbed from the GI tract and rapidly distributed.

Alternative routes available

Parenteral potassium can be used for acute replacement. Concentration and infusion rate should be according to local practice.

Interactions

There is the potential for a physical interaction between the potassium supplement and the enteral feed if the supplement is not sufficiently dilute. This may result in coagulation of the feed. Ensure that the tube is flushed well before and after dosing to ensure that feed does not come into contact with the supplement.

Health and safety

Standard precautions apply.

Suggestions/recommendations

- Sando K tablets and Kloref tablets can be used via feeding tubes. They should be dissolved in a sufficient volume of water to reduce osmotic and irritant effects (50–100 mL).
- Kay-Cee-L liquid can be used but must be diluted with 50–100 mL of water as it is very concentrated. Kay-Cee-L also contains sorbitol: large doses may exacerbate diarrhoea.

Intragastric administration

1. Stop the enteral feed.
2. Flush the enteral feeding tube with the recommended volume of water.
3. Measure 50 mL of water into a measuring pot (a smaller volume may be used in fluid-restricted patients).
4. Add the effervescent tablet and allow to dissolve.
5. Draw into an appropriate size and type of syringe.
6. Flush the medication dose down the feeding tube.
7. Rinse the measure and administer this also to ensure that the total dose is given.
8. Finally, flush with the recommended volume of water.
9. Re-start the feed, unless a prolonged break is required.

Intrajejunal administration

See note above regarding use of Kay-Cee-L syrup. Administer dispersible tablets using the above method. Monitor for increased gastrointestinal side-effects.

References

1. *BNF* 50, September 2005.
2. Adams D. Administration of drugs through a jejunostomy tube. *Br J Intensive Care.* 1994; 4(1): 10–17.
3. Personal communication, Geistlich; July 2005.
4. Personal communication, Alpharma; 21 November 2002.

Pravastatin sodium

Formulations available[1]

Brand name (Manufacturer)	Formulation and strength	Product information/Administration information
Lipostat (Squibb)	Tablets 10 mg, 20 mg, 40 mg	Uncoated tablets.[2] Pravastatin is very soluble in water (1 : 3)[3] All strengths of tablets do not disperse readily in water, but do disperse within 5 minutes if shaken in 10 mL of water for 5 minutes to give a very fine, pale yellow dispersion that flushes easily down an 8Fr NG tube.[4]
Pravastatin (nonproprietary)	Tablets 10 mg, 20 mg, 40 mg	No specific data relating to the enteral tube administration of these formulations.

Site of absorption (oral administration)

Specific site of absorption is not documented. Absorption is rapid with peak plasma concentrations occurring 1–1.5 hours after dosing.[2]

Alternative routes available

No alternative routes are available for any of the 'statins'.

Interactions

Food reduces the systemic bioavailability of the drug by 35–40%;[5] however, the lipid-lowering effect is unaffected.[2] Peak cholesterol synthesis is influenced by meal intake, hence the recommendation that pravastatin be taken in the evening to coincide with peak cholesterol synthesis activity.[6] However, if patients are on an overnight feed it may be prudent to dose in the morning at the end of the feed regimen.

Health and safety

Standard precautions apply

Suggestions/recommendations

- Disperse tablet in water immediately before administration. No prolonged break in feeding is required. The dose is usually administered at bedtime;[2] see note above.

Intragastric administration

1. Stop the enteral feed.
2. Flush the enteral feeding tube with the recommended volume of water.
3. Place the tablet in the barrel of an appropriate size and type of syringe.
4. Draw 10 mL of water into the syringe and allow the tablet to disperse, shaking if necessary.
5. Flush the medication dose down the feeding tube.
6. Draw another 10 mL of water into the syringe and also flush this via the feeding tube (this will rinse the syringe and ensure that the total dose is administered).
7. Finally, flush with the recommended volume of water.
8. Re-start the feed if necessary.

Alternatively, at step (3) place the tablet into a medicine pot, add 10 mL of water and allow the tablet to disperse. Draw this into an appropriate syringe. Ensure that the measure is rinsed and that this rinsing water is administered also to ensure that the total dose is given.

Intrajejunal administration

No specific data are available, so monitor cholesterol levels and titrate to effect. Administer as above.

References

1. *BNF* 50, September 2005.
2. Lipitor (Bristol-Myers Squibb), Summary of Product Characteristics; April 2003.
3. Personal communication, Bristol-Myers Squibb; 24 January 2003.
4. BPNG Data on File, 2004.
5. Dollery C. *Therapeutic Drugs*, 2nd edn. London: Churchill Livingstone; 1998.
6. Cella LK, Cauter E, Schoeller DA. Effect of meal timing on diurnal rhythm of human cholesterol synthesis. *Am J Physiol*. 1995; 269 (Endocrine Metab. 32): E878–E883.

Prednisolone

Formulations available[1]

Brand name (Manufacturer)	Formulation and strength	Product information/Administration information
Prednisolone (Alpharma, APS, Arrow, Beacon, CP, Hillcross, IVAX)	Tablets 1 mg, 5 mg, 25 mg	Beacon brand 25 mg tablets disperse in water within 2 minutes to give a coarse dispersion that settles quickly but flushes via an 8Fr NG tube without blockage.[2]
Prednisolone (Alpharma, APS, Berk, IVAX, Pfizer)	E/C tablets 2.5 mg, 5 mg	Do not crush tablets. Not suitable for administration via the feeding tube.
Prednisolone (Sovereign)	Soluble tablets 5 mg	Prednisolone sodium phosphate. Tablet dissolves within 2 minutes to give a clear pink solution.[2]

Site of absorption (oral administration)

Specific site of absorption is not documented. Prednisolone is rapidly absorbed with peak plasma concentrations occurring within 1–2 hours.[3]

Alternative routes available

Parenteral prednisolone acetate i.m. injection is available for once- or twice-weekly use. Parenteral hydrocortisone can also be used. Suppositories and enemas are available for treatment of local disease only; although there may be some systemic effect, it is not predictable enough for use as an alternative route.

Interactions

No specific interaction with food is documented.[3]

Health and safety

Standard precautions apply.

Suggestions/recommendations

- Use soluble tablets for enteral tube administration. For doses below 5 mg, dissolve one soluble tablet in 5 mL of water (1 mg/mL) and give the appropriate volume.
- For high doses (> 50 mg), use the 25 mg tablets dispersed in water immediately prior to administration.
- A prolonged break in feeding is not required.
- Prednisolone sodium phosphate is less likely to cause local gastric irritation than is prednisolone alcohol.[3]

Intragastric administration

1. Stop the enteral feed.
2. Flush the enteral feeding tube with the recommended volume of water.
3. Measure a suitable quantity of water into a measuring pot; 20–30 mL should be sufficient for most doses.
4. Add the soluble tablet and allow to dissolve.
5. Draw into an appropriate size and type of syringe.
6. Flush the medication dose down the feeding tube.
7. Rinse the measure and administer this also to ensure that the total dose is given.
8. Finally, flush the enteral feeding tube with the recommended volume of water.
9. Re-start the feed, unless a prolonged break is required.

Intrajejunal administration

There are no specific data relating to jejunal administration of prednisolone but, as there is an enteric coated formulation, it can be assumed that sufficient absorption occurs beyond the stomach, and therefore bioavailability will not be significantly affected by jejunal administration.

Follow the above method.

References

1. *BNF* 50, September 2005.
2. BPNG data on file, 2004.
3. Soluble Prednisolone Tablets 5 mg (Sovereign), Summary of Product Characteristics; June 2003.

Primidone

Formulations available[1]

Brand name (Manufacturer)	Formulation and strength	Product information/Administration information
Mysoline (Acorus)	Tablets 250 mg	Scored. Primidone is poorly soluble in water.[2] Tablets disperse rapidly when placed in 10 mL of water to form a milky dispersion that flushes via an 8Fr NG tube without blockage.[3]
Primidone (specials manufacturers)	Suspension 250 mg/5 mL	Available on request only.

Site of absorption (oral administration)

No specific site is documented. Peak plasma concentration occurs 0.5–7 hours following oral dose.[2, 4]

Alternative routes available

No alternative routes available for primidone.
Parenteral route is available for phenobarbital.

Interactions

No specific interaction with food is documented.[2, 4]

Health and safety

Standard precautions apply.

Suggestions/recommendations

- There are reports in the literature of primidone being administered via enteral feeding tubes in neonates, with no reports of treatment failure.
- Disperse the tablets in water immediately prior to administration.
- A prolonged break in feeding is not required.

Intragastric administration

1. Stop the enteral feed.
2. Flush the enteral feeding tube with the recommended volume of water.
3. Place the tablet in the barrel of an appropriate size and type of syringe.
4. Draw 10 mL of water into the syringe and allow the tablet to disperse, shaking if necessary.
5. Flush the medication dose down the feeding tube.
6. Draw another 10 mL of water into the oral syringe and also flush this via the feeding tube (this will rinse the syringe and ensure that the total dose is administered).
7. Finally, flush with the recommended volume of water.
8. Re-start the feed, unless a prolonged break is required.

Alternatively, at step (3) place the tablet into a medicine pot, add 10 mL of water and allow the tablet to disperse. Draw this into an appropriate syringe. Ensure that the measure is rinsed and that this rinsing water is administered also to ensure that the total dose is given.

Intrajejunal administration

There are no specific data on jejunal administration. Administer using the above method. Monitor for increased side-effects or loss of efficacy.

References

1. *BNF* 50, September 2005.
2. Dollery C. *Therapeutic Drugs*, 2nd edn. London: Churchill Livingstone; 1998.
3. BPNG data on file, 2005.
4. Mysoline (AstraZeneca), Summary of Product Characteristics; October 2001.

Prochlorperazine

Formulations available[1]

Brand name (Manufacturer)	Formulation and strength	Product information/Administration information
Prochlorperazine (Alpharma, APS, Ashbourne, Generics, Hillcross, IVAX)	Tablets 5 mg	Prochlorperazine maleate. Alpharma tablets can be crushed, but alternative formulations are available.[2] APS and Meridian brands of tablets disperse in 10 mL of water within 5 minutes, IVAX brand requires shaking; the resulting fine dispersion flushes via an 8Fr NG tube without blockage.[3]
Stemetil (Castlemead)	Tablets 5 mg, 25 mg	Prochlorperazine maleate. No specific data on enteral tube administration are available for this formulation.
Stemetil (Castlemead)	Syrup 5 mg/mL	Prochlorperazine mesilate. Contains sucrose; does not contain sorbitol.[4] Orange, slightly viscous liquid; some resistance to flushing, mixes well with an equal volume of water.[5]
Stemetil (Castlemead)	Effervescent granules 5 mg/sachet	Prochlorperazine mesilate. No specific data on enteral tube administration are available for this formulation.
Stemetil (Castlemead)	Injection 12.5 mg/mL (1 mL)	Prochlorperazine mesilate. Deep i.m. injection only. No specific data on enteral tube administration are available for this formulation.
Stemetil (Castlemead)	Suppositories 5 mg, 25 mg	Prochlorperazine maleate. Rectal administration.
Buccastem (R&C)	Buccal tablets 3 mg	Prochlorperazine maleate. Buccal administration only.

Site of absorption (oral administration)

Site of absorption is unknown; peak plasma concentration occurs 1.8 hours following oral dosing of Stemetil Syrup.[4]

Alternative routes available

Parenteral (i.m.), buccal and rectal routes are available.

Interactions

No interaction with food has been identified, although pharmacokinetic data on prochlorperazine are lacking.[4,6]

Health and safety

Standard precautions apply.

Suggestions/recommendations

- Use buccal tablets or suppositories rectally where clinically practical.
- Syrup can be used via the feeding tube but should be diluted with an equal quantity of water immediately prior to administration. Effervescent sachets can also be used. If administering via jejunostomy, use tablets dispersed in water or effervescent sachets as these have a lower osmolarity.
- A prolonged break in feeding is not required.

Intragastric administration

Liquid preparation

1. Stop the enteral feed.
2. Flush the enteral feeding tube with the recommended volume of water.
3. Draw the medication liquid into an appropriate size and type of syringe.
4. Draw an equal volume of water and a little air into the syringe and shake to mix thoroughly.
5. Flush the medication dose down the feeding tube.
6. Draw an equal volume of water into the syringe and also flush this via the feeding tube (this will rinse the syringe and ensure that the total dose is administered).
7. Finally, flush with the recommended volume of water.
8. Re-start the feed, unless a prolonged break is required.

Alternatively, at step (3) measure the medicine in a suitable container and then add an equal volume of water and mix thoroughly. Draw this into an appropriate syringe. Ensure that the measure is rinsed and that this rinsing water is administered also to ensure that the total dose is given. **Do not** measure liquid medicines using a catheter-tipped syringe as this results in excessive dosing owing to the volume of the tip.

Intrajejunal administration

Tablets

1. Stop the enteral feed.
2. Flush the enteral feeding tube with the recommended volume of water.
3. Place the tablet in the barrel of an appropriate size and type of syringe.
4. Draw 10 mL of water into the syringe and allow the tablet to disperse, shaking if necessary.
5. Flush the medication dose down the feeding tube.
6. Draw another 10 mL of water into the syringe and also flush this via the feeding tube (this will rinse the syringe and ensure that the total dose is administered).
7. Finally, flush with the recommended volume of water.
8. Re-start the feed, unless a prolonged break is required.

Alternatively, at step (3) place the tablet into a medicine pot, add 10 mL of water and allow the tablet to disperse. Draw this into an appropriate syringe. Ensure that the measure is rinsed and that this rinsing water is administered also to ensure that the total dose is given.

References

1. *BNF 50*, September 2005.
2. Personal communication, Alpharma; 21 January 2003.
3. BPNG data on file, 2004.
4. Stemetil Syrup (Castlemead), Summary of Product Characteristics; July 2002.
5. BPNG data on file, 2005.
6. Dollery C. *Therapeutic Drugs*, 2nd edn. London: Churchill Livingstone; 1998.

Procyclidine hydrochloride

Formulations available[1]

Brand name (Manufacturer)	Formulation and strength	Product information/Administration information
Procyclidine (Alpharma, APS, Opus)	Tablets 5 mg	No specific data on enteral tube administration are available for this formulation.
Arpicolin (Rosemont)	Syrup 2.5 mg/5 mL, 5 mg/5 mL	Does not contain sorbitol. Clear nonviscous liquid. Flushes easily via tube without further dilution. Mixes with water if needed.[2]
Kemadrin (GSK)	Tablets 5 mg	Scored. GSK has no information relating to the administration of Kemadrin via enteral feeding tubes.[3]
Kemadrin (Auden McKenzie)	Injection 5 mg/mL (2 mL)	Administered via i.v. or i.m. routes. Rapid onset of action; licensed for acute dystonic reactions.

Site of absorption (oral administration)

No documented site of absorption.[3] Peak plasma concentration occurs 1–2 hours following oral administration in fasted subjects.[4]

Alternative routes available

Parenteral route is available. Only licensed for acute dystonic reactions.

Interactions

There is no documented interaction with food.

Health and safety

Standard precautions apply.

Suggestions/recommendations

- Use a liquid preparation.
- A prolonged break in feeding is not required.

Intragastric administration

1. Stop the enteral feed.
2. Flush the enteral feeding tube with the recommended volume of water.
3. Draw the medication solution into an appropriate size and type of syringe.
4. Flush the medication dose down the feeding tube.
5. Finally, flush with the recommended volume of water.
6. Re-start the feed, unless a prolonged break is required.

Alternatively, at step (3) measure the medicine in a suitable container and then draw into an appropriate syringe. Ensure that the measure is rinsed and that this rinsing water is administered also to ensure that the total dose is given. **Do not** measure liquid medicines using a catheter-tipped syringe as this results in excessive dosing owing to the volume of the tip.

Intrajejunal administration

No specific data are available relating to jejunal administration. Administer using the above method. Monitor for increased side-effects or loss of efficacy.

References

1. *BNF 50*, September 2005.
2. BPNG data on file, 2005.
3. Personal communication, GSK; 22 January 2003.
4. Dollery C. *Therapeutic Drugs*, 2nd edn. London: Churchill Livingstone; 1998.

Promethazine hydrochloride

Formulations available[1]

Brand name (Manufacturer)	Formulation and strength	Product information/Administration information
Phenergan (Rhône-Poulenc Rorer)	Tablets 10 mg, 25 mg	Tablets do not disperse readily in water, but will disintegrate if shaken in water for 5 minutes; the resulting dispersion flushes via an 8Fr NG tube without blockage.[2]

Formulations available [1] (continued)

Brand name (Manufacturer)	Formulation and strength	Product information/Administration information
Phenergan (Rhône-Poulenc Rorer)	Elixir 5 mg/5 mL	Pale orange liquid, slightly viscous with some resistance to flushing. Mixes easily with an equal volume of water to reduce viscosity and resistance to flushing. [2] Contains glucose syrup; does not contain sorbitol. [3]
Phenergan (Rhône-Poulenc Rorer)	Injection 25 mg/mL (1 mL)	For use as slow i.v. infusion or deep i.m. injection.

Site of absorption (oral administration)

No specific site is documented. [4] Peak plasma concentration occurs 2–3 hours following oral administration. [5]

Alternative routes available

Injection is available for parenteral administration.

Interactions

No specific interaction with food is documented. [5]

Health and safety

Standard precautions apply.

Suggestions/recommendations

- Use the liquid preparation; no further dilution is necessary for intragastric administration.
- Dilute the liquid with at least an equal volume of water prior to intrajejunal administration.
- A prolonged break in feeding is not required.

Intragastric administration

1. Stop the enteral feed.
2. Flush the enteral feeding tube with the recommended volume of water.
3. Draw the medication solution into an appropriate size and type of syringe.
4. Flush the medication dose down the feeding tube.
5. Finally, flush with the recommended volume of water.
6. Re-start the feed, unless a prolonged break is required.

Alternatively, at step (3) measure the medicine in a suitable container and then draw into an appropriate syringe. Ensure that the measure is rinsed and that this rinsing water is administered also to ensure that the total dose is given. **Do not** measure liquid medicines using a catheter-tipped syringe as this results in excessive dosing owing to the volume of the tip.

Intrajejunal administration

1. Stop the enteral feed.
2. Flush the enteral feeding tube with the recommended volume of water.
3. Draw the medication liquid into an appropriate size and type of syringe.
4. Draw an equal volume of water and a little air into the syringe and shake to mix thoroughly.
5. Flush the medication dose down the feeding tube.
6. Finally, flush with the recommended volume of water.
7. Re-start the feed, unless a prolonged break is required.

Alternatively, at step (3) measure the medicine in a suitable container and then add an equal volume of water and mix thoroughly. Draw this into an appropriate syringe. Ensure that the measure is rinsed and that this rinsing water is administered also to ensure that the total dose is given. **Do not** measure liquid medicines using a catheter-tipped syringe as this results in excessive dosing owing to the volume of the tip.

References

1. *BNF* 50, September 2005.
2. BPNG data on file, 2005.
3. Phenergan (RPR), Summary of Product Characteristics; April 2002.
4. Personal communication, Aventis Pharma; 13 February 2003.
5. Dollery C. *Therapeutic Drugs*, 2nd edn. London: Churchill Livingstone; 1998.

Propranolol hydrochloride

Formulations available[1]

Brand name (Manufacturer)	Formulation and strength	Product information/Administration information
Inderal (AstraZeneca)	Tablets 10 mg, 40 mg, 80 mg	Tablets are very slow to disperse in water: 10 mg tablet takes 5 minutes to disperse in 10 mL water when shaken continuously.[3]
Inderal (AstraZeneca)	Injection 1 mg/mL (1 mL)	No specific data on enteral tube administration are available for this formulation.
Syprol (Rosemont)	Oral solution 5 mg/5 mL, 10 mg/5 mL, 50 mg/5 mL	5 mg/5 mL and 10 mg/5 mL are clear liquids. 50 mg/5 mL is an orange liquid. Does not contain sorbitol. Contains maltitol.[4] 50 mg/5 mL is an orange, slightly viscous liquid; there is some resistance when flushed via an 8Fr NG tube; the liquid mixes well with an equal volume of water and this reduces the osmolarity and viscosity.[5]
Propranolol (Alpharma, APS, DDSA, Hillcross)	Tablets 10 mg, 40 mg, 80 mg, 160 mg	Alpharma brand is very slow to disperse in water: 10 mg takes 5 minutes to disperse in 10 mL water when shaken continuously.[3] Tablets can be crushed.[6]

Formulations available [1] (continued)

Brand name (Manufacturer)	Formulation and strength	Product information/Administration information
Half-Inderal LA (AstraZeneca)	M/R capsules 80 mg	Swallow whole; do not crush or chew. [1]
Inderal-LA (AstraZeneca)	M/R capsules 160 mg	Swallow whole; do not crush or chew. [1]
Propranolol (APS, Generics, Hillcross, Sandoz, Opus, Tillomed)	M/R capsules 80 mg, 160 mg	Swallow whole; do not crush or chew. [1] (Not all manufacturers make all strengths.)

Site of absorption (oral administration)

Specific site of absorption is not documented. Propranolol is rapidly absorbed with the peak plasma concentration occurring within 1–2 hours. [2]

Alternative routes available

Parenteral route can be used, but is usually reserved for conditions requiring acute beta-blockade. Consult SPC for dosing information.

Interactions

No specific interaction with food is documented.

Health and safety

Standard precautions apply.

Suggestions/recommendations

- As the conventional-release tablets and oral solution of propranolol require twice- to four-times daily administration (depending on indication), consider changing to atenolol (see monograph) to simplify the regimen, if clinically appropriate.
- If continued therapy with propranolol via the feeding tube is indicated, use the appropriate strength of the oral solution; consider mixing with an equal volume of water immediately prior to dosing to reduce viscosity. Flush well before and after dosing.
- If converting from modified-release capsules, give the total daily dose in two to three divided doses.

Intragastric administration

1. Stop the enteral feed.
2. Flush the enteral feeding tube with the recommended volume of water.
3. Shake the medication bottle thoroughly to ensure adequate mixing.
4. Draw the medication suspension into an appropriate size and type of syringe.
5. Draw an equal volume of water and a little air into the syringe and shake to mix thoroughly.
6. Flush the medication dose down the feeding tube.
7. Finally, flush with the recommended volume of water.
8. Re-start the feed.

Alternatively, at step (4) measure the medicine in a suitable container and then add an equal volume of water and mix thoroughly. Draw this into an appropriate syringe. Ensure that the measure is rinsed and that this rinsing water is administered also to ensure that the total dose is given. **Do not** measure liquid medicines using a catheter-tipped syringe as this results in excessive dosing owing to the volume of the tip.

Intrajejunal administration

No specific data are available relating to the jejunal administration of propranolol. Monitor for loss of efficacy. Administer as above.

References

1. *BNF* 50, September 2005.
2. Propranolol Tablets (AstraZeneca), Summary of Product Characteristics; June 2003.
3. BPNG data on file, 2004.
4. Syprol (Rosemont), Summary of Product Characteristics; December 2000.
5. BPNG data on file, 2005.
6. Personal communication, Alpharma; 21 January 2003.

Pyrazinamide

Formulations available[1]

Brand name (Manufacturer)	Formulation and strength	Product information/Administration information
Pyrazinamide (available from IDIS)	Tablets 500 mg	Pharma Wernigerode Brand tested. Tablets do not disperse readily in water; can be crushed and mixed with water.[2]
Pyrazinamide (extemporaneous preparation)	Suspension 100 mg/mL	*Extemporaneous pyrazinamide suspension 100 mg/mL:* Pyrazinamide 500 mg tablets 24 tablets Simple syrup to 120 mL Sixty-day expiry at room temperature or refrigerated.[3]

Site of absorption (oral administration)

Specific site is not documented. Peak plasma concentration occurs 1–2 hours following oral administration.[4]

Alternative routes available

No parenteral route is available for pyrazinamide. Other tuberculosis therapy is available in parenteral form; seek microbiological advice.

Interactions

No interaction documented.[4]

Health and safety

Standard precautions apply.

Suggestions/recommendations

- Obtain a manufactured 'special' or make an extemporaneous suspension. Seek microbiological advice regarding alternative therapy.
- A prolonged break in feeding is not required.

Intragastric administration

Liquid preparation

1. Stop the enteral feed.
2. Flush the enteral feeding tube with the recommended volume of water.
3. Draw medication liquid into appropriate size and type of syringe.
4. Flush the medication dose down the feeding tube.
5. Finally, flush with the recommended volume of water.
6. Re-start the feed, unless a prolonged break is required.

Alternatively, at step (3) measure the medicine in a suitable container and then draw into an appropriate syringe. Ensure that the measure is rinsed and that this rinsing water is administered also to ensure that the total dose is given. **Do not** measure liquid medicines using a catheter-tipped syringe as this results in excessive dosing owing to the volume of the tip.

Intrajejunal administration

Tablet administration (crushing tablets should be considered a last resort)

1. Stop the enteral feed.
2. Flush the enteral feeding tube with the recommended volume of water.
3. Place the tablet in a mortar and crush to a fine powder using the pestle.
4. Add a few millilitres of water and mix until the coating dissolves, to form a paste.
5. Add up to 15 mL of water and mix thoroughly, ensuring that there are no large particles of tablet.
6. Draw this into an appropriate size and type of syringe.
7. Flush the medication dose down the feeding tube.
8. Add another 15 mL of water to the mortar and stir to ensure that any remaining drug is rinsed from the container. Draw this water into the syringe and also flush this via the feeding tube (this will rinse the mortar and syringe and ensure that the total dose is administered).
9. Finally, flush the enteral feeding tube with the recommended volume of water.
10. Re-start the feed, unless a prolonged break is required.

References

1. *BNF 50*, September 2005.
2. BPNG data on file, 2005.
3. Nahata MC, Morosco RS, Peritore SP. Stability of pyrazinamide in two suspensions. *Am J Health Syst Pharm*. 1995; 52: 1558–1560.
4. Dollery C. *Therapeutic Drugs*, 2nd edn. London: Churchill Livingstone; 1998.

Pyridoxine hydrochloride

Formulations available[1]

Brand name (Manufacturer)	Formulation and strength	Product information/Administration information
Pyridoxine (BR, CP, Hillcross)	Tablets 10 mg, 20 mg, 50 mg	CP brand tablets disintegrate within 5 minutes when placed in 10 mL of water but give a very coarse dispersion that is difficult to draw up. When crushed, the powder mixes with water but settles quickly, with risk of leaving some of the dose in the container if it is not rinsed thoroughly.[2]

Site of absorption (oral administration)

Specific site of absorption is not documented. Pyridoxine is readily absorbed from the GI tract.[3]

Alternative routes available

Pabrinex injection contains 50 mg pyridoxine (see Thiamine monograph).

Interactions

No specific interaction.

Health and safety

Standard precautions apply.

Suggestions/recommendations

- Nutritionally complete enteral feeds will contain some pyridoxine. Additional doses should only be used when additional supplementation is required.
- The tablets can be crushed and mixed with water immediately prior to administration.
- A prolonged break in feeding is not required.

Intragastric administration

1. Stop the enteral feed.
2. Flush the enteral feeding tube with the recommended volume of water.
3. Place the tablet in a mortar and crush to a fine powder using the pestle.
4. Add a few millilitres of water and mix to form a paste.
5. Add up to 15 mL of water and mix thoroughly ensuring that there are no large particles of tablet.
6. Draw this into an appropriate syringe.
7. Flush the medication dose down the feeding tube.
8. Add another 15 mL of water to the mortar and stir to ensure that any remaining drug is rinsed from the container. Draw this water into the syringe and also flush this via the feeding tube (this will rinse the mortar and syringe and ensure that the total dose is administered).
9. Finally, flush the enteral feeding tube with the recommended volume of water.
10. Re-start the feed, unless a prolonged break is required.

Intrajejunal administration

Intrajejunal administration should not reduce the bioavailability of pyridoxine. Administer using the above method.

References

1. *BNF* 50, September 2005.
2. BPNG data on file, 2004.
3. Dollery C. *Therapeutic Drugs*, 2nd edn. London: Churchill Livingstone; 1998.

Pyrimethamine

Formulations available[1]

Brand name (Manufacturer)	Formulation and strength	Product information/Administration information
Daraprim (GSK)	Tablets 25 mg	Roche has no data to support the administration of Daraprim via enteral feeding tubes.[2]

Site of absorption (oral administration)

Specific site of absorption is not documented. Peak plasma concentration occurs 2–4 hours following oral administration.[3]

Alternative routes available

None available for daraprim.

Interactions

No specific interaction with food is documented. In-vitro data suggests that absorption may be decreased by antacid salts.[3]

Health and safety

Standard precautions apply.

Suggestions/recommendations

- Seek specialist advice concerning alternative therapy.

References

1. *BNF* 50, September 2005.
2. Personal communication, GSK; 22 January 2003.
3. Daraprim (GSK), Summary of Product Characteristics; July 2003.

Quinapril

Formulations available[1]

Brand name (Manufacturer)	Formulation and strength	Product information/Administration information
Accupro (Parke-Davis)	Tablets 5 mg, 10 mg, 20 mg, 40 mg	Film-coated tablets.[1] Solubility in water > 1 : 10.[2] No specific data on enteral tube administration are available for this formulation.
Accuretic (Parke-Davis)	Tablets Quinapril 10 mg, hydrochlorothiazide 12.5 mg	Film coated tablets.[1] No specific data on enteral tube administration are available for this formulation.
Quinapril (nonproprietary)	Tablets 5 mg, 10 mg, 20 mg, 40 mg	Quinapril hydrochloride. No specific data on enteral tube administration are available for this formulation.

Site of absorption (oral administration)

Specific site of absorption is not documented. Peak plasma concentrations occur within 1 hour.[3]

Alternative routes available

None available.

Interactions

The extent of absorption is not influenced by food,[2] but peak plasma concentration may be delayed by approximately 30 minutes.[2]

Health and safety

Standard precautions apply.

Suggestions/recommendations

- Owing to lack of data, consider changing to an alternative ACE inhibitor for administration via an enteral feeding tube.

References

1. *BNF 50*, September 2005.
2. Dollery C. *Therapeutic Drugs*, 2nd edn. London: Churchill Livingstone; 1998.
3. Accupro (Pfizer), Summary of Product Characteristics; September 2003.

Rabeprazole sodium

Formulations available[1]

Brand name (Manufacturer)	Formulation and strength	Product information/Administration information
Pariet (Eisai)	Tablet 10 mg, 20 mg	Gastro-resistant coating[2]. Rabeprazole is acid-labile and therefore tablets should not be crushed. [3]

Site of absorption (oral administration)

Rabeprazole absorption occurs in the small bowel, the formulation is enteric coated.[2] Peak plasma concentration occurs 3.5 hours after oral dosing.

Alternative routes available

Parenteral route is not available for rabeprazole, parenteral route is available for esomeprazole, omeprazole and pantoprazole.

Interactions

Absorption is unaffected by food.[2]

Health and safety

Standard precautions apply.

Suggestions/recommendations

- No suitable formulation is available for administration via an enteral feeding tube; consider using omeprazole or pantoprazole parenterally or use lansoprazole or omeprazole (see monographs).
- Alternatively, ranitidine may be used if a step-down approach is appropriate (see monograph).

References

1. *BNF* 50, September 2005.
2. Pariet (Eisai), Summary of Product Characteristics; July 2003.
3. Personal Communication, Eisai Ltd; 15 January 2003.

Ramipril

Formulations available[1]

Brand name (Manufacturer)	Formulation and strength	Product information/Administration information
Tritace (Aventis)	Tablets 1.25 mg, 2.5 mg, 5 mg, 10 mg	Tablets disperse quickly (2–5 minutes) in water to give a fine dispersion that settles quickly but draws up and flushes easily down an 8Fr NG tube.[3] Ramipril has poor solubility in water.[6]

Formulations available[1] (*continued*)

Brand name (Manufacturer)	Formulation and strength	Product information/Administration information
Tritace Titration Pack (Aventis)	Capsules 2.5 mg, 5 mg, 10 mg	Anecdotal data suggest that Tritace capsules can be opened and the contents dissolved in water or placed directly into the mouth or on bread. The contents of the capsule are reportedly unpleasant.[4]
Ramipril (various manufacturers)	Capsules 2.5 mg, 5 mg, 10 mg	No specific data on enteral administration are available for this formulation.
Triapin (Aventis)	Tablets Ramipril 2.5 mg/felodipine 2.5 mg, Ramipril 5 mg/felodipine 5 mg	Combination product. Modified release,; tablets must not be divided, crushed or chewed.[5] Unsuitable for enteral tube administration.

Site of absorption (oral administration)

Specific site of absorption is not documented. Peak plasma concentration of ramipril occurs within 1 hour of oral dosing.[2]

Alternative routes available

No alternative route is available for any of the ACE inhibitors.

Interactions

Delay in absorption by food is small and clinically unimportant.[6]

Health and safety

Standard precautions apply.

Suggestions/recommendations

- Reduce dosing frequency to once daily where possible. Ramipril is licensed for once-daily dosing for all indications with the exception of prophylaxis after myocardial infarction.[1]
- Disperse the tablets in water immediately prior to administration.
- A prolonged break in feeding is not required.

Intragastric administration

1. Stop the enteral feed.
2. Flush the enteral feeding tube with the recommended volume of water.
3. Place the tablet in the barrel of an appropriate size and type of syringe.
4. Draw 10 mL of water into the syringe and allow the tablet to disperse, shaking if necessary.
5. Flush the medication dose down the feeding tube.
6. Draw another 10 mL of water into the syringe and also flush this via the feeding tube (this will rinse the syringe and ensure that the total dose is administered).
7. Finally, flush with the recommended volume of water.
8. Re-start the feed, unless a prolonged break is required.

Alternatively, at step (3) place the tablet into a medicine pot, add 10 mL of water and allow the tablet to disperse. Draw this into an appropriate syringe. Ensure that the measure is rinsed and that this rinsing water is administered also to ensure that the total dose is given.

Intrajejunal administration

There is no specific information relating to jejunal administration. Monitor for loss of therapeutic effect. Administer as above.

References

1. *BNF 50*, September 2005.
2. Tritace Tablets (Aventis), Summary of Product Characteristics; September 2003.
3. BPNG data on file, 2004.
4. Personal communication, Aventis Pharma; 2 January 2003.
5. Triapin & Triapin Mite (Aventis), Summary of Product Characteristics; April 2002.
6. Dollery C. *Therapeutic Drugs*, 2nd edn. London: Churchill Livingstone; 1998.

Ranitidine hydrochloride

Formulations available[1]

Brand name (Manufacturer)	Formulation and strength	Product information/Administration information
Zantac (GSK)	Tablets 150 mg, 300 mg	Tablets do not disperse readily in water.[4]
Zantac (GSK)	Effervescent tablets 150 mg, 300 mg	150 mg tablet contains 14.3 mmol sodium/tablet.[1] 300 mg tablet contains 20.8 mmol sodium/tablet.[1]
Zantac (GSK)	Syrup 75 mg/5 mL	Contains alcohol 8%. Contains sorbitol.[2]
Zantac (GSK)	Injection 25 mg/mL	Can be administered enterally.[3]
Ranitidine (Rosemont)	Oral solution 75 mg/5 mL	Contains alcohol 8%. Contains sorbitol 0.7 g/5 mL.[5] Clear, nonviscous liquid; flushes easily via a fine-bore tube without resistance.[4]
Ranitidine (Lagap)	Effervescent tablets 150 mg, 300 mg	Dissolves completely in 10 mL of water. Contains ~ 5 mmol sodium in 150 mg tablet.[4]
Ranitidine (Alpharma, Ratiopharm, Sandoz)	Effervescent tablets 150 mg, 300 mg	Alpharma and Ratiopharm brands contain 5 mmol sodium in 150 mg tablet and 10 mmol sodium in 300 mg tablet.
Ranitidine (Alpharma, APS, Ashbourne, Berk, CP, Generics, Genus, Goldshield, Hillcross, IVAX, PLIVA, Ranbaxy, Sovereign, Sterwin, Tillomed)	Tablets 150 mg, 300 mg	No specific data on enteral tube administration are available for these formulations.

Site of absorption (oral administration)

There is minimal absorption of ranitidine from the stomach; it is predominantly absorbed in the duodenojejunal and distal jejunal areas.[3]

Alternative routes available

Injection is available for parenteral administration.

Interactions

Bioavailability of ranitidine is not affected by food.[2]

Health and safety

Standard precautions apply.

Suggestions/recommendations

- Use ranitidine effervescent tablets as first choice, unless sodium restriction is necessary.
- Liquid preparation can also be used for gastric administration.

Intragastric administration

Effervescent tablets

1. Stop the enteral feed.
2. Flush the enteral feeding tube with the recommended volume of water.
3. Measure 20–30 mL of water into a suitable container.
4. Add the effervescent tablet and allow to dissolve.
5. Draw into an appropriate size and type of syringe.
6. Flush the medication dose down the feeding tube.
7. Rinse the measure and administer this also to ensure that the total dose is given.
8. Finally, flush with the recommended volume of water.
9. Re-start the feed, unless a prolonged break is required.

Liquid preparation

1. Stop the enteral feed.
2. Flush the enteral feeding tube with the recommended volume of water.
3. Draw the medication solution into an appropriate size and type of syringe.
4. Flush the medication dose down the feeding tube.
5. Finally, flush with the recommended volume of water.
6. Re-start the feed, unless a prolonged break is required.

Alternatively, at step (3) measure the medicine in a suitable container and then draw into an appropriate syringe. Ensure that the measure is rinsed and that this rinsing water is administered also to ensure that the total dose is given. **Do not** measure liquid medicines using a catheter-tipped syringe as this results in excessive dosing owing to the volume of the tip.

Intrajejunal administration

Ranitidine is well absorbed following jejunal administration; however, the effervescent tablets or injection should be used for this route as the osmolarity of the liquid preparation is likely to be too high.[3, 6] Administer using the above method.

References

1. *BNF* 50, September 2005.
2. Zantac (GSK), Summary of Product Characteristics; January 2003.
3. Personal communication, GSK; 22 January 2003.
4. BPNG data on file, 2004/2005.
5. Personal communication, Rosemont Pharma; 20 January 2005.
6. Adams D. Administration of drugs through a jejunostomy tube. *Br J Intensive Care.* 1994; 4(1): 10–17.

Reboxetine

Formulations available [1]

Brand name (Manufacturer)	Formulation and strength	Product information/Administration information
Edronax (Pharmacia)	Tablets 4 mg	Scored. Reboxetine mesilate. [2] Tablets can be crushed and dispersed in water. There are no stability data and therefore this should be done immediately prior to dosing. [3]

Site of absorption (oral administration)

Site of absorption is not documented. Peak plasma concentration occurs 2 hours following oral dosing. [2]

Alternative routes available

None available for reboxetine.

Interactions

Food intake delayed the absorption of reboxetine but did not significantly influence the extent of absorption. [2]

Health and safety

Standard precautions apply.

Suggestions/recommendations

- Owing to the limited amount of data, consideration should be given to alternative therapy.
- If continued therapy with reboxetine is indicated, the tablets can be crushed and suspended in water immediately prior to dosing.
- A prolonged break in feeding is not necessary.

Intragastric administration

1. Stop the enteral feed.
2. Flush the enteral feeding tube with the recommended volume of water.
3. Place the tablet in a mortar and crush to a fine powder using the pestle.
4. Add a few millilitres of water and mix to form a paste.
5. Add up to 15 mL of water and mix thoroughly, ensuring that there are no large particles of tablet.
6. Draw this into an appropriate size and type of syringe.
7. Flush the medication dose down the feeding tube.
8. Add another 15 mL of water to the mortar and stir to ensure that any remaining drug is rinsed from the container. Draw this water into the syringe and also flush this via the feeding tube (this will rinse the mortar and syringe and ensure total dose is administered).
9. Finally, flush the enteral feeding tube with the recommended volume of water.
10. Re-start the feed, unless a prolonged break is required.

Intrajejunal administration

There are no specific data relating to the jejunal administration of reboxetine. Administer as above and monitor for loss of efficacy or increased side-effects.

References

1. *BNF* 50, September 2005.
2. Edronax (Pharmacia), Summary of Product Characteristics; September 2004.
3. Personal communication, Pharmacia; 11 March 2003.

Rifabutin

Formulations available[1]

Brand name (Manufacturer)	Formulation and strength	Product information/Administration information
Mycobutin (Pharmacia)	Capsules 150 mg	Pharmacia has anecdotal reports of the capsules being opened and mixed with a small quantity of water immediately prior to administration.[2]
Mycobutin (extemporaneous preparation)	Suspension	*Extemporaneous rifabutin solution 20 mg/mL:* Rifabutin 150 mg capsules 16 capsules Cherry syrup to 120 mL Store in a refrigerator; 84 days' shelf life.[3]

Site of absorption (oral administration)

Specific site of absorption is not documented. Peak plasma concentration occurs 2–4 hours following oral dosing.[4]

Alternative routes available

No alternative available for rifabutin.

Interactions

There is no specific documented interaction with food.

Health and safety

Minimise exposure to drug powder. Standard precautions apply.

Suggestions/recommendations

- Disperse the contents of the capsules in water immediately prior to administration.
- Alternatively, an extemporaneous suspension can be prepared.
- A prolonged break in feeding is not required.

Intragastric administration

Where possible use extemporaneous preparation to minimise operator exposure to antibiotic powder.

Suspension

1. Stop the enteral feed.
2. Flush the enteral feeding tube with the recommended volume of water.
3. Shake the medication bottle thoroughly to ensure adequate mixing.
4. Draw the medication suspension into an appropriate size and type of syringe.
5. Draw an equal volume of water and a little air into the syringe and shake to mix thoroughly.
6. Flush the medication dose down the feeding tube.
7. Finally, flush with the recommended volume of water.
8. Re-start the feed, unless a prolonged break is required.

Alternatively, at step (4) measure the medicine in a suitable container and then add an equal volume of water and mix thoroughly. Draw this into an appropriate syringe. Ensure that the measure is rinsed and that this rinsing water is administered also to ensure that the total dose is given. **Do not** measure liquid medicines using a catheter-tipped syringe as this results in excessive dosing owing to the volume of the tip.

Intrajejunal administration

Capsule contents dispersed in water have a lower osmolarity than the syrup formulation. However, the practicalities of opening the capsules should be borne in mind.

1. Stop the enteral feed.
2. Flush the enteral feeding tube with the recommended volume of water.
3. Open the capsule and pour the contents into a medicine pot.
4. Add 15 mL of water.
5. Stir to disperse the powder.
6. Draw into an appropriate syringe and administer via the feeding tube.
7. Add a further 15 mL of water to the medicine pot; stir to ensure that any powder remaining in the pot is mixed with water.
8. Draw up this dispersion and flush down the tube. This will ensure that the whole dose is given.
9. Flush the tube with water.

References

1. *BNF 50*, September 2005.
2. Personal communication, Alpharma; 21 January 2003.
3. Haslam JL, Egodage KL, Chen Y, Rajewski RA, Stella V. Stability of rifabutin in two extemporaneously compounded oral liquids. *Am J Health Syst Pharm.* 1999; 56: 333–336.
4. Mycobutin (Pharmacia), Summary of Product Characteristics; January 2003.

Rifampicin

Formulations available[1]

Brand name (Manufacturer)	Formulation and strength	Product information/Administration information
Rifampicin (Generics)	Capsules 150 mg, 300 mg	Do not open, see below.
Rifadin (Aventis Pharma)	Capsules 150 mg, 300 mg	Do not open, see below.
Rifadin (Aventis Pharma)	Syrup 100 mg/5 mL	pH 4.5–4.8.[2] Syrup contains sucrose; does not contain sorbitol.[3] Dark red opaque liquid. Some resistance to flushing via an 8Fr NG tube; mixes easily with water.[4]
Rifadin (Aventis Pharma)	Infusion 600 mg	Serum concentrations following infusion are comparable to those achieved following oral administration of the same dose.[5]
Rimactane (Sandoz)	Capsules 150 mg, 300 mg	Do not open, see below.

Site of absorption (oral administration)

Specific site of absorption is not documented.

Alternative routes available

Rifampicin can be given parenterally as an i.v infusion. The dose remains the same.

Interactions

Optimal absorption of rifampicin is achieved if the dose is given 30 minutes before food or 2 hours after.[3]

Health and safety

Do not open capsules owing to the risk of contact sensitisation.

Suggestions/recommendations

- Use the liquid preparation.
- Stop feed at least 2 hours before the dose; do not re-start feed for 30 minutes after dose.

Intragastric administration

1. Stop the enteral feed.
2. Flush the enteral feeding tube with the recommended volume of water.
3. Wait for 2 hours before administering dose.
4. Shake the medication bottle thoroughly to ensure adequate mixing.
5. Draw the medication suspension into an appropriate size and type of syringe.
6. Draw an equal volume of water and a little air into the syringe and shake to mix thoroughly.
7. Flush the medication dose down the feeding tube.
8. Finally, flush with the recommended volume of water.
9. Re-start the feed, unless a prolonged break is required.

Alternatively, at step (4) measure the medicine in a suitable container and then add an equal volume of water and mix thoroughly. Draw this into an appropriate syringe. Ensure that the measure is rinsed and that this rinsing water is administered also to ensure that the total dose is given. **Do not** measure liquid medicines using a catheter-tipped syringe as this results in excessive dosing owing to the volume of the tip.

Jejunal administration

Administer using the above method. Monitor for decreased plasma concentration.

References

1. *BNF* 50, September 2005.
2. Personal communication, Aventis; 2 January 2003.
3. Rifadin (Aventis), Summary of Product Characteristics; February 2000.
4. BPNG data on file, 2005.
5. Rifadin for Infusion (Aventis), Summary of Product Characteristics; April 2003.

Riluzole

Formulations available[1]

Brand name (Manufacturer)	Formulation and strength	Product information/Administration information
Rilutek (Aventis Pharma)	Tablets 50 mg	Film-coated tablets. The manufacturer has anecdotal reports that the tablets can be crushed and mixed with water. The 'suspension' should be administered within 15 minutes.[2]

Site of absorption (oral administration)

Specific site of absorption is unknown. Peak plasma concentration occurs 60–90 minutes following an oral dose.[3]

Alternative routes available

None available for riluzole.

Interactions

Specific interactions with enteral feeds are unknown. The rate and extent of absorption are reduced when riluzole is administered with a high-fat meal, with a decrease in C_{max} of 44% and decrease in AUC of 17%.[4]

Health and safety

Standard precautions apply.

Suggestions/recommendations

- Owing to the limited data available, consider alternative therapy.
- If enteral administration of riluzole is indicated, crush the tablets and disperse in water immediately prior to administration.

Intragastric administration

1. Stop the enteral feed.
2. Flush the enteral feeding tube with the recommended volume of water.
3. Place the tablet in a mortar and crush to a fine powder using the pestle.
4. Add a few millilitres of water and mix to form a paste.
5. Add up to 15 mL of water and mix thoroughly, ensuring that there are no large particles of tablet.
6. Draw this into an appropriate size and type of syringe.
7. Flush the medication dose down the feeding tube.
8. Add another 15 mL of water to the mortar and stir to ensure that any remaining drug is rinsed from the container. Draw this water into the syringe and also flush this via the feeding tube (this will rinse the mortar and syringe and ensure total dose is administered).
9. Finally, flush the enteral feeding tube with the recommended volume of water.
10. Re-start the feed, unless a prolonged break is required.

Intrajejunal administration

There are no specific data relating to jejunal administration of riluzole. Administer using the above method. Monitor for increased side-effect or loss of efficacy.

References

1. *BNF* 50, September 2005.
2. Personal communication, Procter & Gamble; 22 January 2003.
3. Dollery C. *Therapeutic Drugs*, 2nd edn. London: Churchill Livingstone; 1998.
4. Rilutek (Aventis Pharma), Summary of Product Characteristics; December 2002.

Risedronate sodium

Formulations available[1]

Brand name (Manufacturer)	Formulation and strength	Product information/Administration information
Actonel (Procter & Gamble)	Tablet 5 mg, 30 mg	The manufacturers advise that risedronate should not be administered via a feeding tube owing to the risk of interaction with the feed and the tube.[4] The 30 mg tablets disperse in 10 mL of water within 2 minutes to give a fine dispersion that flushes down an 8Fr NG tube without blockage.[5]
Actonel Once a Week (Procter & Gamble)	Tablet 35 mg	The 35 mg tablets disperse in 10 mL of water within 5 minutes (the coating takes a few minutes to dissolve) to give a very fine dispersion that flushes down an 8Fr NG tube without blockage.[5] In a small retrospective chart review (4 patients), 35 mg risedronate was administered via feeding tubes for an average of 18 months; a reduction in bone turnover markers was noted and there were no reported adverse effects. The authors conclude that alendronate and risedronate delivered through feeding tubes in developmentally disabled patients appear to be well tolerated.[6]

Site of absorption (oral administration)

The site of absorption is mainly the duodenum, jejunum and ileum, although there is some absorption in the stomach.[4] Maximum concentrations occur within 1 hour after oral dosing.[2]

Alternative routes available

None available for risedronate. Alternative bisphosphonates are available in parenteral formulations.

Interactions

Bioavailability is decreased when risedronate is administered with food.[2]

Health and safety

Standard precautions apply.

Suggestions/recommendations

- Risedronate tablets have been dispersed in water and successfully administered via enteral feeding tubes with no loss of drug.[7]
- Risedronate should be used with caution in patients with oesophageal disease. Owing to the risks of oesophageal damage, risedronate should be used with caution via an enteral feeding tube, especially in patients with delayed gastric emptying at risk of oesophageal reflux and in those patients unable to sit or stand upright.
- If risedronate is administered via a feeding tube, the once-weekly preparation should be used, owing to the lower incidence of GI related side-effects.[3] The tablet should be dispersed in 10 mL of water and administered immediately, then flushed with at least 50 mL of water. This should be administered first thing in the morning after rising and the patient should remain sitting upright or standing for 30 minutes after the dose is given. Enteral feed should be stopped 2 hours prior to administration, and should not be re-started for at least 2 hours after the dose.

Intragastric administration

1. Stop the enteral feed.
2. Flush the enteral feeding tube with the recommended volume of water.
3. Wait 2 hours.
4. Place the tablet in the barrel of an appropriate size and type of syringe.
5. Draw 10 mL of water into the syringe and allow the tablet to disperse, shaking if necessary.
6. Flush the medication dose down the feeding tube.
7. Draw another 10 mL of water into the syringe and also flush this via the feeding tube (this will rinse the syringe and ensure that the total dose is administered).
8. Finally, flush with at least 50 mL of water.
9. Ensure that the patient is sitting upright or standing.
10. Re start the feed after at least 2 hours.

Alternatively, at step (4) place the tablet into a medicine pot, add 10 mL of water and allow the tablet to disperse. Draw this into an appropriate syringe. Ensure that the measure is rinsed and that this rinsing water is administered also to ensure that the total dose is given.

Intrajejunal administration

There are no specific data relating to jejunal administration of risedronate. The drug is absorbed throughout the small bowel. Administer using the above method.

References

1. *BNF 50*, September 2005.
2. Actonel 5 mg (Procter & Gamble), Summary of Product Characteristics; September 2002.
3. Actonel Once a Week (Procter & Gamble), Summary of Product Characteristics; January 2003.
4. Personal communication, Procter & Gamble; 22 January 2003.
5. BPNG data on file, 2004.
6. Tanner S, Taylor HM. Feeding tube administration of bisphosphonates for treating osteoporosis in institutionalised patients with developmental disabilities. *Bone*. 2004; 34(Suppl 1): S97–98.
7. Dansereau RJ, Crail DJ. Extemporaneous procedures for dissolving risedronate tablets for oral administration and for feeding tubes. *Ann Pharmacother*. 2005; 39: 63–67.

Risperidone

Formulations available[1]

Brand name (Manufacturer)	Formulation and strength	Product information/Administration information
Risperdal (Janssen-Cilag)	Tablets 500 microgram, 1 mg, 2 mg, 3 mg, 4 mg, 6 mg	Film-coated. Scored. Tablets disintegrate within 5 minutes when placed in water. The resulting dispersion flushes easily via an 8Fr NG tube without blockage.[2]
Risperdal Quicklet (Janssen-Cilag)	Orodispersible tablets 0.5 mg, 1 mg, 2 mg	No specific data on enteral tube administration are available for this formulation.
Risperdal (Janssen-Cilag)	Liquid 1 mg/mL	Clear liquid; draws up and flushes easily down the tube without further dilution.[2] The liquid can be diluted with water immediately prior to administration.[3]
Risperdal Consta (Janssen-Cilag)	Injection 25 mg, 37.5 mg, 50 mg	Deep i.m. injection; injection at 2-week intervals

Site of absorption (oral administration)

Specific site is not documented. Peak plasma concentration occurs 1–2 hours following oral administration.[4]

Alternative routes available

Depot injection is suitable for use in patients on doses above 4 mg daily (see SPC).

Interactions

Absorption is unaffected by food.[4]

Health and safety

Standard precautions apply.

Suggestions/recommendations

- Use the liquid preparation; no further dilution is necessary.
- A prolonged break in feeding is not required.
- Consider changing to depot injection for patients on high doses.

Intragastric administration

1. Stop the enteral feed.
2. Flush the enteral feeding tube with the recommended volume of water.
3. Draw the medication solution into an appropriate size and type of syringe.
4. Flush the medication dose down the feeding tube.
5. Finally, flush with the recommended volume of water.
6. Re-start the feed, unless a prolonged break is required.

Alternatively, at step (3) measure the medicine in a suitable container and then draw into an appropriate syringe. Ensure that the measure is rinsed and that this rinsing water is administered also to ensure that the total dose is given. **Do not** measure liquid medicines using a catheter-tipped syringe as this results in excessive dosing owing to the volume of the tip.

Intrajejunal administration

There are no specific data relating to jejunal administration of risperidone. Administer using the above method. Monitor for loss of efficacy or increased side-effects.

References

1. *BNF* 50, September 2005.
2. BPNG data on file, 2004.
3. Personal communication, Janssen-Cilag; 22 January 2003.
4. Risperdal (Janssen-Cilag), Summary of Product Characteristics; May 2005.

Ropinirole

Formulations available[1]

Brand name (Manufacturer)	Formulation and strength	Product information/Administration information
Requip (GSK)	Tablets 0.25 mg, 0.5 mg, 1 mg, 2 mg, 5 mg	Ropinirole hydrochloride. Tablets disintegrate rapidly when placed in 10 mL of water to give fine dispersion that flushes via an 8Fr NG tube without blockage.[2]

Site of absorption (oral administration)

Specific site is not documented. Peak plasma concentration occurs 1.5 hours after oral dosing.[3]

Alternative routes available

No alternative route available.

Interactions

No specific interaction with food is documented. It is recommended that ropinirole be taken with food to improve GI tolerability.

Health and safety

Standard precautions apply

Suggestions/recommendations

- Disperse the tablets in water immediately prior to administration. A prolonged break in feeding is not required.
- Where practical, administer the dose after feed.

Intragastric administration

1. Stop the enteral feed.
2. Flush the enteral feeding tube with the recommended volume of water.
3. Place the tablet in the barrel of an appropriate size and type of syringe.
4. Draw 10 mL of water into the syringe and allow the tablet to disperse, shaking if necessary.
5. Flush the medication dose down the feeding tube.
6. Draw another 10 mL of water into the syringe and also flush this via the feeding tube (this will rinse the syringe and ensure that the total dose is administered).
7. Finally, flush with the recommended volume of water.
8. Re-start the feed, unless a prolonged break is required.

Alternatively, at step (3) place the tablet into a medicine pot, add 10 mL of water and allow the tablet to disperse. Draw this into an appropriate syringe. Ensure that the measure is rinsed and that this rinsing water is administered also to ensure that the total dose is given.

Intrajejunal administration

There are no specific data relating to jejunal administration of ropinirole. Administer using the above method and monitor for increased side-effects or loss of efficacy.

References

1. *BNF* 50, September 2005.
2. BPNG data on file, 2004.
3. Requip (GSK), Summary of Product Characteristics; August 2002.

Rosiglitazone

Formulations available[1]

Brand name (Manufacturer)	Formulation and strength	Product information/Administration information
Avandia (GSK)	Tablets 4 mg, 8 mg	Rosiglitazone maleate. Film-coated tablet. Pharmacological effect is to increase insulin sensitivity. As rosiglitazone does not cause hypoglycaemia, there is no requirement to take it with food.[2] Tablets disperse in 10 mL of water when shaken for 5 minutes to form a very fine, even dispersion that flushes via an 8Fr NG tube without blockage.[3]
Avandamet (GSK)	Tablets 1 mg + 500 mg, 2 mg + 500 mg, 4 mg + 1 g	Film-coated Rosiglitazone + metformin. No specific data on enteral administration are available for this formulation.

Site of absorption (oral administration)

Specific site of absorption is not documented. Peak plasma concentration occurs 1 hour after oral dosing.[2]

Alternative routes available

None available for rosiglitazone. Insulin is available for parenteral therapy.

Interactions

Absorption is not significantly affected by food.[2]

Health and safety

Standard precautions apply.

Suggestions/recommendations

- Disperse the tablet in water immediately prior to administration.
- The dose can be administered at any time during the day, a prolonged break in feeding is not required, and equally there is no requirement to administer at the same time as the feed.

Intragastric administration

1. Stop the enteral feed.
2. Flush the enteral feeding tube with the recommended volume of water.
3. Place the tablet in the barrel of an appropriate size and type of syringe.
4. Draw 10 mL of water into the syringe and allow the tablet to disperse, shaking if necessary.
5. Flush the medication dose down the feeding tube.
6. Draw another 10 mL of water into the oral syringe and also flush this via the feeding tube (this will rinse the syringe and ensure that the total dose is administered).
7. Finally, flush with the recommended volume of water.
8. Re-start the feed, unless a prolonged break is required.

Alternatively, at step (3) place the tablet into a medicine pot, add 10 mL of water and allow the tablet to disperse. Draw this into an appropriate syringe. Ensure that the measure is rinsed and that this rinsing water is administered also to ensure that the total dose is given.

Intrajejunal administration

There are no specific data relating to jejunal administration of rosiglitazone. Monitor blood sugar levels for loss of glycaemic control. Administer as above.

References

1. *BNF* 50, September 2005.
2. Avandia (GlaxoSmtihKline), Summary of Product Characteristics; September 2004.
3. BPNG data on file, 2004.

Rosuvastatin

Formulations available[1]

Brand name (Manufacturer)	Formulation and strength	Product information/Administration information
Crestor (AstraZeneca)	Tablets 10 mg, 20 mg, 40 mg	Film-coated tablets[2] 10 mg tablets disperse in water within 5 minutes to give pale pink, milky dispersion; small white particles are visible but the dispersion flushes down an 8Fr NG tube without blockage.[3]

Site of absorption (oral administration)

Specific site of absorption is not documented. Peak plasma concentrations occur 5 hours after dosing.[2]

Alternative routes available

No alternative route of administration is available for any of the 'statins'.

Interactions

No specific interaction with food is noted in the SPC.[2]

Health and safety

Standard precautions apply.

Suggestions/recommendations

- As limited data are available, consider changing to an alternative statin with more data, e.g. atorvastatin (see monograph).
- Alternatively, if continued treatment with rosuvastatin is considered appropriate, disperse the tablets in water immediately prior to administration.
- A prolonged break in feeding is not required.

Intragastric administration

1. Stop the enteral feed.
2. Flush the enteral feeding tube with the recommended volume of water.
3. Place the tablet in the barrel of an appropriate size and type of syringe.
4. Draw 10 mL of water into the syringe and allow the tablet to disperse, shaking if necessary.
5. Flush the medication dose down the feeding tube.
6. Draw another 10 mL of water into the syringe and also flush this via the feeding tube (this will rinse the syringe and ensure that the total dose is administered).
7. Finally, flush with the recommended volume of water.
8. Re-start the feed, unless a prolonged break is required.

Alternatively, at step (3) place the tablet into a medicine pot, add 10 mL of water and allow the tablet to disperse. Draw this into an appropriate syringe. Ensure that the measure is rinsed and that this rinsing water is administered also to ensure that the total dose is given.

Intrajejunal administration

There are no specific data relating to jejunal administration of rosuvastatin. Monitor cholesterol levels for loss of efficacy of rosuvastatin. Administer using the method detailed above.

References

1. *BNF 50*, September 2005.
2. Crestor 10 mg (AstraZeneca), Summary of Product Characteristics; March 2003.
3. BPNG data on file, 2004.

Saquinavir

Formulations available[1]

Brand name (Manufacturer)	Formulation and strength	Product information/Administration information
Fortovase (Roche)	Capsules 200 mg	Gel-filled capsules. Absorption is greater than with Invirase.[2] Not suitable for administration via enteral feeding tube.
Invirase (Roche)	Capsules 200 mg	Saquinavir mesilate. There is no theoretical reason why the capsules should not be opened and mixed with water immediately prior to administration.[2] Excipients in the hard gelatin capsule shell should disperse in water.

Site of absorption (oral administration)

Saquinavir is absorbed in the proximal small bowel.[2]

Alternative routes available

No alternative route available. Saquinavir is very poorly absorbed rectally.[2]

Interactions

Food increases the bioavailability of saquinavir. It should be taken within 2 hours of a meal. The difference in AUC between fed and fasted state is 5-fold to 10-fold, whereas the difference between a low-calorie, low-fat meal and a high-calorie, high-fat meal is only 2-fold.[2]

Health and safety

Standard precautions apply

Suggestions/recommendations

- Use Invirase capsules. Open capsules and disperse in water immediately prior to administration.
- The dose should be administered within 2 hours of feed.
- Consider changing to protease inhibitor available as liquid preparation e.g. amprenavir, lopinavir, nelfinavir or ritonavir.

Intragastric administration

1. Stop the enteral feed.
2. Flush the enteral feeding tube with the recommended volume of water.
3. Open the capsule and pour the contents into a medicine pot.
4. Add 15 mL of water.
5. Stir to disperse the powder.
6. Draw into an appropriate size and type of syringe and administer via the feeding tube.
7. Add a further 15 mL of water to the medicine pot; stir to ensure that any powder remaining in the pot is mixed with water.
8. Draw up this dispersion and flush down tube. This will ensure that the whole dose is given.
9. Flush the tube with the recommended volume of water.
10. Re-start feed if required, unless a prolonged break is required.

Intrajejunal administration

There are no specific data relating to the jejunal administration of saquinavir. Administer using the above method. Monitor for increased side-effects or loss of efficacy.

References

1. *BNF* 50, September 2005.
2. Personal communication, Roche; 6 February 2003.

Selegiline hydrochloride

Formulations available[1]

Brand name (Manufacturer)	Formulation and strength	Product information/Administration information
Selegiline (Alpharma, APS, Generics, Hillcross, IVAX, Sandoz, Sanofi-Synthelabo, Sterwin)	Tablets 5 mg, 10 mg	No specific data on enteral tube administration are available for this formulation.
Eldepryl (Orion)	Tablets 5 mg, 10 mg	No specific data on enteral tube administration are available for this formulation.
Eldepryl (Orion)	Oral liquid 10 mg/5 mL	Clear, slightly viscous liquid. Some resistance on flushing via an 8Fr NG tube. Mixes easily with an equal volume of water.[2] Does not contain sorbitol.[3]
Zelapar (Athena)	Oral lyophilisates 1.25 mg	Buccal absorption. 1.25 mg lyophilisate = 10 mg oral. Do not administer via enteral feeding tube.[4]

Site of absorption (oral administration)

Selegiline is absorbed through the buccal mucosa (Zelapar) and via GI tract. Following oral administration, peak plasma concentration occurs within 30 minutes; bioavailability is low (10%).

Alternative routes available

Buccal route is available.

Interactions

No specific interaction with food is documented.[3]

Health and safety

Standard precautions apply.

Suggestions/recommendations

- Where clinically possible, use oral lyophilisates. This may not be appropriate for patients with reduced buccal blood flow (extensive maxillofacial surgery) or for patients who cannot hold the tablet in their mouth, e.g. following severe stroke.
- For enteral tube administration, the liquid preparation should be used. For intrajejunal tubes, the liquid should be diluted with an equal volume of water immediately prior to administration to reduce osmolarity.
- A prolonged break in feed is not required.

Intragastric administration

1. Stop the enteral feed.
2. Flush the enteral feeding tube with the recommended volume of water.
3. Draw the medication liquid into an appropriate size and type of syringe.
4. Flush the medication dose down the feeding tube.
5. Finally, flush with the recommended volume of water.
6. Re-start the feed, unless a prolonged break is required.

Alternatively, at step (3) measure the medicine in a suitable container and then draw into an appropriate syringe. Ensure that the measure is rinsed and that this rinsing water is administered also to ensure that the total dose is given. **Do not** measure liquid medicines using a catheter-tipped syringe as this results in excessive dosing owing to the volume of the tip.

Intrajejunal administration

1. Stop the enteral feed.
2. Flush the enteral feeding tube with the recommended volume of water.
3. Draw the medication liquid into an appropriate size and type of syringe.
4. Draw an equal volume of water and a little air into the syringe and shake to mix thoroughly.
5. Flush the medication dose down the feeding tube.
6. Draw an equal volume of water into the syringe and also flush this via the feeding tube (this will rinse the syringe and ensure that the total dose is administered).
7. Finally, flush with the recommended volume of water.
8. Re-start the feed, unless a prolonged break is required.

Alternatively, at step (3) measure the medicine in a suitable container and then add an equal volume of water and mix thoroughly. Draw this into an appropriate syringe. Ensure that the measure is rinsed and that this rinsing water is administered also to ensure that the total dose is given. **Do not** measure liquid medicines using a catheter-tipped syringe as this results in excessive dosing owing to the volume of the tip.

References

1. *BNF* 50, September 2005.
2. BPNG data on file, 2005.
3. Eldepryl (Orion), Summary of Product Characteristics; April 2000/December 1999.
4. Personal communication, Elan Pharma; 16 January 2003.

Senna

Formulations available[1]

Brand name (Manufacturer)	Formulation and strength	Product information/Administration information
Senna (Alpharma, APS, R&C)	Tablets 7.5 mg	No specific data on enteral tube administration are available for this formulation.
Senokot (R&C)	Syrup 7.5 mg/5 mL	Brown, slightly viscous liquid. Flushes down a fine-bore tube with little resistance and no risk of blockage. Mixes with water if further dilution is required.[2]
Manevac (Galen)	Granules	Not suitable for administration via the feeding tube.
Senokot (R&C)	Granules	Not suitable for administration via the feeding tube.

Site of absorption (oral administration)

Senna is not absorbed and the action of the sennasides is colon-specific.[3]

Alternative routes available

Not applicable.

Interactions

No significant interaction with food is documented.

Health and safety

Standard precautions apply.

Suggestions/recommendations

- Use a liquid preparation; flush well before and after dose. A prolonged break in feeding is not required.
- Administration into the jejunum will not affect pharmacological response.

Intragastric administration

1. Stop the enteral feed.
2. Flush the enteral feeding tube with the recommended volume of water.
3. Draw the medication into an appropriate size and type of syringe.
4. Flush the medication dose down the feeding tube.
5. Finally, flush with the recommended volume of water.
6. Re-start the feed, unless a prolonged break is required.

Intrajejunal administration

Therapeutic effect will be unaffected by jejunal administration. Administer using the above method.

References

1. *BNF* 50, September 2005.
2. BPNG data on file, 2004.
3. Senna Tablets (Boots Company plc), Summary of Product Characteristics; November 2004.

Sertraline

Formulations available[1]

Brand name (Manufacturer)	Formulation and strength	Product information/Administration information
Lustral (Pfizer)	Tablets 50 mg, 100 mg	Sertraline hydrochloride.[2] Film-coated tablets.[2] Sertraline is poorly soluble. For administration via a NG or PEG tube, Lustral tablets may be crushed, suspended in sterile water and administered using a suitable syringe. Pfizer does not have any stability data, so this must be done immediately prior to administration.[3] Tablets do not disperse readily in water but do disintegrate if shaken in 10 mL of water for a few minutes; this gives a dispersion with some visible particles that flushes via an 8Fr NG tube without blockage.[4]

Site of absorption (oral administration)

Specific site of absorption is not documented. Peak plasma concentration occurs 4.5–8.4 hours following oral dosing.[2]

Alternative routes available

None available.

Interactions

Food does not significantly affect the bioavailability of Lustral tablets.[2]

Health and safety

Standard precautions apply.

Suggestions/recommendations

- Consider changing to an alternative SSRI available as a liquid preparation.
- If continued therapy with sertraline is indicated, disperse the tablets in water immediately prior to administration; flush well after administration.
- A prolonged break in feeding is not required.

Intragastric administration

1. Stop the enteral feed.
2. Flush the enteral feeding tube with the recommended volume of water.
3. Place the tablet in the barrel of an appropriate size and type of syringe.
4. Draw 10 mL of water into the syringe and allow the tablet to disperse, shaking if necessary.
5. Flush the medication dose down the feeding tube.
6. Draw another 10 mL of water into the oral syringe and also flush this via the feeding tube (this will rinse the syringe and ensure that the total dose is administered).
7. Finally, flush with the recommended volume of water.
8. Re-start the feed, unless a prolonged break is required.

Alternatively, at step (3) place the tablet into a medicine pot, add 10 mL of water and allow the tablet to disperse. Draw this into an appropriate syringe. Ensure that the measure is rinsed and that this rinsing water is administered also to ensure that the total dose is given.

Intrajejunal administration

There are no specific data relating to the jejunal administration of sertraline. Administer using the above method. Monitor for loss of efficacy or increased side-effects.

References

1. *BNF 50*, September 2005.
2. Lustral (Pfizer), Summary of Product Characteristics; December 2003.
3. Personal communication, Pfizer; 23 June 2003.
4. BPNG data on file, 2004.

Sildenafil

Formulations available[1]

Brand name (Manufacturer)	Formulation and strength	Product information/Administration information
Viagra (Pfizer)	Tablets 25 mg, 50 mg, 100 mg	Sildenafil citrate. Tablets can be crushed and dispersed in water to facilitate administration. The formulation of an extemporaneous suspension may be appropriate for accurate administration of paediatric doses.[2] The extemporaneous preparation is stable for 90 days at room temperature.

Site of absorption (oral administration)

The specific site of absorption is not documented. Peak plasma concentration occurs 30–120 minutes following oral administration.[3]

Alternative routes available

None available for sildenafil.

Interactions

The rate but not the extent of absorption of sildenafil is reduced by food. Peak plasma concentrations are reduced by 29% and peak plasma concentration are delayed by 1 hour following a high-fat meal.[2]

Health and safety

Standard precautions apply.

Suggestions/recommendations

- Crush the tablets and disperse in water immediately prior to administration.
- A prolonged break in feeding is not required.

Intragastric administration

1. Stop the enteral feed.
2. Flush the enteral feeding tube with the recommended volume of water.
3. Place the tablet in a mortar and crush to a fine powder using the pestle.
4. Add a few millilitres of water and mix to form a paste.
5. Add up to 15 mL of water and mix thoroughly ensuring that there are no large particles of tablet.
6. Draw this into an appropriate type and size of syringe.
7. Flush the medication dose down the feeding tube.
8. Add another 15 mL of water to the mortar and stir to ensure that any remaining drug is rinsed from the container. Draw this water into the syringe and also flush this via the feeding tube (this will rinse the mortar and syringe and ensure total dose is administered).
9. Finally, flush the enteral feeding tube with the recommended volume of water.
10. Re-start the feed, unless a prolonged break is required.

Intrajejunal administration

There are no specific data relating to jejunal administration of sildenafil. Administer as above and monitor for loss of effect and increased side-effects.

References

1. *BNF 50*, September 2005.
2. Nahata MC, Morosco RS, Brady MT. Extemporaneous sildenafil citrate oral suspensions for the treatment of pulmonary hypertension in children. *Am J Health Syst Pharm.* 2006; 63(3): 254–257.
3. Viagra (Pfizer), Summary of Product Characteristics; July 2003.

Simvastatin

Formulations available[1]

Brand name (Manufacturer)	Formulation and strength	Product information/Administration information
Zocor (MSD)	Tablets 10 mg, 20 mg, 40 mg, 80 mg	Film-coated tablets[2] Simvastatin is almost insoluble in water.[4] 10 mg tablets (other strengths not tested) disperse in 10 mL of water and flush via an 8Fr NG tube.[5]

Formulations available[1] (continued)

Brand name (Manufacturer)	Formulation and strength	Product information/Administration information
Simzal (APS)	Tablets 10 mg, 20 mg, 40 mg, 80 mg	Only 40 mg tested. Tablets do not readily disperse in water, but crush and mix with water to form a dispersion that flushes via an 8Fr NG tube.[5]
Simvastatin (CP Pharma)	Tablets 10 mg, 20 mg, 40 mg, 80 mg	Film-coated tablets. 40 mg strength (other strengths not tested) disperses in 10 mL of water within 5 minutes to give very coarse dispersion that breaks up when drawn into the syringe; this then flushes easily down an 8Fr Ng tube without blockage.[5]
Simvastatin (Dexcel)	Tablets 10 mg, 20 mg, 40 mg, 80 mg	Both 20 mg and 40 mg strength tablets disperse in 10 mL of water within 5 minutes when agitated to form fine dispersion that flushes via an 8Fr NG tube without blockage.[5] Other strengths not tested.
Simvador (Discovery, Generics)	Tablets 10 mg, 20 mg, 40 mg, 80 mg	Film-coated tablets.[3] No specific data on enteral tube administration are available for this formulation.
Simvastatin (Ratiopharm)	Tablets 10 mg, 20 mg, 40 mg, 80 mg	10 mg strength takes almost 5 minutes to disperse in 10 mL water when agitated but the dispersion flushes down an 8Fr NG tube. 20 mg strength does not disintegrate within 5 minutes, but crushes and mixes with water. Other strengths not tested.[5]
Simvastatin (Ranbaxy)	Tablets 10 mg, 20 mg, 40 mg, 80 mg	10 mg, 20 mg and 40 mg (80 mg not tested) strengths of tablets disperse in 10 mL of water, with the length of time and amount of agitation increasing as the strength increases. All produce a dispersion that can be flushed down an 8Fr NG tube, although care should be taken with the 40 mg strength as some of the particles may block a finer tube.[5]

Site of absorption (oral administration)

Specific site of absorption is not documented. Peak plasma concentrations of active metabolite are reached 1–2 hours after administration.[3]

Alternative routes available

No alternative route is available for any of the 'statins'.

Interactions

Food intake does not affect absorption of simvastatin.[3] Peak cholesterol synthesis is influenced by meal intake, hence the recommendation that simvastatin be taken in the evening to coincide with peak cholesterol synthesis activity.[6] However, if patients are on an overnight feed it may be prudent to dose in the morning at the end of the feed regimen.

Health and safety

Standard precautions apply.

Suggestions/recommendations

- All brands of simvastatin tablets are coated and take a significant time to disperse in water, although none appear to block fine-bore tubes once dispersed.
- Alternative therapy with atorvastatin should be considered as this disperses readily in water (see monograph); however, if therapy with simvastatin is to be continued the tablets should be dispersed in water following the method below.
- Note should be taken of the brand used as some disperse better than others (see above).
- See note above regarding timing of dosage.

Intragastic administration

1. Stop the enteral feed.
2. Flush the enteral feeding tube with the recommended volume of water.
3. Place the tablet in the barrel of an appropriate size and type of syringe.
4. Draw 10 mL of water into the syringe and allow the tablet to disperse, shaking if necessary.
5. Flush the medication dose down the feeding tube.
6. Draw another 10 mL of water into the syringe and also flush this via the feeding tube (this will rinse the syringe and ensure that the total dose is administered).
7. Finally, flush with the recommended volume of water.
8. Re-start the feed if necessary, unless a prolonged break is required.

Alternatively, at step (3) place the tablet into a medicine pot, add 10 mL of water and allow the tablet to disperse. Draw this into an appropriate syringe. Ensure that the measure is rinsed and that this rinsing water is administered also to ensure that the total dose is given.

Intrajejunal administration

There are no specific data relating to the administration of simvastatin via jejunal tubes, so cholesterol levels should be monitored and dose titrated to effect.
Use the above method for administration.

References

1. *BNF 50*, September 2005.
2. Zocor (MSD), Summary of Product Characteristics; November 2003.
3. Simvador (Discovery), Summary of Product Characteristics; July 2003.
4. Dollery C. *Therapeutic Drugs*, 2nd edn. London: Churchill Livingstone; 1998.
5. BPNG data on file, 2004.
6. Cella LK, Cauter E, Schoeller DA. Effect of meal timing on diurnal rhythm of human cholesterol synthesis. *Am J Physiol*. 1995; 269(Endocrine Metab. 32): E878–E883.

Sodium clodronate

Formulations available[1]

Brand name (Manufacturer)	Formulation and strength	Product information/Administration information
Bonefos (Boehringer Ingelheim)	Capsules 400 mg	Bonefos capsules and tablets are almost bioequivalent and therefore no dosage adjustment is necessary when changing between Bonefos preparations.[2] Capsules can be opened and flushed via enteral feeding tube.[3]

Formulations available[1] (continued)

Brand name (Manufacturer)	Formulation and strength	Product information/Administration information
Bonefos (Boehringer Ingelheim)	Tablets 800 mg	Tablets will disperse in water.[3]
Bonefos (Boehringer Ingelheim)	Intravenous solution 60 mg/mL (5 mL)	No specific data on enteral tube administration are available for this formulation.
Loron 520 (Roche)	Tablets 520 mg	Owing to a greater bioavailability, one Loron 520 mg tablet is equivalent to two Loron 400 mg capsules. It is not recommended that the tablets be crushed as the bioavailability is likely to be affected.[4]

Site of absorption (oral administration)

Specific site of absorption is not documented.

Alternative routes available

Parenteral route available for acute management of hypercalcaemia of malignancy.

Interactions

Absorption is reduced by calcium ions. Food should be avoided for 1 hour before and 1 hour after dosing.[2]

Health and safety

Standard precautions apply.

Suggestions/recommendations

- It is possible that bioavailability will be adversely affected by administration via enteral feeding tube. The preferred formulation is to open the capsules and mix with water immediately prior to administration.
- Consideration should be given to using alternative therapy such as alendronate or residronate (see monographs) or using maintenance parenteral therapy.

Intragastric administration

1. Stop the enteral feed.
2. Flush the enteral feeding tube with the recommended volume of water.
3. Wait at least 1 hour before administering the dose.
4. Open the capsule and pour the contents into a medicine pot.
5. Add 15 mL of water.
6. Stir to disperse the powder.
7. Draw into an appropriate size and type of syringe and administer via the feeding tube.
8. Add a further 15 mL of water to the medicine pot; stir to ensure that any powder remaining in the pot is mixed with water.
9. Draw up this dispersion and flush down the tube. This will ensure that the whole dose is given.
10. Flush the tube with the recommended volume of water.
11. Wait for at least 1 hour before restarting the feed.

Jejunal administration

There are no specific data relating to jejunal administration of clodronate. Administer as above. Monitor for loss of efficacy or increased side-effects.

References

1. *BNF* 50, September 2005.
2. Bonefos Capsules (Boehringer Ingelheim), Summary of Product Characteristics; July 2002.
3. Personal communication, Boehringer Ingelheim; 6 March 2003.
4. Personal communication, Roche; 6 February 2003.

Sodium picosulfate

Formulations available[1]

Brand name (Manufacturer)	Formulation and strength	Product information/Administration information
Sodium picosulfate (Boehringer Ingelheim)	Elixir 5 mg/5 mL	Can be diluted with water.[2] Contains alcohol.[2] (Laxoberal and Dulco-lax.)
Dulco-lax Perles (Boehringer Ingelheim)	Capsules 2.5 mg	No specific data on enteral tube administration are available for this formulation.
Picolax® (Nordic)	Oral Powder 10 mg/sachet	Licensed for bowel cleansing prior to procedures. Contents of one sachet should be reconstituted in approximately 150 mL of water.[3] Anecdotal evidence supports administration via enteral feeding tubes; however, it should be ensured that the reconstituted solution is stirred well and has cooled before administration.[4]

Site of absorption (oral administration)

Sodium picosulfate reaches the colon without any significant absorption;[2] therefore, the therapeutic response will be unaffected by jejunal administration.

Alternative routes available

Not applicable.

Interactions

No significant interaction with food is documented.

Health and safety

Standard precautions apply.

Suggestions/recommendations

- Use the liquid preparation; dilute with an equal volume of water prior to administration. No prolonged break in feeding is required.
- See notes above for Picolax administration.

Intragastric administration

1. Stop the enteral feed.
2. Flush the enteral feeding tube with the recommended volume of water.
3. Draw the medication into an appropriate size and type of syringe.
4. Flush the medication dose down the feeding tube.
5. Finally, flush with the recommended volume of water.
6. Re-start the feed, unless a prolonged break is required.

Alternatively, at step (3) measure the medicine in a suitable container and then add an equal volume of water and mix thoroughly. Draw this into an appropriate syringe. Ensure that the measure is rinsed and that this rinsing water is administered also to ensure that the total dose is given. **Do not** measure liquid medicines using a catheter-tipped syringe as this results in excessive dosing owing to the volume of the tip.

Intrajejunal administration

The pharmacological affect is unlikely to be affected by jejunal administration. Administer as above.

References

1. *BNF 50*, September 2005.
2. Dulco-Lax Liquid (Boehringer), Summary of Product Characteristics; March 2003.
3. Picolax (Ferring), Summary of Product Characteristics; May 2003.
4. Personal communication, Ferring Pharmaceuticals; 20 January 2003.

Sotalol hydrochloride

Formulations available[1]

Brand name (Manufacturer)	Formulation and strength	Product information/Administration information
Beta-Cardone (Celltech)	Tablets 40 mg, 80 mg, 200 mg	Scored. Tablets are uncoated and can be crushed.[2] Sotalol tablets have been formulated into an extemporaneous preparation that was stable for 8 weeks;[4] therefore, suspending crushed tablets in water will not cause stability concerns. Tablets do not disintegrate readily but will disperse when shaken in 10 mL of water for 3–5 minutes; this forms a very fine suspension that flushes via an 8Fr NG tube without blockage (colour dependent on strength of tablet)[6].

Formulations available[1] (continued)

Brand name (Manufacturer)	Formulation and strength	Product information/Administration information
Sotacor (Bristol-Myers Squibb)	Tablets 80 mg, 160 mg	Sotalol is freely soluble in water.[3] No specific data on enteral tube administration are available for this formulation.
Sotacor (Bristol-Myers Squibb)	Injection 10 mg/mL (4 mL)	No specific data on enteral tube administration are available for this formulation.
Sotalol (Generics, Hillcross, Taro, Tillomed)	Tablets 40 mg, 80 mg, 160 mg	No specific data on enteral tube administration are available for this formulation.

Site of absorption (oral administration)

Specific site of absorption is not documented. Peak plasma concentration occurs 2–3 hours after oral dosing.[5]

Alternative routes available

Parenteral route is available; see SPC for dosing guidelines.

Interactions

No documented interaction with food.

Health and safety

Standard precautions apply.

Suggestions/recommendations

- Disperse the tablets in water immediately prior to dosing.
- A prolonged break in feeding is not necessary.

Intragastric administration

1. Stop the enteral feed.
2. Flush the enteral feeding tube with the recommended volume of water.
3. Place the tablet in the barrel of an appropriate size and type of syringe.
4. Draw 10 mL of water into the syringe and allow the tablet to disperse, shaking if necessary.
5. Flush the medication dose down the feeding tube.
6. Draw another 10 mL of water into the syringe and also flush this via the feeding tube (this will rinse the syringe and ensure that the total dose is administered).
7. Finally, flush with the recommended volume of water.
8. Re-start the feed, unless a prolonged break is required.

Alternatively, at step (3) place the tablet into a medicine pot, add 10 mL of water and allow the tablet to disperse. Draw this into an appropriate syringe. Ensure that the measure is rinsed and that this rinsing water is administered also to ensure that the total dose is given.

Intrajejunal administration

There are no specific data relating to jejunal administration. Monitor for loss of effect. Administer as above.

References

1. *BNF 50*, September 2005.
2. Personal communication, Celltech; 31 March 2003.
3. Personal communication, Bristol-Myers Squibb; 24 January 2003.
4. Dupis LL, James G, Bacola G. Stability of a sotalol hydrochloride oral liquid formulation. *Can J Hosp Pharm.* 1988; 41(3): 121–123.
5. Beta-Cardone Tablets (Celltech), Summary of Product Characteristics; April 2001.
6. BPNG data on file, 2005.

Spironolactone

Formulations available[1]

Brand name (Manufacturer)	Formulation and strength	Product information/Administration information
Spironolactone (Alpharma, APS, Ashbourne, Hillcross, IVAX)	Tablets 25 mg, 50 mg, 100 mg	Alpharma tablets can be crushed and dispersed in water immediately prior to administration.[2] Most brands of tablets will disperse in water if shaken for 2–5 minutes. The resulting dispersion will flush via an 8Fr NG tube without blockage.[3]
Spironolactone (Rosemont)	Oral suspension 5 mg/5 mL, 10 mg/5 mL, 25 mg/5 mL, 50 mg/5 mL, 100 mg/5 mL	Special order manufactured 'special', 12 months' expiry. Contains 0.68 g sorbitol/5 mL dose.[4] Very viscous liquid that is resistant to flushing via fine-bore tubes; however, it mixes with water when shaken vigorously. The diluted liquid is less resistant to flushing.[9]
Aldactone (Searle)	Tablets 25 mg, 50 mg, 100 mg	Film-coated tablets. If necessary a suspension can be prepared by crushing the tablets[8]
Spironolactone (extemporaneous preparation)	Suspension Various strengths	Spironolactone is stable for 28 days when suspended in cherry syrup[6,7] or syrup and carboxymethylcellulose base,[8] at a range of strengths.

Site of absorption (oral administration)

Specific site of absorption is not documented. Spironolactone is well absorbed orally,[5] with peak plasma concentrations occurring 2.6 hours after oral administration.

Alternative routes available

None available for spironolactone. Potassium canreonate injection is available as an unlicensed product.

Interactions

No specific interaction with food is documented. The SPC recommends taking the dose with food.

Health and safety

Standard precautions apply.

Suggestions/recommendations

- Use suspension formulation for enteral administration; alternatively, disperse the tablets in water immediately prior to administration.
- A prolonged break in feeding is not required.

Intragastric administration

1. Stop the enteral feed.
2. Flush the enteral feeding tube with the recommended volume of water.
3. Shake the medication bottle thoroughly to ensure adequate mixing.
4. Draw the medication suspension into an appropriate size and type of syringe.
5. Flush the medication dose down the feeding tube.
6. Finally, flush with the recommended volume of water.
7. Re-start the feed, unless a prolonged break is required.

Alternatively, at step (4) measure the medicine in a suitable container and then add an equal volume of water and mix thoroughly. Draw this into an appropriate syringe. Ensure that the measure is rinsed and that this rinsing water is administered also to ensure that the total dose is given. **Do not** measure liquid medicines using a catheter-tipped syringe as this results in excessive dosing owing to the volume of the tip.

Intrajejunal administration

1. Stop the enteral feed.
2. Flush the enteral feeding tube with the recommended volume of water.
3. Place the tablet in the barrel of an appropriate size and type of syringe.
4. Draw 10 mL of water into the syringe and allow the tablet to disperse, shaking as required.
5. Flush the medication dose down the feeding tube.
6. Draw another 10 mL of water into the syringe and also flush this via the feeding tube (this will rinse the syringe and ensure that the total dose is administered).
7. Finally, flush with the recommended volume of water.
8. Re-start the feed, unless a prolonged break is required.

Alternatively, at step (3) place the tablet into a medicine pot, add 10 mL of water and allow the tablet to disperse. Draw this into an appropriate syringe. Ensure that the measure is rinsed and that this rinsing water is administered also to ensure that the total dose is given.

References

1. *BNF* 50, September 2005.
2. Personal communication, Alpharma; 21 January 2003.
3. BPNG data on file, 2004.
4. Personal communication, Rosemont Pharma; 21 January 2005.
5. Aldactone (Pharmacia), Summary of Product Characteristics; September 2004.
6. Mathur LK, Wickman A. Stability of extemporaneously compounded spironolactone suspensions. *Am J Hosp Pharm.* 1989; 46: 2040–2042.
7. Allen LV, Erickson MA. 1996) Stability of ketoconazole, metolazone, metronidazole, procainamide hydrochloride, and spironolactone in extemporaneously compounded oral liquids. *Am J Health Syst Pharm.* 1996; 53: 2073–2078.
8. Personal communication, Pharmacia; March 11 2003.
9. BPNG data on file, 2005.

Stavudine

Formulations available [1]

Brand name (Manufacturer)	Formulation and strength	Product information/Administration information
Zerit (Bristol-Myers Squibb)	Capsules 15 mg, 20 mg, 30 mg	For optimal absorption stavudine should be administered on an empty stomach; however, if necessary the capsules can be opened and mixed with food. [2] The contents of the capsules pour freely, mix with water when stirred, and flush via an 8Fr NG tube without blockage. [4]
Zerit (Bristol-Myers Squibb)	Oral solution 1 mg/mL	Powder for reconstitution. [3] There is no theoretical reason why this cannot be administered via a feeding tube.

Site of absorption (oral administration)

Specific site of absorption is not documented.

Alternative routes available

None available for stavudine.

Interactions

A high-fat meal reduces and delays peak plasma concentration; [2] there are no reports of this interaction having clinical significance.

Health and safety

Standard precautions apply.

Suggestions/recommendations

- Use the oral solution.
- Where possible allow a break before dosing.
- Flush well after dose and allow 30-minute break before restarting feed.

Intragastric administration

1. Stop the enteral feed.
2. Flush the enteral feeding tube with the recommended volume of water.
3. Allow a break prior to dosing if practical.
4. Draw the medication solution into an appropriate size and type of syringe.
5. Flush the medication dose down the feeding tube.
6. Finally, flush with the recommended volume of water.
7. Wait at least 30 minutes before restarting the feed.

Alternatively, at step (4) measure the medicine in a suitable container and then draw into an appropriate syringe. Ensure that the measure is rinsed and that this rinsing water is administered also to ensure that the total dose is given. **Do not** measure liquid medicines using a catheter-tipped syringe as this results in excessive dosing owing to the volume of the tip.

Intrajejunal administration

There are no specific data relating to the jejunal administration of stavudine. Administer using the above method and monitor for increased side-effects or loss of efficacy.

References

1. *BNF* 50, September 2005.
2. Zerit Capsules (Bristol-Myers), Summary of Product Characteristics; June 2003.
3. Zerit Powder for oral solution (Bristol-Myers), Summary of Product Characteristics; June 2003.
4. BPNG data on file, 2005.

Sucralfate

Formulations available[1]

Brand name (Manufacturer)	Formulation and strength	Product information/Administration information
Antepsin (Chugai)	Tablets 1 g	Tablets may be dispersed in 10–15 mL of water.[2] It is not known whether this is suitable for administration via an enteral tube.
Antepsin (Chugai)	Suspension 1 g/5 mL	Viscous white liquid. Viscosity is reduced by mixing with an equal volume of water; as there are no stability data to support dilution, this must be done immediately prior to administration.[4]

Site of absorption (oral administration)

Sucralfate is only minimally absorbed;[2] its mode of action is local. Increased absorption of aluminium may occur in renal patients.

Alternative routes available

None.

Interactions

Bezoar formation: Following reports of bezoar formation associated with sucralfate, the CSM has advised caution in seriously ill patients, especially those receiving concomitant enteral feeds or those with predisposing conditions such as delayed gastric emptying.[1]

Sucralfate forms an insoluble protein–aluminium complex with enteral feeds, resulting in solid or semi-solid agglomerates that can block feeding tubes, or even the stomach or oesophagus.[3]

Health and safety

Standard precautions apply.

Suggestions/recommendations

• Enteral feed should be stopped at least 1 hour before dose and not restarted for 1 hour post-dose.[2] A longer break may be prudent in patients with delayed gastric emptying.

Intragastric administration

1. Stop the enteral feed.
2. Flush the enteral feeding tube with the recommended volume of water.
3. Wait for at least 1 hour.
4. Shake the medication bottle thoroughly to ensure adequate mixing.
5. Draw the medication suspension into an appropriate size and type of syringe.
6. Draw an equal volume of water and a little air into the syringe and shake to mix thoroughly.
7. Flush the medication dose down the feeding tube.
8. Finally, flush with the recommended volume of water.
9. Wait at least an hour before restarting the feed.

Alternatively, at step (5) measure the medicine in a suitable container and then add an equal volume of water and mix thoroughly. Draw this into an appropriate syringe. Ensure that the measure is rinsed and that this rinsing water is administered also to ensure that the total dose is given. **Do not** measure liquid medicines using a catheter-tipped syringe as this results in excessive dosing owing to the volume of the tip.

Intrajejunal administration

Not appropriate for jejunal administration as the site of action is gastric and duodenal.

References

1. *BNF 50*, September 2005.
2. Antepsin Suspension (Chugai), Summary of Product Characteristics; April 2003.
3. Stockley IH. *Stockley's Drug Interactions*, 6th edn. London: Pharmaceutical Press; 2002.
4. BPNG data on file, 2004.

Sulfasalazine

Formulations available[1]

Brand name (Manufacturer)	Formulation and strength	Product information/Administration information
Salazopyrin (Pharmacia)	Tablets 500 mg	Tablets can be crushed.[2]
Salazopyrin (Pharmacia)	EN-Tabs 500 mg	EN-Tabs cannot be crushed. Not suitable for enteral tube administration.
Salazopyrin (Pharmacia)	Suspension 250 mg/5 mL	Suspension does not contain sorbitol.[3] Viscous orange suspension.
Salazopyrin (Pharmacia)	Suppositories 500 mg	Effective for topical therapy only.
Salazopyrin (Pharmacia)	Retention enema 3 g	Effective for topical therapy only.

Formulations available [1] (continued)

Brand name (Manufacturer)	Formulation and strength	Product information/Administration information
Sulfasalazine (Generics, Hillcross)	Tablets 500 mg	No specific data on enteral tube administration are available for this formulation.
Sulfasalazine (Alpharma)	E/C tablets 500 mg	Do not crush. Not suitable for enteral tube administration.

Site of absorption (oral administration)

Approximately 90% of an oral dose of sulfasalazine reaches the colon, where it is cleaved to release mesalazine.[3]

Alternative routes available

Topical therapy using a rectal 5-ASA preparation should be used first line in local rectal disease.

Interactions

There is no documented interaction with food.[3]

Health and safety

Standard precautions apply.

Suggestions/recommendations

- Use the suspension and flush the tube well before and after administration.
- A prolonged break in feeding is not necessary.

Intragastric administration

1. Stop the enteral feed.
2. Flush the enteral feeding tube with the recommended volume of water.
3. Shake the medication bottle thoroughly to ensure adequate mixing.
4. Draw the medication suspension into an appropriate size and type of syringe.
5. Flush the medication dose down the feeding tube.
6. Finally, flush with the recommended volume of water.
7. Re-start the feed, unless a prolonged break is required.

Alternatively, at step (4) measure the medicine in a suitable container. Draw this into an appropriate syringe. Ensure that the measure is rinsed and that this rinsing water is administered also to ensure that the total dose is given. **Do not** measure liquid medicines using a catheter-tipped syringe as this results in excessive dosing owing to the volume of the tip.

Intrajejunal administration

As the effect of sulfasalazine is topical within the colon, jejunal administration is not expected to affect therapeutic response to treatment.

References

1. *BNF 50*, September 2005.
2. Personal communication, Pharmacia; 11 March 2003.
3. Salazopyrin Suspension (Pharmacia), Summary of Product Characteristics; July 2001.

Sulpiride

Formulations available [1]

Brand name (Manufacturer)	Formulation and strength	Product information/Administration information
Sulpiride (APS, Arrow, CP, Generics, IVAX)	Tablets 200 mg, 400 mg	No specific data on enteral tube administration are available for this formulation.
Dolmatil (Sanofi-Synthelabo)	Tablets 200 mg, 400 mg	Scored tablets. Tablets can be crushed. [2] 200 mg tablets (400 mg not tested) disperse within 2 minutes to form a fine dispersion that settles quickly but that can be drawn up and flushes via an 8Fr NG tube without blockage. [3]
Sulpitil (Pharmacia)	Tablets 200 mg	Scored. There is no theoretical reason why the tablets cannot be crushed and dispersed in water. Pharmacia does not have any stability data to support this. [4]
Sulpor (Rosemont)	Oral solution 200 mg/5 mL	Does not contain sorbitol. [5]

Site of absorption (oral administration)

Specific site of absorption is not documented. Peak plasma concentration occurs 3–6 hours following oral dosing. [5]

Alternative routes available

None available for sulpiride.

Interactions

There is no documented interaction with food.

Health and safety

Standard precautions apply.

Suggestions/recommendations

- Use the liquid preparation.
- Alternatively, the tablets can be dispersed in 10 mL of water immediately prior to administration. This should be considered for intrajejunal administration owing to its lower osmolarity.
- A prolonged break in feeding is not required.

Intragastric administration

1. Stop the enteral feed.
2. Flush the enteral feeding tube with the recommended volume of water.
3. Shake the medication bottle thoroughly to ensure adequate mixing.
4. Draw the medication suspension into an appropriate size and type of syringe.
5. Flush the medication dose down the feeding tube.
6. Finally, flush with the recommended volume of water.
7. Re-start the feed, unless a prolonged break is required.

Alternatively, at step (4) measure the medicine in a suitable container. Draw this into an appropriate syringe. Ensure that the measure is rinsed and that this rinsing water is administered also to ensure that the total dose is given. **Do not** measure liquid medicines using a catheter-tipped syringe as this results in excessive dosing owing to the volume of the tip.

Intrajejunal administration

Use the above method or alternatively disperse tablets in water.

1. Stop the enteral feed.
2. Flush the enteral feeding tube with the recommended volume of water.
3. Place the tablet in the barrel of an appropriate size and type of syringe.
4. Draw 10 mL of water into the syringe and allow the tablet to disperse, shaking if necessary.
5. Flush the medication dose down the feeding tube.
6. Draw another 10 mL of water into the oral syringe and also flush this via the feeding tube (this will rinse the syringe and ensure that the total dose is administered).
7. Finally, flush with the recommended volume of water.
8. Re-start the feed, unless a prolonged break is required.

Alternatively, at step (4) place the tablet into a medicine pot, add 10 mL of water and allow the tablet to disperse. Draw this into an appropriate syringe. Ensure that the measure is rinsed and that this rinsing water is administered also to ensure that the total dose is given.

References

1. *BNF* 50, September 2005.
2. Personal communication, Sanofi; 3 February 2003.
3. BPNG data on file, 2004.
4. Personal communication, Pharmacia; 11 March 2003.
5. Sulpor (Rosemont), Summary of Product Characteristics; August 2001.

Tamoxifen citrate

Formulations available[1]

Brand name (Manufacturer)	Formulation and strength	Product information/Administration information
Tamoxifen (Alpharma, APS, CP, Hillcross, IVAX, Kent)	Tablets 10 mg, 20 mg	No specific data on enteral tube administration are available for this formulation.

Formulations available [1] (continued)

Brand name (Manufacturer)	Formulation and strength	Product information/Administration information
Tamoxifen (Rosemont)	Oral solution 10 mg/5 mL	Contains 0.7 g sorbitol per 5 mL dose.[2]
Nolvadex (AstraZeneca)	Tablets 10 mg, 20 mg	No specific data on enteral tube administration are available for this formulation.

Site of absorption (oral administration)

Specific site is not documented. Peak plasma concentration occurs 4–7 hours following oral dosing.[3]

Alternative routes available

None available for tamoxifen.

Interactions

There is no documented interaction with food.

Health and safety

Tamoxifen is a nonsteroidal anti-oestrogen. Crushing tablets should be avoided to minimise operator exposure.

Suggestions/recommendations

- Use the liquid preparation.
- A prolonged break in feeding is not required.

Intragastric administration

1. Stop the enteral feed.
2. Flush the enteral feeding tube with the recommended volume of water.
3. Draw the medication solution into an appropriate size and type of syringe.
4. Flush the medication dose down the feeding tube.
5. Finally, flush with the recommended volume of water.
6. Re-start the feed, unless a prolonged break is required.

Alternatively, at step (3) measure the medicine in a suitable container and then draw into an appropriate syringe. Ensure that the measure is rinsed and that this rinsing water is administered also to ensure that the total dose is given. **Do not** measure liquid medicines using a catheter-tipped syringe as this results in excessive dosing owing to the volume of the tip.

Intrajejunal administration

There are no specific data relating to jejunal administration of tamoxifen; however, the late peak plasma concentration indicates that significant gastric absorption is unlikely.
Administer using the above method.

References

1. *BNF 50*, September 2005.
2. Personal communication, Rosemont; 20 January 2005.
3. Nolvadex (AstraZeneca), Summary of Product Characteristics; September 2001.

Tamsulosin hydrochloride

Formulations available[1]

Brand name (Manufacturer)	Formulation and strength	Product information/Administration information
Flomax MR (Yamanouchi)	M/R capsule 400 microgram	Capsule contains small, modified-release granules. These clump together when mixed with water, are very difficult to draw into the syringe, and block feeding tubes.[2]

Site of absorption (oral administration)

Specific site of absorption is not documented. Peak plasma concentration occurs 6 hours following oral administration of the M/R preparation.[3]

Alternative routes available

None.

Interactions

Absorption of tamsulosin is reduced by a recent meal.[3]

Health and safety

Standard precautions apply.

Suggestions/recommendations

- Formulation is unsuitable for administration via the feeding tube; consider changing to an alternative drug such as doxazosin (see monograph).

References

1. *BNF* 50, September 2005.
2. BPNG data on file, 2004.
3. Flomax MR (Yamanouchi), Summary of Product Characteristics; July 2001.

Telmisartan

Formulations available[1]

Brand name (Manufacturer)	Formulation and strength	Product information/Administration information
Micardis (Boehringer Ingelheim)	Tablets 20 mg, 40 mg, 80 mg	Tablets contain a small quantity of sorbitol, unlikely to cause GI side-effects.[2] Tablets can be crushed.[3] Tablets disperse in water if shaken for 5 minutes to give a very fine dispersion that flushes via an 8Fr NG tube without blockage.[4]

Formulations available [1] (*continued*)

Brand name (Manufacturer)	Formulation and strength	Product information/Administration information
Micardis Plus (Boehringer Ingelheim)	Tablets 40 mg/12.5 mg, 80 mg/12.5 mg	40/12.5 tablets contain 40 mg telmisartan + 12.5 mg hydrochlorothiazide. 80/12.5 tablets contain 80 mg telmisartan + 12.5 mg hydrochlorothiazide. No specific data on enteral tube administration are available for this formulation.

Site of absorption (oral administration)

Specific site of absorption is not documented.

Alternative routes available

No other routes of administration are available for any of the angiotensin II antagonists.

Interactions

Food delays but does not significantly reduce telmisartan absorption.[2]

Health and safety

Standard precautions apply.

Suggestions/recommendations

- Disperse the tablets in water immediately prior to administration.
- A prolonged break in feeding is not required.

Intragastric administration

1. Stop the enteral feed.
2. Flush the enteral feeding tube with the recommended volume of water.
3. Place the tablet in the barrel of an appropriate size and type of syringe.
4. Draw 10 mL of water into the syringe, shaking if necessary until the tablet disintegrates.
5. Flush the medication dose down the feeding tube.
6. Draw another 10 mL of water into the oral syringe and also flush this via the feeding tube (this will rinse the syringe and ensure that the total dose is administered).
7. Finally, flush with the recommended volume of water.
8. Re-start the feed, unless a prolonged break is required.

Alternatively, at step (3) place the tablet into a medicine pot, add 10 mL of water and allow the tablet to disperse; this may take a considerable length of time without agitation. Draw this dispersion into an appropriate syringe. Ensure that the measure is rinsed and that this rinsing water is administered also to ensure that the total dose is given.

Intrajejunal administration

There are no specific data relating to jejunal administration. Administer using the above method. Monitor for increased side-effects or loss of efficacy.

References

1. *BNF* 50, September 2005.
2. Micardis (Boehringer Ingelheim), Summary of Product Characteristics; June 2002.
3. Personal communication, Boehringer Ingelheim; 6 March 2003.
4. BPNG data on file, 2005.

Temazepam

Formulations available[1]

Brand name (Manufacturer)	Formulation and strength	Product information/Administration information
Temazepam (various manufacturers)	Tablets 10 mg	Alpharma brand tablets can be crushed.[2]
Oral solution (Generics, Hillcross, Pharmacia, Rosemont)	Oral solution 10 mg/5 mL	Rosemont brand contains 0.91 g sorbitol/5 mL dose.[3] Pharmacia brand contains sorbitol.[4] Sugar-free formulations are available.

Site of absorption (oral administration)

Specific site of absorption is not documented. Peak plasma concentration occurs within 50 minutes following oral administration.[4]

Alternative routes available

None available for temazepam. Diazepam (which is metabolised to a number of metabolically active compounds including temazepam) is available as suppositories and injection.

Interactions

There is no documented interaction with food.

Health and safety

Standard precautions apply.

Suggestions/recommendations

- Use the liquid preparation.
- A prolonged break in feeding is not required.

Intragastric administration

1. Stop the enteral feed.
2. Flush the enteral feeding tube with the recommended volume of water.
3. Draw the medication into an appropriate size and type of syringe.
4. Flush the medication dose down the feeding tube.
5. Finally, flush with the recommended volume of water.
6. Re-start the feed, unless a prolonged break is required.

Alternatively, at step (3) measure the medicine in a suitable container. Draw this into an appropriate syringe. Ensure that the measure is rinsed and that this rinsing water is administered also to ensure that the total dose is given. **Do not** measure liquid medicines using a catheter-tipped syringe as this results in excessive dosing owing to the volume of the tip.

Intrajejunal administration

Administer using the above method. Monitor for loss of efficacy or increased side-effects.

References

1. *BNF* 50, September 2005.
2. Personal communication, Alpharma; 21 January 2003.
3. Personal communication, Rosemont; 20 January 2005.
4. Temazepam Elixir (Pharmacia), Summary of Product Characteristics; September 2002.

Tenofovir disoproxil

Formulations available[1]

Brand name (Manufacturer)	Formulation and strength	Product information/Administration information
Viread (Gilead)	Tablets 245 mg	Film-coated tablets. For patients with swallowing difficulties, the tablets can be dispersed in 100 mL of water, orange juice or grape juice.[2] Tablets disperse within 5 minutes when placed in 10 mL of water and flush via an 8Fr NG tube without blockage.[3]

Site of absorption (oral administration)

Specific site of absorption is not documented. Peak plasma concentrations of tenofovir occur within 1 hour in the fasted state and 2 hours in the fed state.[2]

Alternative routes available

None available for tenofovir.

Interactions

Co-administration with food delays the peak plasma concentration by approximately 1 hour. A high-fat meal enhanced tenofovir absorption by 40% when compared to the fasted state. A light meal had no significant effect on pharmacokinetics.[2] The SPC recommends that tenofovir be taken with food.

Health and safety

Standard precautions apply.

Suggestions/recommendations

- Disperse the tablets in water immediately prior to administration.
- A prolonged break in feeding is not necessary.

Intragastric administration

1. Stop the enteral feed.
2. Flush the enteral feeding tube with the recommended volume of water.
3. Place the tablet in the barrel of an appropriate size and type of syringe.
4. Draw 10 mL of water into the syringe and allow the tablet to disperse, shaking if necessary.
5. Flush the medication dose down the feeding tube.
6. Draw an equal volume of water into the syringe and also flush this via the feeding tube (this will rinse the syringe and ensure that the total dose is administered).
7. Finally, flush with the recommended volume of water.
8. Re-start the feed, unless a prolonged break is required.

Alternatively, at step (4) place the tablet into a medicine pot, add 10 mL of water and allow the tablet to disperse. Draw this into an appropriate syringe. Ensure that the measure is rinsed and that this rinsing water is administered also to ensure that the total dose is given.

Jejunal administration

There are no specific data relating to the jejunal administration of tenofovir. Monitor for loss of efficacy or increased side-effects. Use the same method as for intragastric administration.

References

1. *BNF 50*, September 2005.
2. Viread (Gilead), Summary of Product Characteristics; July 2003.
3. BPNG data on file, 2005.

Terbinafine

Formulations available[1]

Brand name (Manufacturer)	Formulation and strength	Product information/Administration information
Lamisil (Novartis)	Tablets 250 mg	Terbinafine hydrochloride. Scored tablets. Soluble 1 : 160 in water.[3] No specific data on enteral tube administration are available for this formulation.
Extemporaneous preparation	Suspension 25 mg/mL	*Extemporaneous terbinafine suspension 25 mg/mL:* Terbinafine 250 mg tablets 10 tablets Ora-Sweet/Ora-Plus (1 : 1) to 100 mL Store in a refrigerator or at room temperature; 42-day expiry.[2]

Site of absorption (oral administration)

Specific site of absorption is not documented. Peak plasma concentration occurs 2 hours following oral dosing.[3]

Alternative routes available

Topical terbinafine is only indicated for mild disease.[1]

Interactions

Absorption is unaffected by food.[3]

Health and safety

Standard precautions apply.

Suggestions/recommendations

- Tablets are scored and therefore there is no reason why the tablets cannot be crushed and dispersed in water immediately prior to administration; alternatively, an extemporaneous preparation can be made, although the viscosity and osmolarity of this is likely to be high.
- A prolonged break in feeding is not required.

Intragastric administration

1. Stop the enteral feed.
2. Flush the enteral feeding tube with the recommended volume of water.
3. Place the tablet in a mortar and crush to a fine powder using the pestle.
4. Add a few millilitres of water and mix to form a paste.
5. Add up to 15 mL of water and mix thoroughly, ensuring that there are no large particles of tablet.
6. Draw this into an appropriate syringe.
7. Flush the medication dose down the feeding tube.
8. Add another 15 mL of water to the mortar and stir to ensure that any remaining drug is rinsed from the container. Draw this water into the syringe and also flush this via the feeding tube (this will rinse the mortar and syringe and ensure total dose is administered).
9. Finally, flush the enteral feeding tube with the recommended volume of water.
10. Re-start the feed, unless a prolonged break is necessary.

Intrajejunal administration

There are no specific data relating to jejunal administration of terbinafine. Administer using the above method. Monitor for increased side-effects or loss of efficacy.

References

1. *BNF 50*, September 2005.
2. Abdel-Rahman SM, Nahata MC. Stability of terbinafine hydrochloride in an extemporaneously prepared oral suspension at 25 and 4 °C. *Am J Health Syst Pharm*. 1999; 56: 243–245.
3. Dollery C. *Therapeutic Drugs*, 2nd edn. London: Churchill Livingstone; 1998.

Theophylline

Formulations available[1]

Brand name (Manufacturer)	Formulation and strength	Product information/Administration information
Nuelin (3M)	Liquid 60 mg/5 mL	Product discontinued March 2004. Brown viscous liquid. Quite resistant to flushing. Mixes easily with an equal quantity of water to reduce osmolarity and resistance to flushing.[2] Contains sucrose, does not contain sorbitol.[3]

Formulations available[1] (continued)

Brand name (Manufacturer)	Formulation and strength	Product information/Administration information
Nuelin SA (3M)	M/R tablets 175 mg, 250 mg	Modified-release tablets; do not crush. To convert to liquid, divide the total daily dose by 3 and administer as three-times-daily liquid preparation.
Slo-Phyllin (Merck)	M/R capsules 60 mg, 125 mg, 250 mg	Modified-release capsules; do not crush modified-release pellets.[4] Capsule can be opened and pellets could be administered via an enteral tube. Pellets may get stuck within the tube, especially in smaller sized tubes.[4] To convert to liquid, divide the total daily dose by 3 and administer as three-times-daily liquid preparation.
Uniphyllin Continuous (Napp)	M/R tablets 200 mg, 300 mg, 400 mg	Modified-release tablets; do not crush.[5] To convert to liquid, divide the total daily dose by 3 and administer as three-times-daily liquid preparation.
Theophylline (Rosemont)	Oral solution 10 mg/5 mL	Manufactured 'special'. Contains 1.14 g sorbitol/5 mL.[6]
Aminophylline Injection (various manufacturers)	Injection 25 mg/mL (10 mL)	Sterile solution of theophylline 2.11% w/v and ethylenediamine 0.52% w/v in water for injection (211 mg theophylline/10 mL). The injection has a pH of 8.6–9 and an osmolality of 170 mOsm/kg.[7] This solution is suitable for oral/enteral administration.

Site of absorption (oral administration)

Specific site of absorption is not documented.

Alternative routes available

Aminophylline injection is available for parenteral use; there are also anecdotal reports of enteral administration of the injection.

Interactions

The effect of food, enteral feed and nutrition per se on the pharmacokinetics of theophylline is complex and largely undefined. A single small study of the co-administration of theophylline with enteral feed reported reduced absorption.[8] There have also been reports of hepatic enzyme induction by high-protein diets.[9] The clinical consequence of the interactions may be variable and therefore close monitoring should be undertaken until plasma concentration and regimen are stabilised.

Health and safety

Standard precautions apply.

Suggestions/recommendations

- Use a liquid special preparation. Convert sustained-released preparations to three or four times daily dosing.
- Dilute the liquid with an equal volume of water immediately prior to administration.
- If necessary, aminophylline injection can be given orally/enterally; note the dose as above.
- Despite the lack of consistent data, it is currently recommended[10] to give theophylline during a break in feeding where possible. If this is not practical, ensure that doses are given consistently with respect to feed times.
- Monitor plasma concentration closely during transition to liquid preparation and during any changes in feeding regimens.

Intragastric administration

1. Stop the enteral feed.
2. Flush the enteral feeding tube with the recommended volume of water.
3. Give during break in feeding if practical; see notes above.
4. Draw the medication into an appropriate size syringe.
5. Flush the medication dose down the feeding tube.
6. Finally, flush with the recommended volume of water.
7. Re-start the feed, unless a prolonged break is required.

Alternatively, at step (4) measure the medicine in a suitable container and then add an equal volume of water and mix thoroughly. Draw this into the syringe with appropriate adapter for tube connector. Ensure that the measure is rinsed and that this rinsing water is administered also to ensure that the total dose is given. **Do not** measure liquid medicines using a catheter-tipped syringe as this results in excessive dosing owing to the volume of the tip.

Intrajejunal administration

No specific data are available. Administer using the above method.

References

1. *BNF* 50, September 2005.
2. BPNG data on file, 2005.
3. Nuelin Liquid (3M), Summary of Product Characteristics; June 2000. (Discontinued 2004.)
4. Personal communication, Merck; 23 January 2003.
5. Personal communication, Napp; 29 January 2003.
6. Personal communication, Rosemont; 20 January 2005.
7. Trissel LA, ed. *Stability of Compounded Formulations*, 2nd edn. Washington, DC: American Pharmaceutical Association; 2000.
8. Gal P, Layson R. Interference with oral theophylline absorption by continuous nasogastric feedings. *Ther Drug Monit.* 1986; 8: 421–423.
9. Welling PG, Lyons LL, Craig WA, Trochta GA. Influence of diet and fluid on bioavailability of theophylline. *Clin Pharmacol Ther.* 1975; 7: 45–480.
10. Stockley IH. *Stockley's Drug Interactions*, 6th edn. London: Pharmaceutical Press; 2002.

Tiagabine

Formulations available [1]		
Brand name (Manufacturer)	**Formulation and strength**	**Product information/Administration information**
Gabitril (Cephalon)	Tablets 5 mg, 10 mg, 15 mg	Tiagabine hydrochloride. Film-coated, scored tablets. Tablets disintegrate if shaken in 10 mL of water for 7 minutes to give a fine dispersion that flushes down an 8Fr NG tube without blockage. Tablets also crush easily and mix well with water. [3]

Site of absorption (oral administration)

Specific site of absorption is not documented.

Alternative routes available

None available for tiagabine.

Interactions

Administration with food results in a reduced rate but not extent of absorption. [2]

Health and safety

Standard precautions apply.

Suggestions/recommendations

- The tablets can be dispersed in water or crushed and suspended in water immediately prior to administration. A prolonged break in feeding is not required.

Intragastric administration

1. Stop the enteral feed.
2. Flush the enteral feeding tube with the recommended volume of water.
3. Place the tablet in the barrel of an appropriate size and type of syringe.
4. Draw 10 mL of water into the syringe and allow the tablet to disperse, shaking vigorously.
5. Flush the medication dose down the feeding tube.
6. Draw another 10 mL of water into the syringe and also flush this via the feeding tube (this will rinse the syringe and ensure that the total dose is administered).
7. Finally, flush with the recommended volume of water.
8. Re-start the feed, unless a prolonged break is required.

Intrajejunal administration

There are no specific data relating to the jejunal administration of tiagabine. For administration via this route, the above method can be used.

References

1. *BNF* 50, September 2005.
2. Gabitril (Cephalon), Summary of Product Characteristics; September 2002.
3. BPNG data on file, 2004.

Timolol maleate

Formulations available[1]

Brand name (Manufacturer)	Formulation and strength	Product information/Administration information
Betim (Valeant)	Tablets 10 mg	Scored. Tablets disperse rapidly in 10 mL of water to give a fine, even dispersion that flushes via an 8Fr NG tube without blockage.[2]

Site of absorption (oral administration)

Specific site of absorption is not documented. Peak plasma concentration occurs 1–2 hours after an oral dose;[4] beta-blocking activity is evident within 30 minutes of dosing.[3]

Alternative routes available

None available for timolol; other beta-blockers are available in parenteral form.

Interactions

There is no documented interaction with food.[3, 4]

Health and safety

Standard precautions apply.

Suggestions/recommendations

- Owing to the limited data, consider changing to an alternative beta-blocker available in liquid formulation.
- If continued therapy with timolol is indicated, disperse the tablets in water immediately prior to dosing.
- A prolonged break in feeding is not necessary.
- Owing to the lack of data relating to this route of administration, monitor the patient for signs of loss of efficacy of therapy.

Intragastric administration

1. Stop the enteral feed.
2. Flush the enteral feeding tube with the recommended volume of water.
3. Place the tablet in the barrel of an appropriate size and type of syringe.
4. Draw 10 mL of water into the syringe and allow the tablet to disperse, shaking if necessary.
5. Flush the medication dose down the feeding tube.
6. Draw another 10 mL of water into the oral syringe and also flush this via the feeding tube (this will rinse the syringe and ensure that the total dose is administered).
7. Finally, flush with the recommended volume of water.
8. Re-start the feed, unless a prolonged break is required.

Alternatively, at step (3) place the tablet into a medicine pot, add 10 mL of water and allow the tablet to disperse. Draw this into an appropriate syringe. Ensure that the measure is rinsed and that this rinsing water is administered also to ensure that the total dose is given.

Intrajejunal administration

There are no specific data relating to jejunal administration; therefore, patient should be monitored. The above method of administration can be used.

References

1. *BNF* 50, September 2005.
2. BPNG data on file, 2005.
3. Betim (ICN), Summary of Product Characteristics; December 2000.
4. Dollery C. *Therapeutic Drugs*, 2nd edn. London: Churchill Livingstone; 1998.

Tizanidine hydrochloride

Formulations available[1]

Brand name (Manufacturer)	Formulation and strength	Product information/Administration information
Zanaflex (Elan)	Tablets 2 mg, 4 mg	Tablets can be crushed and dispersed in water at the time of administration.[2] Tablets do not disperse readily, but will disintegrate if shaken in 10 mL of water for 5 minutes. The resulting dispersion will flush via an 8Fr NG tube without blockage.[3]
Tizanidine (nonproprietary)	Tablets 2 mg, 4 mg	No specific data are available on enteral tube administration of this formulation.

Site of absorption (oral administration)

Specific site of absorption is not documented. Peak plasma concentration occurs within 1 hour following oral dosing.[4]

Alternative routes available

No alternative route available for tizanidine. Diazepam is available in parenteral and rectal formulation.

Interactions

Food has no effect on the pharmacokinetic profile of tizanidine.[4]

Health and safety

Standard precautions apply

Suggestions/recommendations

- Disperse the tablets in water immediately prior to administration.
- A prolonged break in feeding is not required.

Intragastric administration

1. Stop the enteral feed.
2. Flush the enteral feeding tube with the recommended volume of water.
3. Place the tablet in the barrel of an appropriate size and type of syringe.
4. Draw 10 mL of water into the syringe and allow the tablet to disperse, shaking if necessary.
5. Flush the medication dose down the feeding tube.
6. Draw another 10 mL of water into the syringe and also flush this via the feeding tube (this will rinse the syringe and ensure that the total dose is administered).
7. Finally, flush with the recommended volume of water.
8. Re-start the feed, unless a prolonged break is required.

Alternatively, at step (3) place the tablet into a medicine pot, add 10 mL of water and allow the tablet to disperse. Draw this into an appropriate syringe. Ensure that the measure is rinsed and that this rinsing water is administered also to ensure that the total dose is given.

Intrajejunal administration

There are no specific data. Administer using the above method. Monitor for increased side-effects or loss of efficacy.

References

1. *BNF 50*, September 2005.
2. Personal communication, Elan Pharma; 16 January 2003.
3. BPNG data on file, 2005.
4. Zanaflex (Elan), Summary of Product Characteristics; February 2001.

Tolbutamide

Formulations available[1]

Brand name (Manufacturer)	Formulation and strength	Product information/Administration information
Tolbutamide (Alpharma, APS, Hillcross)	Tablets 500 mg	Alpharma brand tablets do not disperse readily and do not mix well with water when crushed.[2]

Site of absorption (oral administration)

Specific site of absorption is not documented. Peak plasma concentration occurs 3–4 hours after oral dosing.[3]

Alternative routes available

None available for tolbutamide. Insulin is available for parenteral administration.

Interactions

No specific interaction with food or feed is documented.[3]

Health and safety

Standard precautions apply.

Suggestions/recommendations

- Owing to limited data, consider changing to an alternative sulphonylurea. Seek specialist advice.

References

1. *BNF* 50, September 2005.
2. BPNG data on file, 2005.
3. Dollery C. *Therapeutic Drugs*, 2nd edn. London: Churchill Livingstone; 1998.

Tolterodine tartrate

Formulations available[1]

Brand name (Manufacturer)	Formulation and strength	Product information/Administration information
Detrusitol (Pharmacia)	Tablets 1 mg, 2 mg	Film-coated. Tablets can be crushed and mixed with water and taken immediately. However, as tolterodine is relatively insoluble in water, the crushed tablets are unlikely to go into solution.[2] Tablets disperse within 2 minutes when placed in 10 mL of water to form a coarse dispersion that settles quickly but draws up and flushes via an 8Fr NG tube without blockage.[3]
Detrusitol XL (Pharmacia)	Capsules 4 mg	Modified-release capsules. Capsules contain modified-release granules that do not disperse well in water and do not draw up into a syringe.[3]

Site of absorption (oral administration)

Specific site of absorption is not documented; however, as a modified-release preparation is available, significant absorption must occur in the small bowel. Peak plasma concentration occurs 1–3 hours following oral dosing of the immediate-release product.[4]

Alternative routes available

None available for tolterodine.

Interactions

Food does not significantly affect bioavailability.[4]

Health and safety

Standard precautions apply.

Suggestions/recommendations

- Consider an alternative therapy available in a suitable formulation.
- If continued therapy with tolterodine is indicated, disperse the tablets in water immediately prior to administration.
- A prolonged break in feeding is not required.

Intragastric administration

1. Stop the enteral feed.
2. Flush the enteral feeding tube with the recommended volume of water.
3. Place the tablet in the barrel of an appropriate size and type of syringe.
4. Draw 10 mL of water into the syringe and allow the tablet to disperse, shaking if necessary.
5. Flush the medication dose down the feeding tube.
6. Draw another 10 mL of water into the syringe and also flush this via the feeding tube (this will rinse the syringe and ensure that the total dose is administered).
7. Finally, flush with the recommended volume of water.
8. Re-start the feed, unless a prolonged break is required.

Alternatively, at step (3) place the tablet into a medicine pot, add 10 mL of water and allow the tablet to disperse. Draw this into an appropriate syringe. Ensure that the measure is rinsed and that this rinsing water is administered also to ensure that the total dose is given.

Intrajejunal administration

There are no specific data relating to the jejunal administration of tolterodine; however, the modified-release preparation is designed to release the drug through the small bowel and therefore jejunal administration is unlikely to affect bioavailability. Administer as above. Monitor for lack of efficacy and increased side-effects.

References

1. *BNF* 50, September 2005.
2. Personal communication, Pharmacia; 11 March 2003.
3. BPNG data on file, 2004.
4. Detrusitol (Pharmacia), Summary of Product Characteristics; April 2003.

Topiramate

Formulations available[1]

Brand name (Manufacturer)	Formulation and strength	Product information/Administration information
Topamax (Janssen-Cilag)	Tablets 25 mg, 50 mg, 100 mg, 200 mg	Film-coated. The only option for enteral feeding tube administration is to crush the tablets and suspend the fine particles in water, making a slurry and administering immediately.[2] Tablets do not disperse readily in water owing to the coating but will disintegrate if shaken in 10 mL of water for 5 minutes; the resulting dispersion flushes down an 8Fr NG tube without blockage.[4]
Topamax (Janssen-Cilag)	Sprinkle capsules 15 mg, 25 mg, 50 mg,	Contents can be sprinkled onto soft food. Administration of the beads through an enteral feeding tube does not work well as the beads readily stick to the tubing and block the tube.[2]

Site of absorption (oral administration)

Rapidly and well absorbed; no specific site of absorption is documented.[3]

Alternative routes available

None for topiramate.

Interactions

There is no clinically significant effect of food on absorption.[3]

Health and safety

Standard precautions apply.

Suggestions/recommendations

- Consider changing to an alternative therapy available in a suitable formulation. If continued therapy with topiramate is indicated, disperse the tablets in water immediately prior to administration.
- A prolonged break in feeding is not required.

Intragastric administration

1. Stop the enteral feed.
2. Flush the enteral feeding tube with the recommended volume of water.
3. Place the tablet in the barrel of an appropriate size and type of syringe.
4. Draw 10 mL of water into the syringe and allow the tablet to disperse, shaking vigorously.
5. Flush the medication dose down the feeding tube.
6. Draw another 10 mL of water into the syringe and also flush this via the feeding tube (this will rinse the syringe and ensure that the total dose is administered).
7. Finally, flush with the recommended volume of water.
8. Re-start the feed, unless a prolonged break is required.

Intrajejunal administration

There are no specific data relating to jejunal administration of topiramate; therefore, monitor for signs of loss of efficacy. Administer by the method detailed above.

References

1. *BNF* 50, September 2005.
2. Personal communication, Janssen-Cilag; 22 January 2003.
3. Topamax (Janssen-Cilag), Summary of Product Characteristics; September 2003.
4. BPNG data on file, 2004.

Tramadol hydrochloride

Formulations available[1]

Brand name (Manufacturer)	Formulation and strength	Product information/Administration information
Tramadol (Alpharma, APS, Arrow, Galen, Generics, Genus, IVAX, PLIVA, Sovereign, Sterwin, Tillomed)	Capsules 50 mg	Alpharma recommends using alternative preparations, rather than opening the capsules.[2] Ranbaxy capsules open easily and the contents mix easily with water to form a fine suspension that flushes easily via an 8Fr NG tube without blockage.[3]
Tramadol (Aurum, Sterwin, Viatris, Searle)	Injection 50 mg/mL (2 mL)	Sterwin brand licensed for i.v. use only. No specific data on enteral administration are available for this formulation. Zamadol; Zydol.
Tramake Insts (Galen)	Sachets 50 mg, 100 mg	50 mg sachet contains 9.7 mmol sodium per sachet. 100 mg sachet contains 14.6 mmol sodium per sachet. Sachet contents effervesce in 10 mL of water to form a clear solution; this can be administered via fine-bore tube without risk of blockage.[6]
Zamadol (Viatris)	Capsules 50 mg	No specific data on enteral tube administration are available for this formulation.
Zamadol Melt (Viatris)	Orodispersible tablets 50 mg	May also be dispersed in water.
Zydol (Searle)	Capsules 50 mg	Pharmacia recommends using soluble tablets; however, if those are unavailable the capsules can be opened and the contents dispersed in water. Care should be taken to avoid alcoholic drinks and foods or drinks at extreme temperature or pH[4].
Zydol (Searle)	Soluble tablets 50 mg	Tablets disperse in water.[4] Recommended volume is 50 mL[5]. Tablets disintegrate in 10 mL of water to form a dispersion that settles quickly. Care must be taken to administer the complete dose. Flushes via an 8Fr NG tube without blockage, but may block finer tubes.[6]

Modified-release preparations
Not suitable for administration via enteral feeding tube:
Dromadol SR (IVAX) modified-release tablets
Dromadol XL (IVAX) modified-release tablets
Zamadol SR (Viatris) modified-release capsules
Zydol SR (Searle) modified-release tablets
Zydol XL (Searle) modified-released tablets

Site of absorption (oral administration)

Specific site of absorption is not documented. Tramadol is detectable in the plasma within 15 minutes of oral administration; peak plasma concentrations occur at 1.6–2 hours.[5]

Alternative routes available

Parenteral formulation is available. Orodispersible tablet disintegrates in the mouth but is not absorbed sublingually.

Interactions

No specific interaction with food is documented.

Health and safety

Standard precautions apply.

Suggestions/recommendations

- Use dispersible tablets or sachets (note the sodium content).
- A prolonged break in feeding is not required.

Intragastric administration

Soluble tablets

1. Stop the enteral feed.
2. Flush the enteral feeding tube with the recommended volume of water.
3. Place the tablet in the barrel of an appropriate size and type of syringe.
4. Draw 10 mL of water into an appropriate size and type of syringe and allow the tablet to disperse.
5. Flush the medication dose down the feeding tube.
6. Draw an equal volume of water into the syringe and also flush this via the feeding tube (this will rinse the syringe and ensure that the total dose is administered).
7. Finally, flush with the recommended volume of water.
8. Re-start the feed, unless a prolonged break is required.

Alternatively, at step (3) place the tablet into a medicine pot, add 10 mL of water and allow the tablet to disperse. Draw this into an appropriate syringe. Ensure that the measure is rinsed and that this rinsing water is administered also to ensure that the total dose is given.

Sachets

1. Stop the enteral feed.
2. Flush the enteral feeding tube with the recommended volume of water.
3. Measure 10 mL of water into a measuring pot.
4. Add the contents of the sachet and allow to dissolve.
5. Draw into an appropriate syringe.
6. Flush the medication dose down the feeding tube.
7. Rinse the measure and administer this also to ensure that the total dose is given.
8. Finally, flush with the recommended volume of water.
9. Re-start the feed, unless a prolonged break is required.

Intrajejunal administration

There are no specific data relating to jejunal administration, but as modified-release preparations are available it is likely that tramadol is absorbed throughout the small bowel. Administer using the above method and monitor for increased side-effects.

References

1. *BNF* 50, September 2005.
2. Personal communication, Alpharma; 21 January 2003.
3. BPNG data on file, 2004.
4. Personal communication, Pharmacia; 11 March 2003.
5. Zydol soluble tablets (Pharmacia), Summary of Product Characteristics; December 2002.
6. BPNG data on file, 2005.

Trandolapril

Formulations available [1]

Brand name (Manufacturer)	Formulation and strength	Product information/Administration information
Gopten (Abbott)	Capsules 500 microgram, 1 mg, 2 mg	Capsules are small and would require significant manual dexterity to open. Solubility in water 1 : 1000.[4] No specific data on enteral tube administration are available for this formulation.
Odrik (Hoechst Marion Roussel)	Capsules 500 microgram, 1 mg, 2 mg	No specific data on enteral tube administration are available for this formulation.
Tarka (Abbott)	Capsules 2 mg/180 mg	Combination product containing trandolapril 2 mg, verapamil 180 mg M/R. Tarka capsules should be swallowed whole;[3] owing to the inclusion of M/R verapamil this formulation is unsuitable for administration via an enteral feeding tube.

Site of absorption (oral administration)

Specific site of absorption is not documented. Peak plasma concentration of trandolapril is reached within 30 minutes of oral dosing.[2]

Alternative routes available

None available for trandolapril.

Interactions

Food intake delays absorption,[4] but the total absorption of trandolapril and conversion to trandolaprilat are unaffected by food.[2]

Health and safety

Standard precautions apply.

Suggestions/recommendations

- Owing to lack of data, consider changing to an alternative once-daily ACE inhibitor, for example lisinopril liquid (see monograph) or ramipril tablets (see monograph).
- An appropriate method of administration cannot be recommended owing to the lack of data.

References

1. *BNF* 50, September 2005.
2. Gopten (Abbott), Summary of Product Characteristics; December 2001.
3. Tarka (Abbott), Summary of Product Characteristics; March 2002.
4. Dollery C. *Therapeutic Drugs*, 2nd edn. London: Churchill Livingstone; 1998.

Tranexamic acid

Formulations available[1]

Brand name (Manufacturer)	Formulation and strength	Product information/Administration information
Cyklokapron (Pharmacia)	Tablets 500 mg	Film-coated, scored. Tablets can be crushed and suspended in water. Tablets disperse in 2–5 minutes when placed in water.[2]
Tranexamic Acid (Manx)	Tablets 500 mg	Tablets do not disperse readily but will disintegrate when shaken in 10 mL of water; the resulting milky dispersion flushes via an 8Fr NG tube without blockage.[3]
Cyklokapron (Pharmacia)	Injection 100 mg/mL (5 mL)	Injection can be used orally. Keep opened injection no longer than 24 hours in the fridge. pH 6.5–8.[2]

Site of absorption (oral administration)

Specific site of absorption is not documented.[4]

Alternative routes available

Parenteral route is available. Injection can be used topically as mouthwash and bladder irrigation (unlicensed indications).

Interactions

Bioavailability is not reduced by food.[4]

Health and safety

Standard precautions apply.

Suggestions/recommendations

- Disperse the tablets in water immediately prior to administration.
- For very fine-bore tubes the injection could be used.
- A prolonged break in feeding is not required.

Intragastric administration

1. Stop the enteral feed.
2. Flush the enteral feeding tube with the recommended volume of water.
3. Place the tablet in the barrel of an appropriate size and type of syringe.
4. Draw 10 mL of water into the syringe and allow the tablet to disperse, shaking if necessary.
5. Flush the medication dose down the feeding tube.
6. Draw another 10 mL of water into the syringe and also flush this via the feeding tube (this will rinse the syringe and ensure that the total dose is administered).
7. Finally, flush with the recommended volume of water.
8. Re-start the feed, unless a prolonged break is required.

Alternatively, at step (3) place the tablet into a medicine pot, add 10 mL of water and allow the tablet to disperse. Draw this into an appropriate syringe. Ensure that the measure is rinsed and that this rinsing water is administered also to ensure that the total dose is given.

Jejunal administration

Administer as above, or use injection formulation.

References

1. *BNF* 50, September 2005.
2. Personal communication, Pharmacia; 11 March 2003.
3. BPNG data on file, 2005.
4. Dollery C. *Therapeutic Drugs*, 2nd edn. London: Churchill Livingstone; 1998.

Trazodone hydrochloride

Formulations available[1]

Brand name (Manufacturer)	Formulation and strength	Product information/Administration information
Trazodone (APS, Generics, Sterwin)	Capsules 50 mg, 100 mg	No specific data on enteral tube administration are available for this formulation.
Trazodone (APS, Generics, Sterwin)	Tablets 150 mg	No specific data on enteral tube administration are available for this formulation.
Molipaxin (Hoechst Marion Roussel)	Capsules 50 mg, 100 mg	50 mg capsules can be opened and the contents mixed with 10 mL of water; no visible particles; flushes via an 8Fr NG tube without blockage.[2]

Formulations available[1] (continued)

Brand name (Manufacturer)	Formulation and strength	Product information/Administration information
Molipaxin (Hoechst Marion Roussel)	Tablets 150 mg	Film-coated.[3] No specific data on enteral tube administration are available for this formulation.
Molipaxin (Hoechst Marion Roussel)	Liquid 50 mg/5 mL	Sugar-free Clear, colourless solution with an orange odour and taste.[4] Contains sorbitol 1.05 mg/5 mL[5]. Very pale yellow, viscous liquid; some resistance on flushing via a fine-bore NG tube. Mixes easily with an equal volume of water to reduce viscosity and resistance to flushing.[6]

Site of absorption (oral administration)

Specific site of administration is not documented. Peak plasma concentration occurs 1.5 hours after oral administration.[3]

Alternative routes available

None available for trazodone.

Interactions

Absorption is delayed and enhanced slightly by food.[3] Tolerability may be increased by taking with food.[3]

Health and safety

Standard precautions apply.

Suggestions/recommendations

- Use the liquid preparation.
- A prolonged break in feeding is not necessary; tolerability may be improved by administering after feed. Alternatively, the capsules can be opened and the contents mixed with water immediately prior to administration; however, this should be considered a last resort.

Intragastric administration

1. Stop the enteral feed.
2. Flush the enteral feeding tube with the recommended volume of water.
3. Draw the medication into an appropriate size and type of syringe.
4. Flush the medication dose down the feeding tube.
5. Finally, flush with the recommended volume of water.
6. Re-start the feed, unless a prolonged break is required.

Alternatively, at step (3) measure the medicine in a suitable container. Draw this into an appropriate syringe. Ensure that the measure is rinsed and that this rinsing water is administered also to ensure that the total dose is given. **Do not** measure liquid medicines using a catheter-tipped syringe as this results in excessive dosing owing to the volume of the tip.

Intrajejunal administration

Use the liquid preparation as detailed above. The dose can be diluted with water immediately prior to administration to reduce the viscosity. Alternatively, the capsule contents can be dispersed in water immediately prior to administration.

1. Stop the enteral feed.
2. Flush the enteral feeding tube with the recommended volume of water.
3. Open the capsule and pour the contents into a medicine pot.
4. Add 15 mL of water.
5. Stir to disperse the powder.
6. Draw into an appropriate syringe and administer via the feeding tube.
7. Add a further 15 mL of water to the medicine pot; stir to ensure that any powder remaining in the pot is mixed with water.
8. Draw up this dispersion and flush down the tube. This will ensure that the whole dose is given.
9. Flush the tube with the recommended volume of water.
10. Re-start the feed, unless a prolonged break is required.

References

1. *BNF 50*, September 2005.
2. BPNG data on file, 2004.
3. Molipaxin 150 mg Tablets (Sanofi-Aventis), Summary of Product Characteristics; June 2001.
4. Molipaxin Liquid 50 mg/5 mL (Sanofi-Aventis), Summary of Product Characteristics; May 2002.
5. Personal communication, Aventis; 9 February 2005.
6. BPNG data on file, 2005.

Trifluoperazine hydrochloride

Formulations available[1]

Brand name (Manufacturer)	Formulation and strength	Product information/Administration information
Trifluoperazine (various manufacturers)	Tablets 1 mg, 5 mg	Coated. No specific data on enteral tube administration are available for this formulation.
Trifluoperazine (Rosemont)	Oral solution 5 mg/5 mL	Sugar-free. Contains 0.45 g sorbitol/5 mL.[2]
Stelazine (Goldshield)	Tablets 1 mg, 5 mg	Film-coated tablets No specific data on enteral tube administration are available for this formulation.
Stelazine Spansules (Goldshield)	M/R capsules 2 mg, 10 mg, 15 mg	Modified-release preparation. Do not crush. Not suitable for enteral tube administration.
Stelazine (Goldshield)	Syrup 1 mg/5 mL	Pale yellow, nonviscous liquid; flushes easily via a fine-bore NG tube with little resistance. Mixes easily with an equal volume of water.[4]

Formulations available [1] (*continued*)

Brand name (Manufacturer)	Formulation and strength	Product information/Administration information
Stelazine (Goldshield)	Oral solution forte 5 mg/5 mL	Sugar-free.

Site of absorption (oral administration)

Specific site of absorption is not specified. Peak plasma concentration occurs 1–6 hours following oral absorption. [3]

Alternative routes available

No alternative route available for trifluoperazine. Alternative antipsychotic drugs are available in parenteral formulation. Seek specialist advice.

Interactions

No specific interaction with food is documented. [3]

Health and safety

Standard precautions apply.

Suggestions/recommendations

- Use the liquid preparation, no further dilution is necessary for intragastric administration. The liquid can be diluted with at least an equal volume of water prior to administration via jejunal tube to reduce the osmolarity.
- A prolonged break in feeding is not required.

Intragastric administration

1. Stop the enteral feed.
2. Flush the enteral feeding tube with the recommended volume of water.
3. Draw the medication solution into an appropriate size and type of syringe.
4. Flush the medication dose down the feeding tube.
5. Finally, flush with the recommended volume of water.
6. Re-start the feed, unless a prolonged break is required.

Alternatively, at step (4) measure the medicine in a suitable container and then draw into an appropriate syringe. Ensure that the measure is rinsed and that this rinsing water is administered also to ensure that the total dose is given. **Do not** measure liquid medicines using a catheter-tipped syringe as this results in excessive dosing owing to the volume of the tip.

Intrajejunal administration

1. Stop the enteral feed.
2. Flush the enteral feeding tube with the recommended volume of water.
3. Draw the medication into an appropriate size and type of syringe.
4. Draw an equal volume of water and a little air into the syringe and shake to mix thoroughly.
5. Flush the medication dose down the feeding tube.
6. Finally, flush with the recommended volume of water.
7. Re-start the feed, unless a prolonged break is required.

Alternatively, at step (3) measure the medicine in a suitable container and then add an equal volume of water and mix thoroughly. Draw this into an appropriate syringe. Ensure that the measure is rinsed and that this rinsing water is administered also to ensure that the total dose is given. **Do not** measure liquid medicines using a catheter-tipped syringe as this results in excessive dosing owing to the volume of the tip.

References

1. *BNF* 50, September 2005.
2. Personal communication, Rosemont Pharma; 20 January 2005.
3. Dollery C. *Therapeutic Drugs*, 2nd edn. London: Churchill Livingstone; 1998.
4. BPNG data on file, 2005.

Trihexyphenidyl (Benzhexol) hydrochloride

Formulations available[1]

Brand name (Manufacturer)	Formulation and strength	Product information/Administration information
Broflex (Alliance)	Syrup 5 mg/5 mL	A blackcurrant-scented and flavoured clear pink syrup.[2] pH 2.45–2.75.[3]
Trihexyphenidyl (Biorex, Genus)	Tablets 2 mg, 5 mg	Tablets disintegrate rapidly in water to form a fine dispersion that flushes via an 8Fr NG tube without blockage.[4]

Site of absorption (oral administration)

Trihexyphenidyl is readily absorbed from the GI tract; the exact site of absorption is not known.[3]

Alternative routes available

None available for trihexyphenidyl. Procyclidine is available in parenteral formulation.

Interactions

No interaction with food is documented.

Health and safety

Standard precautions apply.

Suggestions/recommendations

- Use the liquid preparation or disperse tablets in water immediately prior to administration.
- A prolonged break in feeding is not required.

Intragastric administration

1. Stop the enteral feed.
2. Flush the enteral feeding tube with the recommended volume of water.
3. Draw the medication solution into an appropriate size and type of syringe.
4. Flush the medication dose down the feeding tube.
5. Finally, flush with the recommended volume of water.
6. Re-start the feed, unless a prolonged break is required.

Alternatively, at step (3) measure the medicine in a suitable container and then draw into an appropriate syringe. Ensure that the measure is rinsed and that this rinsing water is administered also to ensure that the total dose is given. **Do not** measure liquid medicines using a catheter-tipped syringe as this results in excessive dosing owing to the volume of the tip.

Intrajejunal administration

There are no specific data. Administer using the method above or use tablets dispersed in water. Monitor for increased side-effects or loss of efficacy.

References

1. *BNF* 50, September 2005.
2. Broflex, Summary of Product Characteristics; October 2001.
3. Personal communication, Alliance Pharmaceuticals; January 2003.
4. BPNG data on file, 2005.

Trimethoprim

Formulations available [1]

Brand name (Manufacturer)	Formulation and strength	Product information/Administration information
Trimethoprim (Alpharma, APS, Berk, IVAX, Kent)	Tablets 100 mg, 200 mg	Avoid crushing tablets owing to the risk of third-party exposure to the powder. [2]
Monotrim (Solvay)	Suspension 50 mg/5 mL	Solvay does not have any specific information on the administration of Monotrim via enteral feeding tubes. Trimethoprim is well absorbed from the GI tract and therefore the company does not envisage any problems and does not expect any change in bioavailability. [3] The liquid should not be mixed with enteral feed. [3] Contains sorbitol. pH 6.8.

Formulations available[1] (continued)

Brand name (Manufacturer)	Formulation and strength	Product information/Administration information
Trimopan (APS)	Suspension 50 mg/5 mL	White cloudy suspension; some resistance to flushing via a fine-bore tube. Mixes easily with an equal volume of water and this reduces resistance to flushing.[4]
Monotrim	Injection 100 mg/5 mL	Discontinued in UK in April 2003. Available through IDIS.

Site of absorption (oral administration)

Specific site is not documented. Peak plasma concentration occurs 1–4 hours following oral dose.[5]

Alternative routes available

Parenteral route is available.

Interactions

Concomitant administration of trimethoprim with food has resulted in reduced absorption; therefore, trimethoprim should be administered during a break in feed for optimal absorption.[3]

Health and safety

Standard precautions apply when handling the liquid. Avoid crushing the tablets.

Suggestions/recommendations

- Use the liquid preparation.
- Give during a break in feed for optimal absorption if practical.

Intragastric administration

1. Stop the enteral feed.
2. Flush the enteral feeding tube with the recommended volume of water.
3. Give the dose during a break in feeding if practical.
4. Shake the medication bottle thoroughly to ensure adequate mixing.
5. Draw the medication suspension into an appropriate size and type of syringe.
6. Flush the medication dose down the feeding tube.
7. Finally, flush with the recommended volume of water.
8. Re-start the feed, unless a prolonged break is required.

Alternatively, at step (5) measure the medicine in a suitable container. Draw this into an appropriate syringe. Ensure that the measure is rinsed and that this rinsing water is administered also to ensure that the total dose is given. **Do not** measure liquid medicines using a catheter-tipped syringe as this results in excessive dosing owing to the volume of the tip.

Intrajejunal administration

There are no specific data. Administer using the above method.

References

1. *BNF* 50, September 2005.
2. Personal communication, Alpharma; 21 January 2003.
3. Personal communication, Solvay; 19 February 2003.
4. BPNG data on file, 2004.
5. Dollery C. *Therapeutic Drugs*, 2nd edn. London: Churchill Livingstone; 1998.

Trimipramine

Formulations available[1]

Brand name (Manufacturer)	Formulation and strength	Product information/Administration information
Surmontil (Aventis)	Capsules 50 mg	White crystalline powder, pours easily from the capsule. Disperses easily in water but settles quickly; care must be taken to ensure that the entire dose is administered. Flushes via an 8Fr NG tube without blockage.[2]
Surmontil (Aventis)	Tablets 10 mg, 25 mg	Tablets do not disperse readily in water, but can be crushed and mixed with water.[2]

Site of absorption (oral administration)

Specific site of absorption is not documented.[3]

Alternative routes available

None available for trimipramine.

Interactions

No interaction with food is documented.[3]

Health and safety

Standard precautions apply.

Suggestions/recommendations

- For long-term therapy, consider changing to an alternative tricyclic antidepressant available as a liquid.
- If continued therapy with trimipramine is indicated, the tablets can be crushed and mixed with water or the capsule contents can be dispersed in water; this should be considered a last resort.

References

1. *BNF* 50, September 2005.
2. BPNG data on file, 2005.
3. Dollery C. *Therapeutic Drugs*, 2nd edn. London: Churchill Livingstone; 1998.

Ursodeoxycholic acid

Formulations available[1]

Brand name (Manufacturer)	Formulation and strength	Product information/Administration information
Ursodeoxycholic acid (Hillcross)	Tablets 150 mg Capsules 250 mg	No specific data on enteral tube administration are available for this formulation.
Destolit (Norgine)	Tablets 150 mg	The tablets are not a specially coated or slow-release product and in theory can be crushed.[2] Tablets disperse when shaken in 10 mL of water for 4 minutes to give a fine dispersion with some visible particles that flush down an 8Fr tube without blockage.[5]
Urdox (CP)	Tablets 300 mg	It should be acceptable to crush Urdox tablets and suspend in water immediately prior to administration.[3]
Ursofalk (Dr Falk)	Capsules 250 mg	The capsules can be opened and the contents sprinkled onto food. However, the powder is not very soluble and so the suspension is recommended.[4] The capsule contents do not disperse easily in water, and contain some large granules that settle quickly; there is high risk of tube blockage with administration via fine-bore tubes.[5]
Ursofalk (Dr Falk)	Suspension 250 mg/5 mL	Sugar-free suspension does not contain sorbitol.[6]
Ursogal (Galen)	Tablets 150 mg Capsules 250 mg	No specific data on enteral tube administration are available for this formulation.

Site of absorption (oral administration)

Ursodeoxycholic acid is absorbed in the jejunum and ileum, with approximately 20% absorbed in the colon.[4]

Alternative routes available

No alternative route available for ursodeoxycholic acid.

Interactions

There is no specific interaction with food. However, it is recommended that doses be taken after food and/or at night.

Health and safety

Standard precautions apply.

Suggestions/recommendations

- Use the suspension formulation; dilute with an equal volume of water immediately prior to administration. If necessary, Destolit tablets can be dispersed in 10 mL of water immediately prior to administration. Administer after feed.
- Jejunal administration should not reduce bioavailability.

Intragastric administration

1. Stop the enteral feed.
2. Flush the enteral feeding tube with the recommended volume of water.
3. Shake the medication bottle thoroughly to ensure adequate mixing.
4. Draw the medication suspension into an appropriate size and type of syringe.
5. Draw an equal volume of water and a little air into the syringe and shake to mix thoroughly.
6. Flush the medication dose down the feeding tube.
7. Finally, flush with the recommended volume of water.
8. Re-start the feed.

Alternatively, at step (4) measure the medicine in a suitable container and then add an equal volume of water and mix thoroughly. Draw this into an appropriate syringe. Ensure that the measure is rinsed and that this rinsing water is administered also to ensure that the total dose is given. **Do not** measure liquid medicines using a catheter-tipped syringe as this results in excessive dosing owing to the volume of the tip.

Jejunal administration

Administer as above.

References

1. *BNF* 50, September 2005.
2. Personal communication, Norgine Ltd; 24 January 2003.
3. Personal communication, CP Pharma; 20 January 2003.
4. Personal communication, Provalis Healthcare; 5 February 2003.
5. BPNG data on file, 2004.
6. Ursofalk Suspension, Summary of Product Characteristics; October 2001.

Valaciclovir

Formulations available[1]

Brand name (Manufacturer)	Formulation and strength	Product information/Administration information
Valtrex (GSK)	Tablets 500 mg	Valaciclovir hydrochloride. Film-coated tablets. Tablets are very hard and do not disperse readily in water. Tablets are quite difficult to crush and the powder does not suspend well and settles quickly; care must be taken to rinse the crushing device to ensure that the full dose is given.[2] If crushed and suspended in water, the dose must be given immediately owing to the rapid rate of hydrolysis of valaciclovir.[3] A suspension formulation with 21–35 days' expiry, under refrigeration, is available using US suspending agents;[4] the US formulation of Valtrex is similar to the UK formulation and therefore these stability data should be transferable.[3] *Extemporaneous preparation of valaciclovir suspension 50 mg/5 mL:[4]* Valaciclovir tablets 18 tablets / Ora-Plus 40 mL / Ora-Sweet to 180 mL / Expiry 21 Days, Refrigerated. (If Syrpalta is used as suspending agent, an expiration of 35 days, refrigerated storage, can be assigned.)

Site of absorption (oral administration)

The specific site of absorption is not documented. After oral administration, valaciclovir is well absorbed and rapidly converted to aciclovir.[5] peak plasma concentration occurs 30–100 minutes following oral dosing.

Alternative routes available

None available for valaciclovir; parenteral formulation is available for aciclovir.

Interactions

Bioavailability is not affected by food.[5]

Health and safety

Standard precautions apply.

Suggestions/recommendations

- As no liquid preparation is available and tablets are not dispersible, consider using aciclovir.
- Alternatively, an extemporaneous suspension can be formulated using the formula above. Administer as below.
- A prolonged break in feeding is not required.
- Consider using parenteral aciclovir for severe infections.

Intragastric administration

1. Using extemporaneous preparation
2. Stop the enteral feed.
3. Flush the enteral feeding tube with the recommended volume of water.
4. Shake the medication bottle thoroughly to ensure adequate mixing.
5. Draw the medication suspension into an appropriate size and type of syringe.
6. Draw an equal volume of water and a little air into the syringe and shake to mix thoroughly.
7. Flush the medication dose down the feeding tube.
8. Finally, flush with the recommended volume of water.
9. Re-start the feed, unless a prolonged break is required.

Alternatively, at step (4) measure the medicine in a suitable container and then add an equal volume of water and mix thoroughly. Draw this into an appropriate syringe. Ensure that the measure is rinsed and that this rinsing water is administered also to ensure that the total dose is given. **Do not** measure liquid medicines using a catheter-tipped syringe as this results in excessive dosing owing to the volume of the tip.

Intrajejunal administration

There are no specific data relating to the jejunal administration of valaciclovir. Consider changing to parenteral therapy.

References

1. *BNF 50*, September 2005.
2. BPNG data on file, 2005.
3. Personal communication, GlaxoSmithKline UK Ltd; 22 January 2003.
4. Fish DN, Vidaurri VA, Deeter RG. Stability of valaciclovir hydrochloride in extemporaneously prepared oral liquids. *Am J Health Syst Pharm*. 1999; 56: 1957–1960.
5. Valtrex (GSK), Summary of Product Characteristics; April 2002.

Valproate (Sodium valproate)

Formulations available[1]

Brand name (Manufacturer)	Formulation and strength	Product information/Administration information
Epilim (Sanofi-Synthelabo) Sodium Valproate (Hillcross)	Tablets 100 mg	Crushable.[2] Epilim tablets disintegrate if shaken in 10 mL of water for 5 minutes to give a fine dispersion that flushes easily down an 8Fr NG tube.[6]
Epilim (Sanofi-Synthelabo)	Tablets 200 mg, 500 mg	Enteric coated; do not crush[2]
Epilim (Sanofi-Synthelabo)	Liquid 200 mg/5 mL	Sugar-free. Contains sorbitol.[3] Red, clear liquid; resistant to flushing via an 8Fr NG tube; mixes easily with water, which reduces resistance.[4]

Formulations available [1] (continued)

Brand name (Manufacturer)	Formulation and strength	Product information/Administration information
Epilim (Sanofi-Synthelabo)	Syrup 200 mg/5 mL	Contains sorbitol. [3]
Epilim Chrono (Sanofi-Synthelabo)	M/R tablets 200 mg, 300 mg, 500 mg	Modified-release; do not crush.
Epilim Intravenous (Sanofi-Synthelabo)	Injection 400 mg	Not suitable for use via NG tube. [2]
Sodium valproate (Alpharma, APS, CP, Hillcross, IVAX, Sterwin)	Tablets 200 mg, 500 mg	Enteric coated; do not crush
Sodium valproate (CP, Hillcross, IVAX, Sterwin)	Oral solution 200 mg/5 mL	CP brand, Orlept, contains maltitol. [5]

Site of absorption (oral administration)

Specific site of absorption is not documented. Peak plasma concentration occurs 1–2 hours after administration of liquid and immediate-release preparations, and 2–8 hours after enteric coated or modified-release preparations. [7] Absorption is complete. [7]

Alternative routes available

Parenteral route is available.

Interactions

Food may delay the absorption of valproate. [7]

Health and safety

Standard precautions apply.

Suggestions/recommendations

- Use the liquid preparation and dilute with water immediately prior to administration.
- A prolonged break in feeding is not required.
- There are no specific data on jejunal administration; however, if this route is used the tablets dispersed in water should be used.

Intragastric administration

1. Stop the enteral feed.
2. Flush the enteral feeding tube with the recommended volume of water.
3. Shake the medication bottle thoroughly to ensure adequate mixing.
4. Draw the medication suspension into an appropriate size and type of syringe.
5. Flush the medication dose down the feeding tube.
6. Finally, flush with the recommended volume of water.
7. Re-start the feed, unless a prolonged break is required.

Alternatively, at step (4) measure the medicine in a suitable container. Draw this into an appropriate syringe. Ensure that the measure is rinsed and that this rinsing water is administered also to ensure that the total dose is given. **Do not** measure liquid medicines using a catheter-tipped syringe as this results in excessive dosing owing to the volume of the tip.

Intrajejunal administration

There are no specific data relating to jejunal administration. For liquid administration, administer using the above method; dilute the dose with 3–4 times the volume in water to reduce osmolarity. The 100 mg tablets can be used, although this is only practical for doses at the lower end of the range:

1. Stop the enteral feed.
2. Flush the enteral feeding tube with the recommended volume of water.
3. Place the tablets in the barrel of an appropriate size and type of syringe.
4. Draw 10 mL of water for every tablet into the syringe and allow tablet(s) to disperse; this may take up to 5 minutes with vigorous shaking.
5. Flush the medication dose down the feeding tube.
6. Draw another 10 mL of water into the syringe and also flush this via the feeding tube (this will rinse the syringe and ensure that the total dose is administered).
7. Finally, flush with the recommended volume of water.
8. Re-start the feed, unless a prolonged break is required.

Alternatively, at step (3) place tablet(s) into medicine pot and add 10 mL of water per tablet and allow tablet(s) to disperse. This may take more than 5 minutes. Draw this into an appropriate syringe. Ensure that the measure is rinsed and that this rinsing water is administered also to ensure that the total dose is given.

References

1. *BNF* 50, September 2005.
2. Personal communication, Sanofi-Synthelabo; 3 February 2003.
3. Epilim (Sanofi-Synthelabo), Summary of Product Characteristics; April 2003.
4. BPNG data on file, 2005.
5. Personal communication, CP Pharma; 20 January 2003.
6. BPNG data on file, 2004.
7. Dollery C. *Therapeutic Drugs*, 2nd edn. London: Churchill Livingstone; 1998.

Valsartan

Formulations available[1]

Brand name (Manufacturer)	Formulation and strength	Product information/Administration information
Diovan (Novartis)	Capsules 40 mg, 80 mg, 160 mg	Hard gelatin capsules.[2] Capsules can be opened; the white granular contents pour easily and disperse well in 10 mL of water; granules settle quickly, but the dispersion draws into the syringe and flushes down an 8Fr NG tube without blockage.[3]
Diovan (Novartis)	Tablets 40 mg	No specific data are available relating to the enteral tube administration of this formulation.

Site of absorption (oral administration)

Specific site of absorption is not documented.

Alternative routes available

No other routes of administration are available for any of the angiotensin II antagonists.

Interactions

Valsartan may be given with or without food.[2]

Health and safety

Standard precautions apply.

Suggestions/recommendations

- Where clinically indicated, an alternative therapy should be used. Consider changing to irbesartan (see monograph).
- If continued therapy with valsartan is indicated, the capsules can be opened and the contents mixed with water immediately before administration. A prolonged break in feeding is not required.

Intragastric administration

1. Stop the enteral feed.
2. Flush the enteral feeding tube with the recommended volume of water.
3. Open the capsule and pour the contents into a medicine pot.
4. Add 15 mL of water.
5. Stir to disperse the powder.
6. Draw into an appropriate syringe.
7. Add a further 15 mL of water to the medicine pot; stir to ensure that any powder remaining in the pot is mixed with water.
8. Draw up this dispersion and flush down tube. This will ensure that the whole dose is given.
9. Flush the enteral feeding tube with the recommended volume of water.
10. Re-start the feed.

Intrajejunal administration

There are no specific data relating to jejunal administration of valsartan. The patient should be monitored for lack of therapeutic effect of treatment. The above method of administration can be used.

References

1. *BNF* 50, September 2005.
2. Diovan (Novartis), Summary of Product Characteristics; September 2002.
3. BPNG data on file, 2004.

Vancomycin hydrochloride

Formulations available[1]

Brand name (Manufacturer)	Formulation and strength	Product information/Administration information
Vancomycin (Alpharma)	Capsules 125 mg, 250 mg	Contents are gel-formed and are not suitable for administration via the feeding tube.[2] Capsules are almost impossible to open and the contents are not suitable for use.[3]
Vancomycin (Alpharma, Mayne)	Injection 500 mg, 1 g	Injection can be reconstituted for use as an oral solution. When used for the oral route, the reconstituted injection can be stored in a fridge for 24 hours.[2] pH of reconstituted injection is 2.8–4.5.[4]
Vancocin (Flynn)	Injection 500 mg, 1 g	Licensed for use via nasogastric tube. Vial contents can be reconstituted and used for oral or enteral use. Each dose can be further diluted to 30 mL with water if required.[5]

Site of absorption (oral administration)

Vancomycin is not significantly absorbed from the normal gastrointestinal tract.[4]

Alternative routes available

Oral/enteral administration is used for its topical effect in the gut. Although the parenteral route is available, it is not used for the same indications.

Interactions

There is no documented interaction with food.

Health and safety

Standard precautions apply. Ensure that any unused solution is clearly labelled for oral/enteral use.

Suggestions/recommendations

- Use reconstituted injection for oral use.
- A prolonged break in feeding is not required.

Intragastric administration

1. Stop the enteral feed.
2. Flush the enteral feeding tube with the recommended volume of water.
3. Reconstitute injection as directed (the reconstituted solution can be stored in the fridge for 24 hours for enteral use).
4. Draw the medication solution into an appropriate size and type of syringe.
5. Flush the medication dose down the feeding tube.
6. Finally, flush with the recommended volume of water.
7. Re-start the feed.

Intrajejunal administration

Administer as above.

References

1. *BNF 50*, September 2005.
2. Personal communication, Alpharma; 21 January 2003.
3. BPNG data on file, 2004.
4. Vancomycin Powder for infusion (Dumex), Summary of Product Characteristics, January 2002.
5. Vancocin CP Injection (Lilly), Summary of Product Characteristics; May 2000.

Venlafaxine hydrochloride

Formulations available[1]

Brand name (Manufacturer)	Formulation and strength	Product information/Administration information
Efexor (Wyeth)	Tablets 37.5 mg, 50 mg, 75 mg,	37.5 mg tablet disperses within 5 minutes when placed in 10 mL of water to give a fine dispersion that settles quickly but flushes through an 8Fr NG tube without blockage. 75 mg tablet requires shaking in 10 mL of water for 5 minutes; the resulting dispersion contains some larger granules that flush via an 8Fr NG tube but may block finer-bore tubes.[2]
Efexor XL (Wyeth)	Capsules 75 mg, 150 mg	Modified-release preparation; unsuitable for administration via feeding tube. Convert the patient to twice-daily conventional-release tablets.

Site of absorption (oral administration)

Specific site of absorption is not documented. Peak plasma concentration occurs 2.4 hours following oral dosing.[3]

Alternative routes available

None available for venlafaxine.

Interactions

No specific interaction with food is documented; however, it is recommended that venlafaxine be taken with food.[3]

Health and safety

Standard precautions apply.

Suggestions/recommendations

- Disperse the tablets in water immediately prior to administration.
- Administer after feed.

Intragastric administration

1. Stop the enteral feed.
2. Flush the enteral feeding tube with the recommended volume of water.
3. Place the tablet in the barrel of an appropriate size and type of syringe.
4. Draw 10 mL of water into the syringe and allow the tablet to disperse, shaking if necessary.
5. Flush the medication dose down the feeding tube.
6. Draw another 10 mL of water into the syringe and also flush this via the feeding tube (this will rinse the syringe and ensure that the total dose is administered).
7. Finally, flush with the recommended volume of water.
8. Re-start the feed, unless a prolonged break is required.

Alternatively, at step (3) place the tablet into a medicine pot, add 10 mL of water and allow the tablet to disperse. Draw this into an appropriate syringe. Ensure that the measure is rinsed and that this rinsing water is administered also to ensure that the total dose is given.

Intrajejunal administration

Jejunal administration of venlafaxine would not be expected to affect bioavailability as the modified-released preparation is designed to release drug through the small bowel. Administer using the above method.

References

1. *BNF* 50, September 2005.
2. BPNG data on file, 2004.
3. Efexor (Wyeth), Summary of Product Characteristics; July 2000.

Verapamil hydrochloride

Formulations available[1]

Brand name (Manufacturer)	Formulation and strength	Product information/Administration information
Securon (Abbott)	Tablets 40 mg, 120 mg	Verapamil solubility 1 : 20 in water.[7]
Securon (Abbott)	Injection 2.5 mg/mL (2 mL)	pH 4.0–6.5; osmolality 290 mOsm/kg; bitter taste.[2] The injection is suitable for oral/enteral use.

Formulations available[1] (continued)

Brand name (Manufacturer)	Formulation and strength	Product information/Administration information
Cordilox (IVAX)	Tablets 40 mg, 80 mg, 120 mg Injection 2.5 mg/mL (2 mL)	No specific data on enteral tube administration are available for this formulation.
Verapamil (Alpharma, APS, Generics, Hillcross, IVAX)	Tablets 40 mg, 80 mg, 120 mg, 160 mg	Alpharma tablets are difficult to crush owing to the coating, but when crushed do disperse in water and flush easily via an 8Fr NG tube.[4] Generics brand tablets disperse in 10 mL of water within 5 minutes, if agitated, to give a yellow dispersion that flushes down an 8Fr NG tube without blockage.[4]
Zolvera (Rosemont)	Solution 40 mg/5 mL	Contains liquid maltitol, which may cause diarrhoea in high doses.[6]
Half Securon SR (Abbott)	M/R tablet 120 mg	Modified-release preparation. Do not crush. Not suitable for enteral tube administration.
Securon SR (Abbott)	M/R tablet 240 mg	Modified-release preparation. Do not crush. Not suitable for enteral tube administration.
Univer (Zeneus)	M/R capsules 120 mg, 180 mg, 240 mg	These capsules can be opened to facilitate administration providing the enclosed granules are not crushed.[3] No data on risk of tube blockage.
Verapress MR (Dexcel)	M/R tablets 240 mg	Modified-release preparation. Do not crush. Not suitable for enteral tube administration.
Vertab SR 240 (Trinity-Chiesi)	M/R tablets 240 mg	Modified-release preparation. Do not crush. Not suitable for enteral tube administration.

Site of absorption (oral administration)

Specific site of absorption is not documented. Peak plasma concentration occurs within 1–2 hours of oral dosing.[5, 6]

Alternative routes available

Parenteral route is available.

Interactions

No significant interaction with food is documented.[6, 7]

Health and safety

Standard precautions apply.

Suggestions/recommendations

- Use the oral solution. If changing from a modified-release preparation, divide the dose into three equal daily doses. No prolonged break in feeding is necessary.
- Parenteral route is available; consult the product literature for the dose.

Intragastric administration

1. Stop the enteral feed.
2. Flush the enteral feeding tube with the recommended volume of water.
3. Draw the medication solution into an appropriate size and type of syringe.
4. Flush the medication dose down the feeding tube.
5. Finally, flush with the recommended volume of water.
6. Re-start the feed, unless a prolonged break is required.

Alternatively, at step (3) measure the medicine in a suitable container and then draw into an appropriate syringe. Ensure that the measure is rinsed and that this rinsing water is administered also to ensure that the total dose is given. **Do not** measure liquid medicines using a catheter-tipped syringe as this results in excessive dosing owing to the volume of the tip.

Intrajejunal administration

There are no specific data. Administer as above. Monitor for lack of efficacy and increased side-effects.

References

1. *BNF 50*, September 2005.
2. Trissel LA, ed. *Stability of Compounded Formulations*, 2nd edn. Washington, DC: American Pharmaceutical Association; 2000.
3. Personal communication, Elan Pharma; 16 January 2003.
4. BPNG data on file, 2004.
5. Securon (Abbott), Summary of Product Characteristics; August 2003.
6. Zolvera Oral Solution (Rosemont), Summary of Product Characteristics; May 2001.
7. Dollery C. *Therapeutic Drugs*, 2nd edn. London: Churchill Livingstone; 1998.

Vigabatrin

Formulations available[1]

Brand name (Manufacturer)	Formulation and strength	Product information/Administration information
Sabril (Aventis Pharma)	Tablets 500 mg	Film-coated, scored. No specific data on enteral tube administration are available for this formulation.
Sabril (Aventis Pharma)	Powder 500 mg/sachet	The contents of a sachet should be dissolved in water or a soft drink immediately before taking. Aventis has no specific information relating to the administration of vigabatrin via an enteral feeding tube.[2] Sachet contents dissolve completely in 10 mL of water and flush down an 8Fr NG tube without blockage.[4]

Site of absorption (oral administration)

No specific site is documented. Vigabatrin is rapidly and completely absorbed following oral administration.[3]

Alternative routes available

None available for vigabatrin.

Interactions

Food does not affect the absorption of vigabatrin.[3]

Health and safety

Standard precautions apply.

Suggestions/recommendations

- Use the sachet formulation.
- A prolonged break in feeding is not necessary.

Intragastic administration

1. Stop the enteral feed.
2. Flush the enteral feeding tube with the recommended volume of water.
3. Measure 10 mL of water into a measuring pot.
4. Add the sachet contents and allow to dissolve.
5. Draw into an appropriate size and type of syringe.
6. Flush the medication dose down the feeding tube.
7. Rinse the measure and administer this also to ensure that the total dose is given.
8. Finally, flush with the recommended volume of water.
9. Re-start the feed.

Intrajejunal administration

There are no specific data relating to jejunal administration of vigabatrin. The above method can be used for jejunal administration.

References

1. *BNF* 50, September 2005.
2. Personal communication, Aventis Pharma; 2 January 2003.
3. Sabril (Aventis), Summary of Product Characteristics; December 2001.
4. BPNG data on file, 2004.

Vitamin E

Formulations available[1]

Brand name (Manufacturer)	Formulation and strength	Product information/Administration information
Vitamin E (Cambridge)	Suspension 500 mg/5 mL	Alpha-tocopherol acetate 500 mg/5 mL. Contains syrup, does not contain sorbitol.[2] White cloudy liquid, slightly viscous; some resistance to flushing.[3]

Site of absorption (oral administration)

Vitamin E absorption is dependent on the presence of bile and pancreatic enzymes. It enters the bloodstream via the lymphatic system.[3]

Alternative routes available

Parenteral multivitamin preparations are available: Vitlipid and Cernevit.

Interactions

No specific interaction with food is documented.

Health and safety

Standard precautions apply.

Suggestions/recommendations

- Use liquid preparation.
- A prolonged break in feed is not required.

Intragastric administration

1. Stop the enteral feed.
2. Flush the enteral feeding tube with the recommended volume of water.
3. Draw the medication solution into an appropriate size and type of syringe.
4. Flush the medication dose down the feeding tube.
5. Finally, flush with the recommended volume of water.
6. Re-start the feed, unless a prolonged break is required.

Alternatively, at step (3) measure the medicine in a suitable container and then draw into an appropriate syringe. Ensure that the measure is rinsed and that this rinsing water is administered also to ensure that the total dose is given. **Do not** measure liquid medicines using a catheter-tipped syringe as this results in excessive dosing owing to the volume of the tip.

Intrajejunal administration

Jejunal administration should not affect bioavailability providing the patient has sufficient bile and pancreatic enzyme secretion. Administer as above.

References

1. *BNF* 50, September 2005.
2. Vitamin E Suspension (Cambridge), Summary of Product Characteristics; March 2000.
3. BPNG data on file, 2005.
4. Sweetman SC, ed. *Martindale*, 34th edn. London: Pharmaceutical Press; 2005.

Voriconazole

Formulations available[1]

Brand name (Manufacturer)	Formulation and strength	Product information/Administration information
Vfend (Pfizer)	Tablets 50 mg, 200 mg	Film-coated tablets Pfizer has no data relating to the pharmacokinetic or stability effects of breaking or crushing Vfend tablets.[2] There has been one case report of the tablets being crushed and suspended in 50 mL of water and administered via a jejunostomy tube. This gave a similar plasma concentration to oral administration.[3] The dose should be taken 1 hour before food or 1 hour after.[4]
Vfend (Pfizer)	Suspension 40 mg/mL	Powder for oral suspension. Contains sucrose, does not contain sorbitol.[4] Recommended to be taken 1 hour before or 2 hours after food.[4]
Vfend (Pfizer)	Infusion 200 mg	No specific data on enteral tube administration are available for this formulation.

Site of absorption (oral administration)

Peak plasma concentration occurs 1–2 hours post oral dose.[4] The specific site of absorption is not documented; however, the drug appears to be effectively absorbed from the jejunum.[3]

Alternative routes available

Parenteral route is available.

Interactions

The absorption of voriconazole does not appear to be affected by intragastric pH. High-fat meals decrease C_{max} by 34% and AUC by 24%. See notes above for recommendations on dose timing.

Health and safety

Standard precautions apply.

Suggestions/recommendations

- Parenteral therapy should be used for life-threatening infections.
- There are limited data to support administration via enteral feeding tubes. If alternative therapy is not appropriate, the suspension should be used.
- The dose should be administered 1 hour before feed or at least 2 hours after.

Intragastric administration

1. Stop the enteral feed.
2. Flush the enteral feeding tube with the recommended volume of water.
3. Allow at least 1 hour before giving the dose.
4. Shake the medication bottle thoroughly to ensure adequate mixing.
5. Draw the medication suspension into an appropriate size and type of syringe.
6. Flush the medication dose down the feeding tube.
7. Finally, flush with the recommended volume of water.
8. Allow 2 hours before restarting the feed.

Alternatively, at step (5) measure the medicine in a suitable container. Draw this into an appropriate syringe. Ensure that the measure is rinsed and that this rinsing water is administered also to ensure that the total dose is given. **Do not** measure liquid medicines using a catheter-tipped syringe as this results in excessive dosing owing to the volume of the tip.

Intrajejunal administration

Absorption does not appear to be affected by intrajejunal administration, but see notes above. Administer using the method above.

References

1. *BNF 50*, September 2005.
2. Personal communication, Pfizer; 25 January 2005.
3. Martinez V, Le Guillou J, Lamer C, *et al*. Serum voriconazole levels following administration via percutaneous jejunostomy tube. *Antimicrob Agents Chemother*. 2003; 47(10): 3375.
4. Vfend (Pfizer), Summary of Product Characteristics; March 2005.

Warfarin sodium

Formulations available [1]

Brand name (Manufacturer)	Formulation and strength	Product information/Administration information
Warfarin (Alpharma, APS, Generics, Goldshield, Hillcross, IVAX, Taro)	Tablets 0.5 mg, 1 mg, 3 mg, 5 mg	All brands of tablets can be crushed and suspended in water. [3] Most brands of tablets will disperse in water within 5 minutes if shaken; the resulting dispersion flushes easily via a fine bore feeding tube without blockage. [2]

Site of absorption (oral administration)

Specific site of absorption is not documented. Peak plasma concentration occurs 3–9 hours after oral dosing. [4]

Alternative routes available

None for warfarin. Anticoagulation can be provided via the parenteral route using heparin.

Interactions

The variable vitamin K content in the diet and enteral feed can result in fluctuations in INR until the dietary regimen is stabilised. There is evidence of a physicochemical interaction between enteral feed and warfarin.[5]

There are also potential interactions with other food components; the clinical significance of this is uncertain.[6]

Health and safety

Standard precautions apply.

Suggestions/recommendations

- Disperse the tablets in water immediately prior to administration.
- Where possible give the warfarin dose during a break in the feeding regimen; when this is not possible, ensure that the timing of feed and dose are kept as stable as possible.

Intragastric administration

1. Stop the enteral feed.
2. Flush the enteral feeding tube with the recommended volume of water.
3. Where possible, allow a break before dosing.
4. Place the tablet in the barrel of an appropriate size and type of syringe.
5. Draw 10 mL of water into the syringe and allow the tablet to disperse, shaking if necessary.
6. Flush the medication dose down the feeding tube.
7. Draw another 10 mL of water into the syringe and also flush this via the feeding tube (this will rinse the syringe and ensure that the total dose is administered).
8. Finally, flush with the recommended volume of water.
9. Re-start the feed, unless a prolonged break is required.

Alternatively, at step (4) place the tablet into a medicine pot, add 10 mL of water and allow the tablet to disperse. Draw this into an appropriate syringe. Ensure that the measure is rinsed and that this rinsing water is administered also to ensure that the total dose is given.

Intrajejunal administration

There are no specific data relating to the jejunal administration of warfarin. Administer using the above method. Monitor INR and titrate dose to effect.

References

1. *BNF 50*, September 2005.
2. BPNG data on file, 2004.
3. Personal communication, Alpharma; 21 January 2003.
4. Dollery C. *Therapeutic Drugs*, 2nd edn. London: Churchill Livingstone; 1998.
5. Stockley IH. *Stockley's Drug Interactions*, 6th edn. London: Pharmaceutical Press; 2002.
6. Harris JE. Interaction of dietary factors with oral anticoagulant: review and applications. *J Am Diet Assoc.* 95(5): 580–584.

Zalcitabine

Formulations available[1]

Brand name (Manufacturer)	Formulation and strength	Product information/Administration information
Hivid (Roche)	Tablets 375 microgram, 750 microgram	Film-coated tablets. Roche has no data relating to crushing Hivid tablets and administration via enteral feeding tubes.[2]

Site of absorption (oral administration)

Specific site is not documented. Peak plasma concentration occurs 0.8 hours after oral dosing in fasted patients and 1.6 hours in fed patients.[3]

Alternative routes available

None available for zalcitabine.

Interactions

Food decreases the bioavailability of zalcitabine by 14%;[2] this is unlikely to be clinically important.

Health and safety

Zalcitabine powder is irritant to skin and mucous membranes.[2] Avoid crushing.

Suggestions/recommendations

- Seek specialist advice regarding alternative therapy.
- There are no data to support crushing tablets as a method of administration.

References

1. *BNF* 50, September 2005.
2. Personal communication, Roche; 6 February 2003.
3. Hivid (Roche), Summary of Product Characteristics; June 2003.

Zidovudine

Formulations available[1]

Brand name (Manufacturer)	Formulation and strength	Product information/Administration information
Retrovir (GSK)	Capsules 100 mg, 250 mg	No specific data on enteral administration are available for this formulation.

Formulations available [1] (*continued*)

Brand name (Manufacturer)	Formulation and strength	Product information/Administration information
Retrovir (GSK)	Oral solution 50 mg/5 mL	GSK is aware of anecdotal reports of Retrovir oral solution being successfully administered via an enteral feeding tube. [2] Clear, slightly viscous liquid; flushes via tube with little resistance; mixes with an equal volume of water. [3]
Retrovir (GSK)	Injection 10 mg/mL (20 mL)	Licensed for parenteral use in patients unable to take zidovudine by mouth.
Combivir (GSK)	Tablets 300 mg + 150 mg	Zidovudine 300 mg + lamivudine 150 mg. GSK recommends administering the two components separately, using the liquid preparations. [2] Although there are no stability data to support crushing the tablets, as the tablets are not sustained-release, theoretically the tablets could be crushed and dispersed in water immediately prior to administration. [2]

With abacavir and lamivudine – see Abacavir

Site of absorption (oral administration)

Specific site of absorption is not documented.

Alternative routes available

Parenteral route is available.

Interactions

There is no documented interaction with food.

Health and safety

Standard precautions apply.

Suggestions/recommendations

- Use the liquid preparation.
- A prolonged break in feeding is not required.

Intragastric administration

1. Stop the enteral feed.
2. Flush the enteral feeding tube with the recommended volume of water.
3. Draw the medication solution into an appropriate size and type of syringe.
4. Flush the medication dose down the feeding tube.
5. Finally, flush with the recommended volume of water.
6. Re-start the feed, unless a prolonged break is required.

Alternatively, at step (3) measure the medicine in a suitable container and then draw into an appropriate syringe. Ensure that the measure is rinsed and that this rinsing water is administered also to ensure that the total dose is given. **Do not** measure liquid medicines using a catheter-tipped syringe as this results in excessive dosing owing to the volume of the tip.

Intrajejunal administration

Administer using the above method. Monitor for increased side-effects or loss of efficacy.

References

1. *BNF* 50, September 2005.
2. Personal communication, GlaxoSmithKline; 22 January 2003.
3. BPNG data on file, 2005.

Zinc sulphate

Formulations available[1]

Brand name (Manufacturer)	Formulation and strength	Product information/Administration information
Solvazinc (Provalis)	Effervescent tablets 125 mg	125 mg zinc sulphate monohydrate = 45 mg zinc = 700 micromol zinc. Tablets effervesce in 10 mL of water to give a clear solution.[2]
Zinc sulphate (Aurum)	Injection 14.6 mg/mL	50 micromol/mL. No specific data on enteral tube administration are available for this formulation.

Site of absorption (oral administration)

Zinc is absorbed in the stomach and upper small intestine.[3]

Alternative routes available

Parenteral route is available.

Interactions

The absorption of zinc is reduced by high concentrations of copper in the gut lumen. No other specific interactions are documented.

Health and safety

Standard precautions apply.

Suggestions/recommendations

- Disperse the tablet in water immediately prior to administration.
- A prolonged break in feeding is not required.

Intragastric administration

1. Stop the enteral feed.
2. Flush the enteral feeding tube with the recommended volume of water.
3. Measure at least 10 mL of water into a measuring pot.
4. Add the effervescent tablet and allow to dissolve.
5. Draw into an appropriate syringe.
6. Flush the medication dose down the feeding tube.
7. Rinse the measure and administer this also to ensure that the total dose is given.
8. Finally, flush with the recommended volume of water.
9. Re-start the feed.

Intrajejunal administration

Intrajejunal administration may lead to reduced bioavailability of zinc preparations. Monitor plasma concentration and consider using parenteral therapy.

References

1. *BNF* 50, September 2005.
2. BPNG data on file, 2004.
3. Personal communication, Provalis; 5 February 2003.

Zopiclone

Formulations available [1]

Brand name (Manufacturer)	Formulation and strength	Product information/Administration information
Zopiclone (Alpharma, APS, Arrow, CP, Dominion, Generics, IVAX, Opus)	Tablets 3.75 mg, 7.5 mg	Alpharma brand tablets are film-coated to mask the bitter taste. The company does not recommend crushing the tablets as the coating may block the tube. [2]
Zimovane (Rhône-Poulenc Rorer)	Tablets 3.75 mg, 7.5 mg	Aventis recommends that Zimovane tablets are not crushed as the bioavailability may be altered. The tablets are very hard and cannot easily be crushed. [3]

Site of absorption (oral administration)

Specific site is not specified. Peak plasma concentrations occur 1.5–2 hours following oral dosing. [4]

Alternative routes available

None available for zopiclone.

Interactions

Absorption is not affected by food. [4]

Health and safety

Standard precautions apply.

Suggestions/recommendations

- Tablets are not suitable for use. Consider changing to zolpidem or temazepam (see monographs).

References

1. *BNF* 50, September 2005.
2. Personal communication, Alpharma; 21 January 2003.
3. Personal communication, Aventis; 13 February 2003.
4. Zimovane (RPR), Summary of Product Characteristics; July 2003.

Index